Eastern Religions, Spirituality, and Psychiatry

Eastern Religions, Spirituality, and Psychiatry

H. Steven Moffic • Rama Rao Gogineni
John R. Peteet • Neil Krishan Aggarwal
Narpinder K. Malhi • Ahmed Hankir
Editors

Eastern Religions, Spirituality, and Psychiatry

An Expansive Perspective on Mental Health and Illness

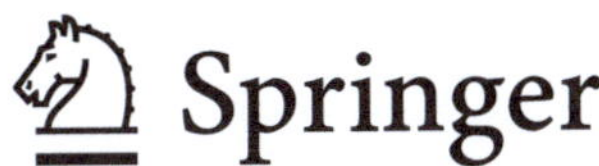

Springer

Editors
H. Steven Moffic
Private Community Psychiatrist
MILWAUKEE, WI, USA

John R. Peteet
Department of Psychiatry
Brigham and Women's Hospital
Boston, MA, USA

Narpinder K. Malhi
Department of Behavioral Health
ChristianaCare
Wilmington, DE, USA

Rama Rao Gogineni
Developmental Psychiatry
Cooper Medical School of Rowan
University
Camden, NJ, USA

Neil Krishan Aggarwal
New York State Psychiatric Institute
Columbia University Medical Center
New York, NY, USA

Ahmed Hankir
Institute of Psychiatry
King's College Hospital
London, UK

ISBN 978-3-031-56746-9   ISBN 978-3-031-56744-5   (eBook)
https://doi.org/10.1007/978-3-031-56744-5

This Springer imprint is published by the registered company Springer Nature Switzerland AG
The registered company address is: Gewerbestrasse 11, 6330 Cham, Switzerland

If disposing of this product, please recycle the paper.

Preface: The Need for a Book on Eastern Religions, Spirituality, and Psychiatry

> For me, the purpose of life is to grow in moral imagination until there is no us versus them and the whole world is my circle of caring.—Mary Pipher, Clinical Psychologist and Author.

What were we thinking, when several of the co-editors of the previous books of Springer on the interaction of psychiatry with Islamophobia (2019), Anti-Semitism (2020), and Christianity (2021) felt that we had finished a job well done, given the very confirming reviews? Gradually, during the worldwide Covid pandemic, it dawned upon us that we were not finished, but only finished with what have been called the Abrahamic religions that came to the Middle East and spread to the West. But if we wanted to be more comprehensive about religion, spirituality, and psychiatry, we needed to attempt an additional volume on what are called the Eastern traditions that came out of Asia, keeping in mind that East and West are convenient psychosocial terms for where something is located in a round and spinning Earth. By now, the followers of Hinduism, Buddhism, and the rest number about a quarter of those with religious beliefs around the world, over a billion people, with increasing immigration to the United States and elsewhere from the East.

Spirituality was added to the title of this latest volume because it seems especially descriptive of the Eastern traditions, given the common understanding that Buddhism is more of a philosophy and spiritual practice than a religion with a focus on divine worship. Whereas religions are organized systems sharing moral beliefs and rituals, spirituality generally refers to an individual's quest for meaning and purpose in life—though of course a given believer can be both religious and spiritual.

Consequently, during the last stages of the pandemic, we proposed this volume and it was accepted. Once again, our core of co-editors—Drs. Moffic, Peteet, and Hankir—were supplemented by other editors of faiths that fit the book's focus. And, once again, as in the volume on Islamophobia, we struggled with the perennial questions in cultural psychiatry and in society: "Does it take one to know one?" And "Who should tell the stories?" about a given culture.

In some ways, the answers to these related questions have never been quite resolved, but have led to a workable creative tension and a unique interfaith volume of editors and authors writing not only about their psychiatric expertise in their own faiths, but conveying what they perceived and were trying to learn cross-culturally about Eastern religions and spirituality. The implied hope was that we could be a model for the world of interfaith cooperation, learning, and healing in psychiatry and mental health, which in turn could be applied to politics and other conflictual situations.

This editing process meant that along the way we needed to be able to adjust and compromise as unsuitable productions were sunk and new ones floated. One example of a late addition was a chapter put together by Dilip Jeste, former President of the American Psychiatric Association and expert in research-based wisdom, who was becoming more and more interested in the social aspects of psychiatry. Of Hindu background himself, he added two colleagues from Brazil with expertise in spirituality, as well as one of the editors, as co-authors for the chapter titled: Spirituality: Relationship with Religion, Health, Wisdom, and Positive Psychiatry.

Although there is a robust literature regarding Eastern religions and spirituality, as well as books on specific psychiatric practices derived from various Eastern traditions, this volume was designed to be unique and necessary in covering the major Eastern religions and spiritual traditions and how psychiatric treatments are adapted to and from them, from the perspectives of psychiatrists of both Eastern and Western religions. The editors and chapter authors came from various faiths and had lived—or are living—in various countries, mainly the United States, and also Canada, England, Ireland, Lebanon, Israel, Italy, India, China, and Brazil.

The subtitle of the book is also quite important, especially the "expansive" perspective suggested by our acquisition editor. Its expansiveness is what makes the book so unique in its diverse coverage of religious and spiritual traditions from psychiatrist experts of diverse religious backgrounds. There is clear coverage of particular traditions, but debatable perspectives of some topics due in part to migration and religious adaptations. There are both complementary and conflictual points of view that readers can resolve for themselves.

To align the specific chapters with the overall intentions, this book is divided into five parts. Part I covers general issues, including principles of culture, religion, and spirituality in psychiatry, spirituality in psychiatry, spirituality across the lifespan, child rearing, practice and faith, and how death and dying is approached in these Eastern traditions. Part II covers specific eastern religions and spiritual traditions, including basic principles and research-based clinical aspects of Hinduism, Buddhism, Sikhism, Taoism, Zoroastrianism, Jainism, as well as Confucian philosophical ideas. Part III attempts to apply the importance of cultural humility to perspectives on the Eastern traditions from Western psychiatry. These include Christian, Muslim, and Jewish perspectives, not of expertise, but of explorations in learning. Part IV covers specific social psychiatric perspectives, including the psychiatric harm that can come from caste divisions and cults posing as religions, but closes with a perspective on the Eastern connections to the relatively unknown, but unifying, Omnist perspective that brings almost all together, perhaps a desired harbinger for the world's future.

Finally, the editors produce an Afterword on lessons learned about the Eastern religions, spirituality, and psychiatry. We hope that all of these will be helpful to mental health clinicians, related academicians, and the large lay public interested in the subject.

<table>
<tr><td>Milwaukee, WI</td><td>H. Steven Moffic</td></tr>
<tr><td>Camden, NJ</td><td>Rama Rao Gogineni</td></tr>
<tr><td>Boston, MA</td><td>John R. Peteet</td></tr>
<tr><td>New York, NY</td><td>Neil Krishan Aggarwal</td></tr>
<tr><td>Wilmington, DE</td><td>Narpinder K. Malhi</td></tr>
<tr><td>London, UK</td><td>Ahmed Hankir</td></tr>
</table>

Contents

Culture, Religion, and Spirituality in Mental Health and Illness

Neil Krishan Aggarwal

Introduction: Religion and Spirituality in Mental Health Settings

Systematic reviews and meta-analyses of clinical studies have consistently demonstrated that patients turn to religion and spirituality to address mental health concerns. Spiritual interventions are significantly associated with lower psychiatric symptoms, greater well-being, and higher levels of spirituality compared to treatments as usual [1]. Religious-based interventions have reduced symptoms of depression among people with chronic medical illnesses, pregnant women, patients on hemodialysis, elderly nursing home residents, people with major depressive disorder or dysthymia, and coronary artery bypass graft surgery patients [2]. Patients with anxiety disorders who receive spiritual based interventions benefit from symptom improvements compared to those receiving treatments as usual [3]. Religiosity is negatively associated with non-suicidal self-harm [4]. Specific practices such as

N. K. Aggarwal (✉)
New York State Psychiatric Institute,
New York, NY, USA

Columbia University Medical Center,
New York, NY, USA

Committee on Global Thought, Columbia University,
New York, NY, USA
e-mail: Neil.Aggarwal@nyspi.columbia.edu

mindfulness meditation decrease ruminative thinking and trait anxiety while increasing empathy and self-compassion even among healthy people not seeking mental health services [5]. Clinical studies of religious and spiritual based interventions are showing promise in the treatment of bipolar and posttraumatic stress disorders [6].

Despite these benefits, mental health providers have traditionally been reluctant to address religion and spirituality. Common reasons for this reluctance include providers being less religiously observant than patients, a lack of knowledge about assessment methods, minimal clinical training, and discomfort with models of care that religious personnel such as clergy use to address mental distress [7]. Federal agencies in high-income countries have not funded researchers who study the relationship between religion/spirituality and mental health outcomes, leading to a paucity of organized research [8]. In line with an emerging clinical, educational, and research agenda to center religion and spirituality in mental health, this chapter adopts the following understanding for these terms with the recognition that exact definitions are contested:

- Religion: specific behavioral, social, doctrinal, and denominational characteristics that involve a belief in a supernatural power or transcendent being, truth, or ultimate reality expressed through rituals [7].

- Spirituality: a concern with ultimate questions about life's meaning as it relates to the transcendent, which may or may not arise from formal religious traditions [7].

This chapter summarizes the evolution of attitudes toward religion and spirituality in mental health. It begins by reviewing the ambivalence toward religion and spirituality in psychoanalysis, the dominant paradigm for mental health in Europe and North America for most of the last century. Afterwards, it examines how considerations of religion and spirituality in patient lives began with greater attention to cross-cultural issues throughout medicine. Finally, it discusses developments in assessment methods for providers to use with patients.

Psychoanalytic Skepticism Toward Religion and Spirituality

Mental health providers could ask why they would benefit from paying attention to religion and spirituality. Revisiting the historical bias of psychiatry helps answer this question. From the 1920s to 1970s, psychoanalysis was the dominant orientation among academic and private psychiatrists in the United States [9]. Understanding psychoanalytic perspectives offers context for ambivalent attitudes toward religion and spirituality among many providers.

Historically, psychoanalysis has taken a skeptical view of religion. The founder of psychoanalysis Sigmund Freud (1856–1939) interpreted religious phenomena through psychological terms. In *The Psychopathology of Everyday Life*, Freud wrote, "I believe that a large part of the mythological view of the world, which extends a long way into the most modern religions, is *nothing but psychology projected into the external world* [original emphasis]. The obscure recognition (the endopsychic perception, as it were) of psychical factors and relations in the unconscious is mirrored" ([10], p. 258). In *Obsessive Actions and Religious Practices*, Freud expanded his views after observing similarities between individuals who performed behaviors compulsively and religious devotees who performed rituals with strict adherence:

> The formation of a religion, too, seems to be based on the suppression, the renunciation, of certain instinctual impulses. These impulses, however, are not, as in the neuroses, exclusively components of the sexual instinct; they are self-seeking, socially harmful instincts, though, even so, they are usually not without a sexual component. A sense of guilt following upon continual temptation and an expectant anxiety in the form of fear of divine punishment have, after all, been familiar to us in the field of religion longer than in that of neurosis. Perhaps because of the admixture of sexual components, perhaps because of some general characteristics of the instincts, the suppression of instinct proves to be an inadequate and interminable process in religious life also. Indeed, complete backslidings into sin are more common among pious people than among neurotics and these give rise to a new form of religious activity, namely acts of penance, which have their counterpart in obsessional neurosis ([11], p. 125).

For Freud, religion represented a "primitive" form of human understanding about the world. According to his *Totem and Taboo*, religion preceded science in human evolution: "The human race, if we are to follow the authorities, have in the course of ages developed three such systems of thought—three great pictures of the universe: animistic (or mythological), religious and scientific" ([12], p. 77)Freud disparaged adherents of religious traditions for their hatred of disbelievers, as *Group Psychology and the Analysis of the Ego* revealed: "Every religion is in this same way a religion of love for all those whom it embraces; while cruelty and intolerance towards those who do not belong to it are natural to every religion. However difficult we may find it personally, we ought not to reproach believers too severely on this account; people who are unbelieving or indifferent are much better off psychologically in this matter" ([13], p. 98). In latter works, Freud took a negative view of religion, claiming in *Civilization and Its Discontents* that "the religions of mankind must be classed among the mass-delusions" ([14], p. 81) and that religion could "spare" individuals from neuroses "by forcibly fixing them in a state of psychical infantilism and by drawing them into a mass-delusion" ([14], pp. 84–85).

Freud acknowledged his lack of interest in religion. In addressing a Jewish organization, he stated, "I was myself a Jew, and it had always seemed to me not only unworthy but positively senseless to deny the fact. What bound me to Jewry was (I am ashamed to admit) neither faith nor national pride, for I have always been an unbeliever and was brought up without any religion though not without a respect for what are called the 'ethical' standards of human civilization" ([15], p. 273). In his writings, Freud professionalized personal discomforts related to religion.

Psychoanalysts since Freud have differed on religion. Two of Freud's early associates, Alfred Adler (1870–1937) and Otto Rank (1884–1939), also viewed religion as the result of pathological unconscious drives that people project onto the external material world [16, 17]. However, Carl Jung (1875–1961) did not see religion in pathological terms. He viewed it as part of what he called "the collective unconscious," which he hypothesized to be universal, impersonal archetypes that all individuals inherit as a natural part of being members in society [18]. Hence, psychoanalysts right from the first generation of Freud's students have not held uniform views about religion. Nonetheless, Freud's theories influenced generations of psychoanalysts who established training institutes in the United States well into the 1980s and subscribed to his original ideas in varying degrees [19].

Attention to Religion and Spirituality in Response to Increasing Global Migration

The rise of cultural initiatives in American medicine can be attributed to two social reforms from the 1960s [20]. First, the Civil Rights Act of 1964 outlawed discrimination on the basis of race, color, religion, sex, and national origin in public institutions funded by the federal government. Second, the Immigration and Nationality Act of 1965 expanded the number of immigrants that the United States accepted each year from Africa, Asia, Eastern Europe, and Southern Europe in the most monumental act of legislation since the Immigration Act of 1964. Subsequently, patients from unfamiliar immigrant and minoritized ethnoracial communities accessed medical services with unprecedented volume, prompting providers to implement federal anti-discrimination laws in local settings [20].

Training in cross-cultural issues within American medical education began in the 1990s. In response to trends in the humanities and social sciences related to multiculturalism, medical schools introduced case studies of patients from minoritized ethnic, linguistic, racial, and religious backgrounds to encourage discussions about how patients explain illness, health, and treatment preferences in ways that differ from secular biomedical explanations [21]. Scholarship appeared on cross-cultural medicine, cultural sensitivity, transcultural nursing, and multicultural counseling [22]. To prepare for DSM-IV's publication in 1994, the American Psychiatric Association (APA) engaged a National Institute of Mental Health (NIMH) Group on Culture and Diagnosis composed mostly of cultural psychiatrists, cross-cultural psychologists, and anthropologists to consider the cross-cultural applicability of diagnostic criteria to minoritized populations in the United States and to non-Americans abroad [23, 24]. Members of this NIMH group held different views about what "culture" meant—some used it interchangeably with ethnicity, race, and religion, whereas others referred to minoritized ethnoracial groups organized around US Census categories [25]. By the late 1990s, researchers demonstrated that minoritized communities face disparities in accessing mental health services, receiving evidence-based treatments, and experiencing improved health outcomes compared to white patients [26]. The question of how mental health services cater to diverse populations has shown that mental health providers often exhibit negative attitudes toward religion despite multiple surveys showing that over two-thirds of all people in the United States believe in an organized religion [27].

Table 1.1 Prevalent models for cross-cultural work in mental health settings

Reference	Model name	Definition	Components
[30]	Cultural competence	"A set of congruent behaviors, attitudes, and policies that come together in a system, agency or among professionals and enable that system, agency or those professions to work effectively in cross-cultural situations" (p. 9)	(1) Valuing patient diversity, (2) assessment, (3) being conscious of dynamics when cultures interact, (4) training in cross-cultural issues, and (5) culturally adapting services
[31]	Cultural humility	"A lifelong commitment to self-evaluation and critique, to redressing power imbalances … and to developing mutually beneficial and non-paternalistic partnerships with communities on behalf of individuals and defined populations" (p. 123)	(1) Learning about patient cultural, ethnic, and racial identities and (2) examining the cultures of the provider and service institution
[32]	Cultural safety	"A process of reflection on his/her cultural identity and [that] will recognize the impact that his/her personal culture has on his/her professional practice. Unsafe cultural practice comprises any action which diminishes, demeans or disempowers the cultural identity and wellbeing of an individual" (p. 7)	(1) Understanding how patients defined themselves and (2) examining the cultures of the provider and service institution
[33]	Cultural formulation	"Systematically evaluating and reporting the impact of the individual's cultural context" (p. 843)	Identifying the (1) cultural identity of the individual, (2) cultural explanation of the individual's illness, (3) cultural factors related to psychosocial environment and functioning, (4) cultural elements of the relationship between the individual and the clinician, (5) overall cultural assessment for diagnosis and care

The need to attend to cross-cultural issues across medicine has led to a proliferation of models for providers. One review from a federal agency uncovered 24 models [28]. To help providers navigate this scholarship, the APA's Division of Diversity & Health Equity has identified the most prevalent models in clinical practice [29], which appear in Table 1.1.

Cultural competence [30] and cultural humility [31] originated in the United States, but other models have international contributors. Cultural safety was developed in New Zealand [32], and the NIMH group creating the cultural formulation for DSM-IV aggregated mental health researchers across several countries [33]. Although attention to cross-cultural issues in mental health began in the United States, providers around the world are now committed to delivering services that respond to patients from diverse religious and spiritual backgrounds [34].

The Recognition of Religion and Spirituality in Cross-Cultural Work

Clinical experience with models for cross-cultural work in mental health settings has led to guidelines for assessing religion and spirituality. At McGill University's Cultural Consultation Service in which medical providers refer patients for a cross-cultural assessment based on the DSM-IV Outline for Cultural Formulation [33], nearly a fifth of referring providers indicated that cultural formulations improved their knowledge about religious beliefs and practices [35]. Teams completing cultural formulations observed that religious practices were important for coping and social support, particularly with grief and anxiety [35]. Others have criticized the cultural formulation approach for only assessing religion and spirituality as elements of psychosocial functioning through social supports and stressors, but not in other domains such as the cultural identity of the patient and cultural explanations of illness [36]. This is a significant shortcoming as people may use religion to define their identities [37] and ascribe explanations to what happens to them throughout life [38]. Religions may have prescriptions and prohibitions pertaining to everyday activities that relate to mental health such as alcohol use, consumption of mind-altering substances such as marijuana, patterns of sexual activity, sleep, and diet, making assessments of religion and spirituality essential [39]. The largest and most conclusive literature on the positive effects of religion and spirituality comes from outcomes with substance use disorders [40], so providers should actively assess for religion and spirituality.

Researchers have identified certain patients for whom religion and spirituality should be assessed. These include patients who say that they are deeply religious and spiritual, those who request religion and spirituality to be incorporated into clinical work, those who use religion and spirituality to cope, those using religious vocabularies with providers, and those whose appearances identify them as observant individuals [41]. Providers can use the social history to understand how religion and spirituality impact living situations, relationships, and lifestyles with specific attention to diet, exercise, and coping with stress [42]. Three techniques for raising these topics include following up on patient vocabularies for clarification or greater explanation, identifying shifts in emotion during conversations about religion and spirituality, and weaving in stories of a tradition that patients and providers may share [43]. A literature review from 2022 has identified clinical assessment tools for providers [44] that are summarized in Table 1.2. The first four [45–48] are mnemonics of domains to assess, and the last two [49, 50] present questions:

Providers have options to assess patient religion and spirituality. Case studies describing experiences with these tools can expand the scientific evidence base on how to implement such assessments, answering key questions such as how assessments should be done, in which settings, at what points in care, with which patients, and how assessments relate to outcomes.

Table 1.2 Assessment tools for religion and spirituality

Reference	Assessment	Assessed domains
[45]	FACT	**F**aith or belief How **A**ctive the person is in their faith community and the **A**vailability, **A**ccessibility, and **A**pplicability of that support **C**oping strategies, their **C**omfort, and potential **C**onflicts or **C**oncerns about treatment Available **T**reatments
[46]	FICA	**F**aith and belief **I**mportance for their life and health **C**ommunity of faith **A**ddress in care (for health and the spiritual journey)
[47]	HOPE	What provides **H**ope, meaning, or comfort **O**rganized religion **P**ersonal spirituality and practices **E**ffects on health care and end-of-life issues
[48]	SPIRIT	**S**piritual belief system **P**ersonal spirituality **I**ntegration in a faith community **R**ituals **I**mplications for medical care **T**erminal event planning

(continued)

Table 1.2 (continued)

Reference	Assessment	Assessed domains
[49]	The Royal College of Psychiatrists' *Spirituality and Mental Health* leaflet	**Beliefs and questions** What is life all about? What gives you a sense of meaning or purpose? If you believe in God— – what is your relationship like? What is God like? What does he think about you? What would you ask God? What do you think happens after death? Do your spiritual beliefs make you uneasy about any parts of your treatment plan? **Spiritual practices** How do spiritual practices help you? Does anything about them create problems for you? **Spirituality and community** What supports and/or difficulties do you get from family, friends, school/work, or your faith community? **Spiritual experiences** Have you had any spiritual experiences? What did they mean? **How does spirituality affect you?** Could you describe your emotions?
[50]	Religion/spirituality assessment guide	**Screening questions** Do you consider yourself a religious or spiritual person or neither? If so, please explain how you are. If not, conclude the interview. If yes, see below: **Assessment questions** Explain how your beliefs provide comfort. Do you have any religious or spiritual beliefs that cause stress? Do you have any spiritual or religious beliefs that might influence your willingness to take medication, receive psychotherapy, or receive other treatments? Are you an active member of a faith community, such as a church, synagogue, or mosque? How supportive has your faith community been in helping you? If not, why has your faith community not been supportive? Tell me about the spiritual or religious environment in which you were raised. Were either of your parents religious? As a child, were your experiences positive or negative ones in this environment? Have you ever had a significant change in your spiritual or religious life, either an increase or a decrease? If so, tell me about the change, and why. Do you wish to incorporate your spiritual or religious beliefs in your treatment? If so, how would you like this to be done? Do you have any other spiritual needs or concerns that you would like to be addressed in your care?

Discussion

This chapter has briefly summarized the evolution of attitudes toward religion and spirituality among mental health practitioners. Despite decades of ambivalence, providers have increasingly situated assessments of religion and spirituality within cross-cultural work. By completing such assessments, providers may better understand how patients make meanings about themselves, health, illness, and their place in the world.

References

1. de Diego-Cordero R, Suárez-Reina P, Badanta B, Lucchetti G, Vega-Escaño J. Appl Nurs Res. 2022;67:151618.
2. Marques A, Ihle A, Souza A, Peralta M, de Matos MG. Religious-based interventions for depression: a systematic review and meta-analysis of experimental studies. J Affect Disord. 2022;309:289–96.
3. Gonçalves JPB, Lucchetti G, Menezes PR, Vallada H. Religious and spiritual interventions in mental health care: a systematic review and meta-analysis of randomized controlled clinical trials. Psychol Med. 2015;45(14):2937–49.
4. Haney AM. Nonsuicidal self-injury and religiosity: a meta-analytic investigation. Am J Orthopsychiatry. 2020;90(1):78–89.
5. Chiesa A, Serretti A. Mindfulness-based stress reduction for stress management in healthy people: a review and meta-analysis. J Altern Complement Med. 2009;15(5):593–600.
6. Lucchetti G, Koenig HG, Lucchetti ALG. Spirituality, religiousness, and mental health: a review of the current scientific evidence. World J Clin Cases. 2021;9(26):7620–31.
7. Huguelet P, Koenig HG. Introduction: key concepts. In: Huguelet P, Koenig HG, editors. Religion and spirituality in psychiatry. Cambridge: Cambridge University Press; 2009. p. 1–5.
8. Rosmarin DH, Pargament KI, Koenig HG. Spirituality and mental health: challenges and opportunities. Lancet Psychiatry. 2021;8(2):92–3.
9. Luhrmann TM. Of two minds: an anthropologist looks at American psychiatry. New York: Knopf Doubleday; 2001.
10. Freud S. The psychopathology of everyday life: forgetting, slips of the tongue, bungled actions, superstitions and errors [1901]. In: Freud S, Strachey J, Freud A, Rothgeb C, Richards A, editors. The standard edition of the complete psychological works of Sigmund Freud 6. London: Hogarth Press; 1953.
11. Freud S. Obsessive actions and religious practices [1907]. In: Freud S, Strachey J, Freud A, Rothgeb C, Richards A, editors. The standard edition of the complete psychological works of Sigmund Freud 9. London: Hogarth Press; 1953.
12. Freud S. Totem and taboo: some points of agreement between the mental lives of savages and neurotics [1913]. In: Freud S, Strachey J, Freud A, Rothgeb C, Richards A, editors. The standard edition of the complete psychological works of Sigmund Freud 13. London: Hogarth Press; 1953.
13. Freud S. Group psychology and the analysis of the ego [1921]. In: Freud S, Strachey J, Freud A, Rothgeb C, Richards A, editors. The standard edition of the complete psychological works of Sigmund Freud 18. London: Hogarth Press; 1953.
14. Freud S. Civilization and its discontents [1930]. In: Freud S, Strachey J, Freud A, Rothgeb C, Richards A, editors. The standard edition of the complete psychological works of Sigmund Freud 21. London: Hogarth Press; 1953.
15. Freud S. Address to the Society of B'Nai B'Rith [1926]. In: Freud S, Strachey J, Freud A, Rothgeb C, Richards A, editors. The standard edition of the complete psychological works of Sigmund Freud 20. London: Hogarth Press; 1953.
16. Rank O, Sachs H, Payne C. The significance of psychoanalysis for the mental sciences. Psychoanal Rev. 1916;3(3):318–35.
17. Adler A. La pulsion d'agression dans la vie et dans la névrose. Rev Fr Psychanal. 1974;38:417–26.
18. Jung CG. The concept of the collective unconscious [1936]. In: Jung CG, Read H, Fordham M, Adler G, Hull RFC, editors. Collected works of CG Jung 9. Princeton: Princeton University Press; 1969.
19. Hale NG Jr. The rise and crisis of psychoanalysis in the United States: Freud and the Americans, 1917–1985. Oxford: Oxford University Press; 1995.
20. Shaw SJ. The politics of recognition in culturally appropriate care. Med Anthropol Q. 2005;19(3):290–309.
21. Taylor JS. The story catches you and you fall down: tragedy, ethnography, and "cultural competence". Med Anthropol Q. 2003;17(2):159–81.
22. Saha S, Beach MC, Cooper LA. Patient centeredness, cultural competence and healthcare quality. J Natl Med Assoc. 2008;100(11):1275–85.
23. Littlewood R. DSM–IV and culture: is the classification internationally valid? Psychiatr Bull. 1992;16:257–61.
24. Mezzich JE, Kirmayer LJ, Kleinman A, Fabrega H Jr, Parron DL, Good BJ, Lin KM, Manson SM. The place of culture in DSM-IV. J Nerv Ment Dis. 1999;187(8):457–64.
25. Aggarwal NK. The evolving culture concept in psychiatric cultural formulation: implications for anthropological theory and psychiatric practice. Cult Med Psychiatry. 2023;47(2):555–75.
26. Santiago-Irizarry V. Culture as cure. Cult Anthropol. 1996;11(1):3–24.
27. Lukoff D, Turner R, Lu F. Transpersonal psychology research review: psychoreligious dimensions of healing. J Transpers Psychol. 1992;24(1):41–60.
28. Butler M, McCreedy E, Schwer N, Burgess D, Call K, Przedworski J, Rosser S, Larson S, Allen M, Fu S, Kane RL. Improving cultural competence to reduce health disparities. Rockville: Agency for Healthcare Research and Quality; 2016.
29. American Psychiatric Association. Diversity, equity, and inclusion: a strategic plan for DEI at APA. https://www.psychiatry.org/getmedia/174552a4-fadf-43f0-b816-4abf3ff81ca2/APA-DEI-Strategic-Plan.pdf.
30. Cross TL, Bazron BJ, Dennis KW, Isaacs MR. Towards a culturally competent system of care: a monograph on effective services for minority children who are severely emotionally disturbed. Washington, DC: CASSP Technical Assistance Center; 1989.

31. Tervalon M, Murray-García J. Cultural humility versus cultural competence: a critical distinction in defining physician training outcomes in multicultural education. J Health Care Poor Underserved. 1998;9(2):117–25.
32. Nursing Council of New Zealand. Guidelines for cultural safety, the treaty of Waitangi, and Maori health in nursing and mid-wifery education and practice. Wellington: Nursing Council of New Zealand; 2005.
33. American Psychiatric Association. Diagnostic and statistical manual of mental disorders, fourth edition: DSM-IV. Washington, DC: American Psychiatric Association; 1994.
34. Kirmayer LJ, Minas H. The future of cultural psychiatry: an international perspective. Can J Psychiatr. 2000;45(5):438–46.
35. Kirmayer LJ, Groleau D, Guzder J, Blake C, Jarvis E. Cultural consultation: a model of mental health service for multicultural societies. Can J Psychiatr. 2003;48(3):145–53.
36. Lukoff D, Lu FG, Turner R. Cultural considerations in the assessment and treatment of religious and spiritual problems. Psychiatr Clin North Am. 1995;18(3):467–85.
37. Boehnlein JK. Religion and spirituality in psychiatric care: looking back, looking ahead. Transcult Psychiatry. 2006;43(4):634–51.
38. Alarcón RD, Bell CC, Kirmayer LJ, Lin KM, Üstün B, Wisner KL. Beyond the funhouse mirrors: research agenda on culture and psychiatric diagnosis. In: Kupfer DJ, First MB, Regier DA, editors. A research agenda for DSM-V. Arlington: American Psychiatric Association; 2002. p. 219–81.
39. Whitley R. Religious competence as cultural competence. Transcult Psychiatry. 2012;49(2):245–60.
40. Dein S, Cook CCH, Koenig H. Religion, spirituality, and mental health: current controversies and future directions. J Nerv Ment Dis. 2012;200(10):852–5.
41. Koenig HG, Peteet JR, VanderWeele TJ. Religion and psychiatry: clinical applications. BJPsych Adv. 2020;26:273–81.
42. Gellerman DM. Religious and spiritual assessment. In: Lim RF, editor. Clinical manual of cultural psychiatry. 2nd ed. Washington, DC: American Psychiatric Publishing; 2015. p. 411–34.
43. Josephson AM, Peteet JR. Talking with patients about spirituality and worldview: practical interviewing techniques and strategies. Psychiatr Clin North Am. 2007;30(2):181–97.
44. Ross L, Grimwade L, Eagger S. Spiritual assessment. In: Cook CCH, Powell A, editors. Spirituality and psychiatry. Cambridge: Cambridge University Press; 2022. p. 23–48.
45. LaRocca-Pitts MA. FACT: taking a spiritual history in a clinical setting. J Health Care Chaplain. 2009;15(1):1–12.
46. Puchalaski C, Romer AL. Taking a spiritual history allows clinicians to understand patients more fully. J Palliat Med. 2000;3(1):129–37.
47. Anandarajah G, Hight E. Spirituality and medical practice: using the HOPE questions as a practical tool for spiritual assessment. Am Fam Physician. 2001;63(1):81–9.
48. Maugans TA. The SPIRITual history. Arch Fam Med. 1996;5(1):11–6.
49. Cook C, Grimwade L. Spirituality and mental health. London: Royal College of Psychiatrists; 2021.
50. Koenig H. Religion and mental health: research and clinical applications. San Diego: Academic Press; 2018.

Eastern Spirituality and Mental Health: Beyond the Mind

2

N. Yoganathan

Introduction

Madness is like energy: it is never lost, it is merely transformed.[1]

Why have I chosen to write about this topic? I do not profess to be an expert on religion or spirituality, but I do know about mental health, and my experience suggests that they are important bedfellows. To understand how my interest in these issues has arisen, I need to tell you a little about my personal and professional journey.

After qualifying as a doctor in my native Sri Lanka, I fled the country and moved to England in 1985 to pursue my postgraduate training, with no specialism in mind, partly due to the insecurities brought about by my immigration status and institutionalised 'isms' (race, class, gender, etc.) within the medical profession. I had always been fascinated by the mind, especially after I had encountered a patient with a conversion syndrome (a woman presenting with paralysis and atrophied muscles though there was no physiological cause of this condition), but it was almost by accident that I came to psychiatry, when I took on a locum psychiatrist position at a time of unprecedented change in mental health care in the UK. Instantly, I had found my calling.

I was confronted by the insidious shadow of stigma still hanging over mental illness. I sensed an idealistic drive—almost a crusade—to move people who were seriously mentally ill into the community, influenced by the work of Erving Goffman[2] and others on asylums and stigma. The buzz word was 'normalisation', which was initially quite seductive, but, as I became more experienced, I began to doubt the effectiveness of what had been a sincere and well-intentioned policy. It begged a recognition: 'norms' are socially constructed and by definition there will be a Gaussian curve, with outliers for whom, in this instance, the community was not the appropriate place for care.[3]

Another inescapable observation was the commodification of health care and the dominance of a market economy for the last 50 years. During my training and, since 1996, as a consul-

---

[1] Yoganathan, N. (2023). WASP/RCPsych Joint Congress London (After Isaac Newton).

In the beginner's mind there are many possibilities, but in the expert's there are few (Suzuki, S. (1970). Zen Mind, Beginner's Mind. Weatherhill. California).

N. Yoganathan (✉)
Kingston Wellbeing Ltd., New Malden, UK

[2] Goffman, E. (1961). Asylums: Essays on the Condition of the Social Situation of Mental Patients and Other Inmates. Anchor Books. New York.

[3] See e.g. Yoganathan, N. https://slidetodoc.com/stigma-and-empowerment-dr-n-yoganathan-mbbs-dpm/.

H. S. Moffic et al. (eds.), *Eastern Religions, Spirituality, and Psychiatry*,
https://doi.org/10.1007/978-3-031-56744-5_2

tant, I have witnessed how scientific advances have enabled us better to understand mental disorders, and there has been a natural tendency to focus on the aspect of 'cure' rather than 'healing', much as we would with a physical condition. Underpinning this has been a welcome effort to remove stigma, something I, too, have been addressing in my own clinical work, teaching[4] and work with Careif, a mental health charity.[5] Psychiatric illness often carries a sense of stigma due to the social component (group dynamics), but I suggest that this stigma cannot be *cured* though it may be *healed* through greater understanding and hence empowerment.

Psychodynamic therapy was initially pioneered by Freudian theories, but it was not effective for all conditions. Some of Freud's successors, neo-Freudians[6] such as Jung, Horney, Perls and Fromm, incorporated in their own therapeutic models of Eastern spiritual, philosophical and mystical concepts from Zen (Buddhism) and Hinduism. Despite the existence of these models, I have been intrigued by how an evidence-based therapy—CBT—recently had to diversify and incorporate Eastern spiritual and religious concepts such as mindfulness, Zen and detachment. These new therapies, what I consider to be 'old wine in new bottles', and which are also now manualised, are inherently prescriptive (religious) and lose their spontaneity, creativity and humaneness (spirituality). I cannot help asking, is the driver clinical effectiveness or a reflection of market economy reductionism and radicalisation?

Since becoming a consultant in 1996, I have been conducting presentations and workshops on confronting and dealing with the effects of stigma at personal and societal levels. In 2015 and 2017, I was part of the team who wrote Careif's[7] position statements on stigma, religion, spirituality,

mental health and diversity.[8] These various experiences inspired me to give a presentation on Eastern spirituality and mental health at a conference in London in 2023.[9] My session attracted positive feedback and led to an invitation to write this chapter, expanding on those ideas. I offer it as a merely personal insight and hope that it will stimulate your own reflections.

Formative Years

Returning to my background, I am originally from Ceylon (Sri Lanka) and was born into its minority Tamil community. Just 1 year before my birth, in 1956, the aspiring Prime Minister had sought to use the majority language—Sinhala—to win his electoral campaign, effectively dividing the indigenous populace. Following his political success, in 1958, the country experienced its first ethnic violence and, for the first time, the Tamils became aware of their being different.

Moving on a few years, schools were segregated by ethnic language groups, reinforcing a sense of minority status for my community, which also experienced some minor incidents of racial discrimination.

By the age of 16, I had begun to read more serious books and come across the Mahabharata, an ancient Hindu epic, translated from Sanskrit. A sanitised version of this text was taught in school and had been reproduced on film: simplistically, it was a tale of a group of good men triumphing over their evil cousins with the winners living happily ever after the version of the book that I read with great interest included additional chapters to those taught in school, one being the lake scene which I discuss below; in these chapters, familial loyalties were in conflict, and even the good succeeded only thanks to some acts of dubious morality. The final chapters in my book

---

[4]See website, N Yoganathan—careif.com.

[5]See e.g. Yoganathan, N. (2015) https://www.researchgate.net/publication/277664468_Careif_Position_Statement_on_STIGMA.

[6]Neo-Freudians see e.g. https://www.verywellmind.com/who-were-the-neo-freudians-2795576.

[7]Careif https://www.careif.org/.

---

[8]Yoganathan, N. et al. (2017) https://www.academia.edu/97479994/Global_Position_Statement_Religion_and_Spirituality_in_Mental_Health_Care.

[9]WASP/RCPsych Joint Congress 2023. London.

addressed not only the loss that the winners, too, suffered but also their eventual demise and the concepts of desire, death, illusion (*maya*) and *dharma* (the order of the world). This left my 16-year-old brain scrambled, but somehow the confusion lodged in my unconscious memory.

The next seminal moments for me were the re-emergence of ethnic violence in my country in 1977 and 1981 and the Jonestown incident/massacre in Guyana[10] in 1978, where a charismatic leader triggered his own and the death of his devoted followers. I was also fascinated by the power of an Indian mystic, Rajneesh,[11] and the mass group following he attracted before the movement imploded. Prompted by these events, I began to reflect on the ability of leaders and groups to be both creative and destructive.

Then in 1983, just before my final medical exams, the ethnic violence in Sri Lanka came to a peak. My family home was looted, damaged, ransacked and burnt, together with my books and our valuables. Many of my fellow Tamil students were temporarily displaced from their residences and had to seek refuge in camps; I was fortunate that, although my family home was no longer habitable, I was able to move in with a friend whose family had escaped the attacks.

This experience had a significant impact on me: whilst I was sad and angry, I wanted to understand why groups of people who had historically lived in harmony had turned against each other. Ceylon had had a succession of foreign rulers in modern times, from the Portuguese (1505–1658) to the Dutch (1658–1796), and briefly the French before the British (1796–1948), yet we had co-existed amicably. Why, only 10 years after the country had been left to forge its own independent identity, had fighting broken out between the indigenous groups to the point of it becoming normalised? My conclusion was that these primitive instincts had come to the fore in the absence of any real comprehension of 'democracy', and I began to

question whether education and 'civilisation' can actually nullify such basic instincts. Latterly, we have seen further evidence of these instincts in the emergence of radicalisation in so-called advanced societies, e.g. the American cult, Heaven's Gate (1974–1997),[12] Waco siege (1993)[13] and the Friedrichshof Commune[14] in Austria (1972–1990).

Beyond Science

Medicine is clearly a science, based on observation, evidence, demonstrable facts and practices. However, during my training as a doctor, I saw conditions where science simply had no answer and I was forced to recognise its limitations, not least in regard to the elusive power of the mind. I realised that there is something beyond 'the medical model'. This was confirmed by my subsequent training in psychiatry, dynamic psychotherapy and groups, specifically Median Groups[15], where I met the late Pat de Maré and his theory of healing through dialogue (koinonia). I began to differentiate between cure (the didactic/medical model) and healing (the dialectic/explorative model), which can be transpersonal and spiritual.

This coincided with my discovery of the works of Joseph Campbell[16] on mythology and cultures, Jungian psychotherapy[17] and Peter Brook's film of the epic Mahabharata.[18] My teenage self had been unable to make sense of this story, but now, with the wisdom born of my professional and personal experience, and seeing the characters brought to life on screen, I had a

---

[10] Jamestown, Guyana. See e.g. https://www.history.com/topics/crime/jonestown.

[11] Rajneesh, see e.g. https://www.learnreligions.com/the-real-rajneesh-cult-4165818.

[12] See e.g. The Story Of Heaven's Gate And Their Infamous Mass Suicide (allthatsinteresting.com).

[13] See e.g. The Waco Siege: a timeline of tragedy | Crime + Investigation UK (crimeandinvestigation.co.uk).

[14] See e.g. https://www.wikiwand.com/en/Friedrichshof_Commune.

[15] De Mare, P. (1991). Koinonia: From Hate, through Dialogue, to Culture in the Larger Group. Karnac Books.

[16] Brooks, P. (1989). The Mahabharata.

[17] Campbell, J. (1991). The Power of Myth. Anchor. New York.

[18] Jung, C. (1964). Man and his Symbols. Doubleday.

new-found understanding of the book. It brought with it a different perspective on the ethnic conflict in my native Ceylon. My group training showed how dialogue is the way to healing, but the difficulty with dialogue is that we need to negotiate our own uncomfortable feelings—such as anxiety, frustration, hate and grief—before we can engage in fruitful discussion with others.[19] These experiences made me become aware of the conscious and unconscious processes underpinning stigmatisation, which is pervasive in its nature.

Another important influence on my evolving thoughts was the UK's mental health policy from the 1970s to close the old mental asylums and replace them with care in the community.[20] Whilst well-intentioned, in practice, this proved to be unrealistic and impracticable. What had been a holistic system for supporting the mentally ill and their carers was superseded by a reductionist model, based on measurement and quasi-evidence. Many individuals found themselves merely moved from one system (health) into another (penal). As I wrote in 2013,

When the asylums closed, madness entered the community—and I do not mean patients! We responded to large group anxiety by imposing new forms of constraint (manuals, guidelines, tick boxes, categorisation).[21]

This situation can be illustrated by some recent UK statistics[22]:

- 71% of female and 43% of male prisoners reported having one or more mental health conditions.
- 998 prisoners were transferred from prison to a secure hospital in 2020.

The trend is not confined to the UK: we see a similar increase in the US penal system:

Serious mental illness has become so prevalent in the US corrections system that jails and prisons are now commonly called "the new asylums.[23]

Mental Illness

For diverse reasons, there has been an immense global increase in those with a mental illness—the WHO[24] declared depression to have the third highest illness burden in the non-communicable category—despite new discoveries and the availability of more forms of treatment (see the DSM[25] and ICD[26] descriptors). For instance, from the original, simple differentiation between insanity (madness) and idiocy (learning disability), by 1994, the DSM listed 297 different psychiatric conditions. It is important to acknowledge that most of the conditions listed in the DSM are based on consensus rather than objective, biological, markers. Had there really been such an exponential expansion in the nature of mental illness in 150 years or is this evidence of a need on the part of professionals and patients alike to draw reassurance from categorisation, from being

---

[19] Some reflections on the Gasi Large Group Experience during the Covid Pandemic, Yoganathan, N. Gasi Issue 19 https://groupanalyticsociety.co.uk/contexts/issue-89/event-reports/some-reflections-on-the-gasi-online-large-group-experience-during-the-covid-19-pandemic/.

[20] Making a Reality of Community Care, Audit Commission for Local Authorities in England and Wales, 1986, ISBN 978-0-11-701323-0.

[21] Yoganathan, N. & Willis, J. (2013). The Madness of Psychiatry. https://www.academia.edu/4404365/THE_MADNESS_OF_PSYCH....

[22] The Prison Reform Trust, Bromley Briefings Summer 2021.

[23] Torey, E.F. et al. (2014). The treatment of persons with mental illness in jails and prisons: a state survey. Arlington, VA. Treatment Advocacy Centre.

[24] WHO https://www.who.int/news-room/fact-sheets/detail/depression.

[25] https://www.thedsm5.com/the-dsm-5/.

[26] ICD-11 (who.int).

recognised as belonging to a group, no longer being 'other'?

Mental illnesses tend to alienate individuals from society (large group). This is essential for mutual existence. Any treatment and rehabilitation which do not aim to reintegrate the individual into wider society are doomed to fail in the long term. Median Groups offer a medium in which the anxieties of carers and patients can be managed more effectively. A process of dialogue encourages impersonal fellowship, helping individuals to discover and accept their own nature (Zen). This in turn aids destigmatisation, healing and recovery.

Since the 1970s, the UK has seen a sociocultural change in psychiatric care provision, with closure of large asylums. Conversely, there has been an exponential increase in beds in low- and medium-secure settings, as well as a disproportionate rise in psychiatric morbidity in prisons (over 60% of inmates).

The recent mantra of Western clinical work is 'evidence-based' practice. Whilst it may be justified for costly medical treatments to be objective, in psychiatry, this has led to CBT being used as a panacea. This and other quasi-scientific approaches and therapies undermine intuitive/interactive clinical practice, its spontaneity, humaneness and potential for healing.

Like the complementary of Yin and Yang, provision of psychiatric care should integrate evidence- and tradition-based (culture) practices. This can only be achieved successfully through a process of dialogue (dialectic) between different agencies. Failure leads to didactic and divisive practices, resulting in further stigmatisation and alienation, as witnessed in the UK.[27]

Religion, Spirituality, Psychiatry and Psychotherapy

So, why am I writing about this and what do psychiatry and mental health have to do with spirituality and religion?

In the past, Western psychotherapy has incorporated Eastern spiritual concepts which evolved in societies unconstrained by the scientific model. We have seized on such practices as offering a panacea, irrespective of their potential incompatibility with their adoptive cultures. Theories have been built upon existing theories, and hence, we saw Jung borrowing from Indian mysticism; some neo-Freudians adopted the ideas of Morita,[28] a Japanese psychiatrist and psychotherapist. The following quotations reflect the nature of such thinking:

Creativity requires the courage to let go of certainties.[29]

Lose your mind and come to your senses.[30]

The didactic model of psychiatry is about helping people to remove or control symptoms/conditions. It is evidence-based (usually quantitative), with strict codes of practice, and focuses on prescription and cure. By contrast, therapies which may have their roots in Eastern belief systems are dialectical and explorative; they seek healing through understanding and integration. Such practices call upon the creativity (art) of the psychiatrist. It is my view that the recent training and practice of psychiatry, based purely on quantitative evidence, are inevitably didactic and prescriptive, and hence, it is 'religious'. This is in contrast to the 'spirituality' of the dialectical model.

---

[27]Yognathan, Y. (2007). 'Zen, Stigma, Mental Health & Mental Illness', WFMH Congress, East Meets West, Hong Kong.

[28]Morita, Masatake; Kondo, Akihisa; Le Vine, Peg (1998). Morita Therapy and the True Nature of Anxiety-Based Disorders (Shinkeishitsu). Albany, NY: SUNY Press. ISBN 9780791437667.

[29]Fromm, E. (1941). Escape from Freedom (US), The Fear of Freedom (UK). ISBN 978-0-8050-3149-2.

[30]Perls, F. (1969). Gestalt Therapy Verbatim (1969) ISBN 0-911226-02-8.

[31]CBT research e.g. https://beckinstitute.org.

Recent research[31] and interest in developing culturally sensitive/responsive CBT may be of interest to many, but when it is manualised, will it truly capture the essence of healing?

Joseph Campbell's writings and film series, *The Power of Myth*, eruditely review how cultures across the globe and time have created stories and myths to make sense of the world, the divine and the struggle of the human mind to comprehend some of our profound experiences. For me, there is a fundamental difference between the Abrahamic and Eastern belief systems: the former mostly makes a clear, binary division between present life on earth and death (in either heaven or hell), symbolised by God and Satan, whereas spirituality, as in some alternative belief systems, is about transcending such duality. This is not to say that Eastern belief systems/religions do not have gods and demon figures; of course they do, but these are symbolic, and, whilst also showing followers how to behave morally and giving them opportunities to act 'mindfully', they enable them to reach 'God' during their lifetime, thereby blurring duality and transcending it.

> *Every religion is true one way or another. It is true when understood metaphorically. But when it gets stuck in its own metaphors, interpreting them as facts, then you are in trouble.*[32]

Before going any further, I should make explicit my use of the terms 'religion' and 'spirituality'. I follow an established differentiation between a belief system (religion) which is formalised and has accepted rituals,

> *A religion is a unified system of beliefs and practices relative to sacred things, that is to say, things set apart and forbidden—beliefs and practices which unite into one single moral community called a church, all those who adhere to them,*[33]

as opposed to 'spirituality', which is broader and non-formalised and may co-exist with religion or be stand-alone (see, e.g., Rethink[34]):

> *Spirituality is more of an individual practice and has to do with having a sense of peace and purpose. It also relates to the process of developing beliefs around the meaning of life and connection with others.*[35]

Qualitative research led by Willis[36] provides some useful insights into lay perceptions of the nature of religion and spirituality and their contribution to creating a sense of personal wellbeing. She concluded from her data:

> *There is considerable overlap of themes, suggesting that for our respondents, at least, religion and spirituality go hand in hand. They both offer moral frameworks for behaviour, provide opportunities for connecting with others, adopt similar practices of prayer or reflection, all of which contribute to a sense of purpose, hence wellbeing. Even though answers cannot be found to the meaning of life, respondents are largely content to accept that these issues are beyond human understanding, and to accept their place in the world.*

We should, however, heed Erich Fromm's words of caution:

> *The danger of the past was that men became slaves. The danger of the future is that men may become robots.*[37]

---

[32] Cambell, J. (1949). The Hero with a Thousand Faces. Pantheon Books.

[33] Durkheim, E. (1915). Elementary forms of the religious life p. 47.

[34] Reachout: www.reachout.com.

[35] Rethink. (2015). Spirituality, Religion and Mental Illness, 2015, v. 4 www.rethink.org.

[36] Willis, J. Persaud, A. Bhugra, D., 2016.The Centre for Applied Research and Evaluation International Foundation/World Psychiatric Association. Global Survey of Wellbeing. Report of Findings. www.careif.org and House of Lords Library. London. UK. (Careif/WPA Wellbeing.2016).

[37] Op cit.

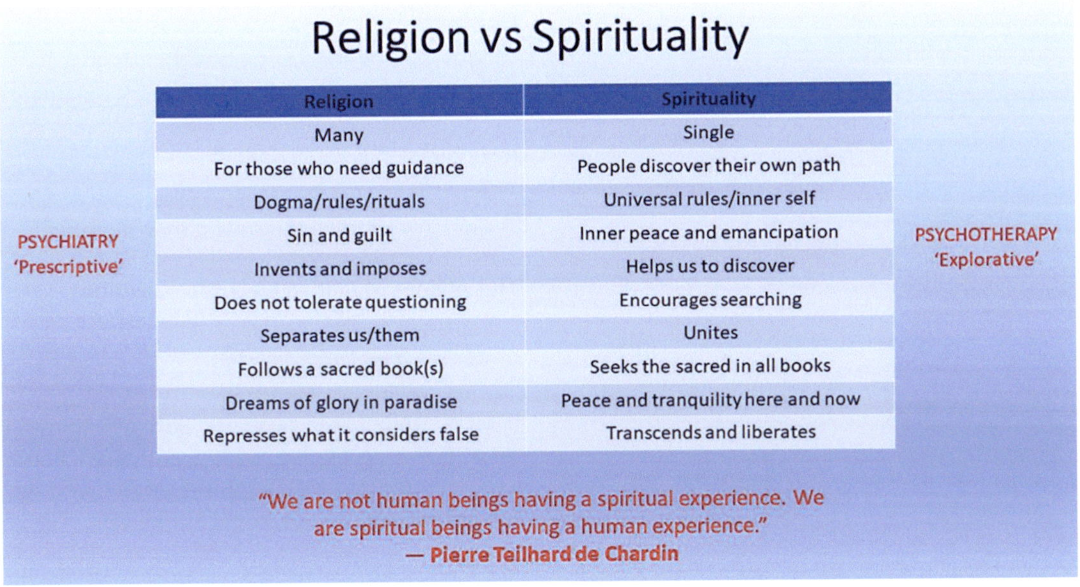

Religion vs Spirituality

	Religion	Spirituality	
	Many	Single	
	For those who need guidance	People discover their own path	
	Dogma/rules/rituals	Universal rules/inner self	
PSYCHIATRY 'Prescriptive'	Sin and guilt	Inner peace and emancipation	**PSYCHOTHERAPY** 'Explorative'
	Invents and imposes	Helps us to discover	
	Does not tolerate questioning	Encourages searching	
	Separates us/them	Unites	
	Follows a sacred book(s)	Seeks the sacred in all books	
	Dreams of glory in paradise	Peace and tranquility here and now	
	Represses what it considers false	Transcends and liberates	

"We are not human beings having a spiritual experience. We are spiritual beings having a human experience."
— Pierre Teilhard de Chardin

Fig. 2.1 Religion and spirituality

Figure 2.1 summarises what I perceive to be the broad differences between religion and spirituality before I explore Eastern spirituality and dharma.

Eastern Spirituality and Dharma

In order to capture the essence of spirituality and humankind's struggle to understand the concept of 'dharma', one meaning of which is 'the order of the world', I draw on the lake scene in Peter Brook's film, Mahabharata, which is transcribed below.

As in many other mythological stories, the heroes in the Mahabharata must overcome adversity during their journey through life. The context of this scene is that the five brothers representing goodness are exiled into the jungle for 13 years before they can leave to reclaim their kingdom. During this period, they encounter a magic lake.

They are thirsty but are only permitted to drink from it if they can answer certain questions. The four younger brothers fail to do so and die in the process; now, the eldest, Yudhishthira (Y) is questioned by the lake (L).

Questions from Lake

L: First answer my questions then I'll let you drink.

Y: Who are you? I don't see you.

L: Answer.

Y: Are you here? Are you in the water?

L: I am neither fish nor bird. I struck down your brothers because they wanted to drink without answering my questions.

Y: Examine me.

L: What is quicker than the wind?

Y: Thought.

L: What can cover the earth?

Y: Darkness.

L: Who are more numerous, the living or the dead?

Y: The living because the dead are no longer.

L: Give me an example of space.

Y: My two hands as one.

L: An example of grief.

Y: Ignorance.

L: Of poison.

Y: Desire.

L: An example of defeat.

Y: Victory.

L: Which came first, day or night?

Y: Day, but it was only a day ahead.

L: What is the cause of the world?

Y: Love.

L: What is your opposite?

Y: Myself.

L: What is madness?

Y: A forgotten way.

L: And revolt? Why do men revolt?

Y: To find beauty, either in life or in death.

L: And what for each of us is inevitable?

Y: Happiness.

L: And what is the greatest wonder?

Y: Each day death strikes and we live as though we were immortal. This is the greatest wonder.

Then the voice from the lake said:

L: May all your brothers come back to life.

Y: Who are you?

L: I am dharma, your father. I am constancy of lightness, the order of the world.

Y: You have taken the form of a lake?

L: I am all forms.

Yudhishthira's responses are paradoxical, yet they reflect the contradictions we find in nature. The punchline of this exchange (*'I am all forms'*) encapsulates the essence of Yin and Yang, the ambivalence of dualism and transcendence. The death and revival of the younger brothers symbolise the need for us to lay to rest our own 'innocence' when having to come to terms with the real world. Carl Jung expressed this when he wrote:

In all chaos, there is cosmos, in all disorder, there is a secret order.[38]

He observed,

The pendulum of the mind alternates between sense and non-sense, not right-wrong.

Joseph Campbell concluded:

It is only when a man tames his own demons that he becomes the king of himself, if not of the world.[39]

This echoes Mahatma Gandhi's[40] caution:

Our greatest ability as humans is not to change the world, but to change ourselves.

Which brings me back to dialogue and the need for us first to recognise our own prejudices before we can enter into meaningful dialogue with others and potentially overcome our biases.

Mindfulness, Eastern Spirituality and Beyond the Mind

The problem for psychiatry (mind medicine) is that it tends to imitate or follow the achievements of other areas of medicine (body medicine), which have benefited from the latest technological advancements. Not surprisingly, recent training and practice in psychiatry have also followed this trend, maybe due to envy, as well as due to the pressures of a market economy and globalisation. Despite this, I am fascinated by the latest fad (mindfulness), which is being packaged and marketed beyond therapeutic realms.

The fundamental difficulty is that the mind is not an organ, but it is essential for our very existence. Despite various models and attempts to define or understand the mind, it is my opinion that it will, and should, remain partly elusive and mystical so that we remain humble, grounded and spiritual. To achieve this is to view the mind not only as a noun but also as a verb. A person with a healthy mind is able to mind not only himself/herself but also the environment and others.

In other words, paradoxically, mindfulness is thinking not only about ourselves, but also about

---

[38] Op cit.

[39] Op cit.

[40] Gandhi, M.K. (1958). The Collected Works of Mahatma Gandhi.

others: minding—caring for them. I proposed at an international conference in Athens in 2009:

> To be truly mindful of others, one has to reach a state of "no mind.[41]

How one reaches a state of 'no mind' is the question that many ask.[42] In my view, the answer may lie in what Robert Oppenheimer, speaking after the first test of the atom bomb in July 1945, remarked:

> We knew the world would not be the same. A few people laughed, a few people cried. Most people were silent. I remembered the line from the Hindu scripture, the Bhagavad-Gita; Vishnu is trying to persuade the Prince that he should do his duty, and to impress him, takes on his multi-armed form and says, "Now I am become Death, the destroyer of worlds." I suppose we all thought that, one way or another[43]

To contextualise his words, here is another extract from the Mahabharata, the encounter between the charioteer, Krishna (K), and Prince Arjuna (A), the warrior, just before the war. Oppenheimer's reference follows the encounter below:

Krishna's Encounter with Arjuna

What is Krishna doing? He is speaking to Arjuna.

What is he saying?

He is telling Arjuna that victory and defeat are the same. He is urging him to act but not to reflect on the fruit of the act. He says to him: Seek detachment, fight without desire.

A: You said forget desire, seek detachment? Yet you urge me to battle, to massacre, your words are ambiguous, I am confused.

Krishna tells him: Don't withdraw into solitude. Renunciation is not enough. You must act, yet action mustn't dominate you. In the heart of action, you must remain free from all attachment.

A: How can I put into practice what you are demanding of me? The mind is capricious, unstable, it's evasive, feverish, turbulent, tenacious; it is harder to subdue than taming the wind.

K: You must learn to see with the same eye a mound of earth, a heap of gold, a cow, a sage, a dog, and a man who eats the dog. There's another intelligence beyond the mind.

In other words, Krishna is reminding Arjuna of humankind's limitations to comprehend the meaning of life and of our need to free ourselves from our man-made values and desires.

Viktor Frankl's unimaginable experience as a concentration camp inmate during the Holocaust led him to find meaning beyond this elusive reality through humble acceptance of our existence. He was thereby able to forge his own meaning by assuming responsibility for how he lived his life:

> Ultimately, man should not ask what the meaning of his life is, but rather must recognize that it is he who is asked. In a word, each man is questioned by life; and he can only answer to life by answering for his own life; to life he can only respond by being responsible.[44]

He proposed:

> Between stimulus and response there is a space. In that space is our power to choose our response. In our response lies our growth and our freedom.

We might equate this with being mindful—thinking before we act whilst having the potential to determine the nature of our actions.

---

[41] Yoganathan, N. (2009). 'From Socrates to Darwin and Beyond.' World Federation of Mental Health Congress. Athens.

[42] 'Moving Beyond Christianity: Islam, Judaism, Hinduism and Mental Health', World Cultural Psychiatry Research Review 2019: 13-19.

[43] Oppenheimer, R. (1945).

[44] Frankl, V. (1946). Man's Search for Meaning. Vienna.

[45] Yoganathan, N. (2015). Stigma, Identity & Radicalisation, WACP, Puerto Vallarta, Mexico.

Conclusion

Following through with my analysis, I suggest that evidence-based psychiatry (the didactic model), which includes not only prescription of drugs but also therapies based on manuals, is comparable to religion, being by definition dualistic or binary. It is science supported by art. By contrast, psychiatric interventions based on a dialectic model which includes not only prescriptions but also cultural/traditional methods and exploration of personal meaning pursue healing through a process which can be spiritual for both the patient and the therapist. This is art supported by science. In effect, this is the difference between prescriptive psychiatry and explorative psychotherapy. Figure 2.1 proposed the differences between the two models. They are challenging and may not be a comfortable proposition for some, as I reminded colleagues in 2015:

> *In the era of evidence-based practice, freedom of thought is heresy; freedom of action is blasphemy.*[45]

It is time for psychiatry to reclaim its identity as an art guided by science!

Spirituality Across the Lifespan, with Emphasis on Eastern Traditions

Andrew J. McLean

Introduction

While one could claim to write a chapter on spiritual and religious development from a totally objective standpoint, implicit bias is a given. The introduction to this chapter is provided through my own background:

My paternal grandfather and uncle were Presbyterian ministers. My father always said that had he not become a physician, he would have become a minister. My siblings and I were raised Roman Catholic, in my mother's tradition. (My father did not "convert.") So, growing up, I experienced a rather ecumenical version of Christianity.

As a preteen altar boy, I experienced the power of religion through all senses: the ring of sanctus bells, the smell of incense, the sight of the crucifix, the taste of the Eucharist, and the feel of the cassock and surplice. Many religious traditions, particularly Eastern, provide similar visceral experiences.

Like many, I look at my teenage years as a time not of solidifying belief, but of trial and discovery, a common passage as will be elucidated in sections below. An older brother, then enrolled in a liberal arts college, introduced me to the Upanishads and Bhagavad Gita. Literature and music provided gateways to religions of the East. During my sophomore year at that same liberal Catholic college, I lived in the seminary. Years later, I married a "Lutheran girl" and joined her church, to which we are still "enrolled."

It was in middle age when I came to acknowledge my agnosticism, a reflection of my limitations in certainty regarding religious doctrine. Perhaps, this correlates with what Medina terms "epistemic humility," defined as "having a humble and self-questioning attitude toward one's cognitive repertoire" [1]. However, based on definitions of spirituality within this chapter, it would be fair to say that I am a spiritual person and one who is enormously grateful for religious experiences and respectful of others of various faiths.

Spirituality and Religion

Books on spirituality have been particularly popular in recent decades. Some of these tie closely to sacred texts; others are quite separate. Many have themes interwoven with health and wellness. With the advent of the Internet, seekers of knowledge and comfort can immediately search for information, ideas, and guidance. Social media has been seen as both a positive and negative force in developing and maintaining one's well-being.

A. J. McLean (✉)
Department of Psychiatry and Behavioral Science, University of North Dakota School of Medicine and Health Sciences, Fargo, ND, USA
e-mail: andrew.mclean@und.edu

For both the public and those in academia, defining spirituality has been a challenge.

Common definitions of the term "spirituality" refer to a personal sense of connection with universal concepts. The University of Minnesota Earl E. Bakken Center for Spirituality & Healing site notes, "People may describe a spiritual experience as sacred or transcendent or simply a deep sense of aliveness and interconnectedness." Typically, definitions include an associated search for meaning and/or purpose in our lives. In fact, some authors see spirituality as part of an individual's "meaning system" [2]. Sinnott describes spirituality as connoting an individualized, inner experience as opposed to that of following a particular faith tradition [3]. Some researchers have been frustrated by the expanded and varied definitions of spirituality, particularly those distant from religion, as it complicates analytic comparisons. Monod et al. [4] found 35 separate instruments used in clinical research on spirituality, concluding that there is a "scarcity of instruments specifically designed to measure a patient's current spiritual state." Many have noted similarities between "religiosity" and "spirituality," though most see them as separate, but often overlapping. While both spirituality and religion may include behaviors and rituals, religion tends to be more organized and group-minded. Koenig et al. defined religion as "a system of beliefs and practices observed by a community, supported by rituals that acknowledge, worship, communicate with, or approach the Sacred, the Divine, Ultimate Truth, Reality, or nirvana" [5].

Religion has often been associated with institutional beliefs and practices, though one can have a personalized set directed toward a higher power/being. Elkind described a "personal" vs. "institutional" religion while studying developmental theory, with the former being more experiential and the latter developing through stages of increasing cognitive capacity [6].

According to King and Boyatzis [7], development of one's own organized system of beliefs can be linked to, or separate from, religious institutions. The term "religiousness" can refer to beliefs and activities tied to an individual's religion. Another term seen in the literature is "religiosity," which encompasses various aspects of religious behavior/thought. A number of studies have looked at intrinsic religiosity (internally oriented religiousness) and extrinsic religiosity (tied to social reward or acceptance) [8, 9]. In reviewing the field of religious research, DeHaan et al. [10] found the most common measure to be that of "religious salience," i.e., the importance of one's religious faith in matters of identity and thought.

Developmental Models and Stages Tied to Critical Time Periods (Table 3.1)

Childhood

It should not be a surprise that theories of development related to religion and spirituality intersect with those of psychology and psychiatry. Erikson's stages of psychosocial development [11] with their associated tasks have been incorporated into a number of developmental paradigms related to spirituality and religion. As the reader may recall, Erikson's stages related not only to the individual, but also to those who influence the individual through their significant relationships—the "counterplayers." In early childhood, these tend to be the mother and the family. Scientific data indicate that parents have the greatest influence on their children's religious and spiritual development [12]. A multicultural survey of parents (including those from Southeast/East Asia—Thailand, China, the Philippines) acknowledged the importance that religion played in their parenting [13].

The most well-known theory of cognitive development is attributed to Piaget [14]. As to the question of focusing on cognitive development when there are so many variables involved in religious development, K. Helmut Reich stated that the reason is "Because cognition is the dimension that generally correlates most clearly with more dimensions of social behavior and development than other personal characteristics" [15].

In Piaget's preoperational stage, symbols for representation of words, images, and ideas are

Table 3.1 Developmental models and stages tied to critical time periods

Age in years	Piaget Cognitive	Erikson Psychosocial	Fowler Religious	Elkind Religious	Kohlberg Moral
0–1.5	Sensorimotor	Trust vs. mistrust	Primal faith		Pre-conventional morality
1.5–3	Pre-	Autonomy vs. shame			1. Obedience/ punishment orientation
3–5	Operational	Initiative vs. guilt	Intuitive-projective		
5–12	Concrete operational	Industry vs. inferiority	Faith Mythic-literal faith	I. Undifferentiated II. Concrete/ behavioral III. Abstract/ reflective	2. Individualism/ exchange
12–18	Formal operational	Identity vs. role confusion	Synthetic-conventional faith		Conventional morality 3. Good interpersonal relationships
18–40		Intimacy vs. isolation	Individuative-reflective faith		4. Maintaining the social order
40–65		Generativity vs. stagnation	Conjunctive faith		Post-conventional morality 5. Social contract/ individual rights 6. Universal principles
65+		Integrity vs. despair	Universalizing faith		

utilized; however, abstract thinking does not occur until the stage of formal operations. Yet, over the entire lifespan, the concept of "schemata" or mental models are being developed through assimilation of new information or experiences. Individuals then change these schemata by accommodation with their world. Many cognitive psychologists feel that this reflects a fifth cognitive stage, the "post-formal." Here, the importance of context and experience comes into play. Cartwright, in her work *Cognitive Developmental Theory and Spiritual Development*, notes, "Piagetian theory made no provision for development of reasoning beyond the level of the single logical system" [16]. Haidt, in "The Happiness Hypothesis" [17], posits that regarding morality and behaviors, emotion plays a significantly larger role than cognitive developmentalists have afforded.

Elkind's three stages of religious identity roughly follow Piaget's cognitive stages of pre/ formal/concrete operations. His research indicated that by the time a child is roughly 5 years old, he or she has a sense of religious identity, though very global and undifferentiated. Around

7 or 8 years old, a child can differentiate between religious and nonreligious categories, not based on personal reflection, but by observation and behavior. According to Elkind, by the time a child leaves his or her preteen years, he or she begins to have his or her own concept of faith and belief.

Lawrence Kohlberg established a theory of moral development based in part on Piaget's cognitive work [18]. He also used Piaget's method of storytelling in gathering research data from subjects. Tied to cognitive development, he posited that individuals advance through moral stages, from a pre-conventional level based on reward/ punishment to a conventional level based on external ethics and to a post-conventional level tied to universal ethical principles. This is consistent with many moral and spiritual/religious theories which follow a progression of inner-directedness (self) to adherence (group) and to universality.

James Fowler was a theologian who incorporated many concepts from Erikson, Kohlberg, and Rizzuto in developing his stages of faith and selfhood. Rizzuto had developed two significant concepts on childhood relationship to God. One was the God Image—the emotional understanding of God, an intrapsychic understanding that impacts one's internal, psychological life. The other was the God Concept—intellectual thoughts which form an individual's conscious, external expression of spirituality and religion [19]. According to Fowler [20], the God Image is formed from infancy to middle childhood by interactions with those close to the child—i.e., Erikson's "counterplayers." (One can see the potential for incorporation of Piaget's theory of object permanence—the ability to know that objects/people exist when they cannot be seen or heard.) As the youth develops logic and a refined search for meaning, the God Concept is formed. As an individual matures and wrestles with paradox and dialectic, an interweaving of the God Image and God Concept becomes more complex and sophisticated, with the last stage reflective of a sense of universality and mission. Universality, the ability to tolerate and even embrace paradox, and dialectic are common to many Eastern religions.

Adolescence

In adolescence, peers become extremely important, and their influence often supplants that of the family. In today's world, social media also has a significant impact [21]. The task at this stage is establishing one's identity. Adolescence, with the development of abstract thinking, is a critical time for pondering, "finding one's-self," as well as a quest for meaning. Good and Willoughby [22] describe this as a "sensitive period" of identity and religious belief, theorizing that impacts last through adulthood due to waning plasticity. Spilka et al. [23] note that changes in religious beliefs and conversions are common in this stage of life. The Child Trends analysis of 2013 indicated that approximately one-fourth of US adolescents felt that religion was "very important" to them, which was a decrease from decades past [24].

It can also be argued that while teens are physically maturing earlier than previous generations, there is a protracted adolescence, particularly among those from higher income families. According to Yi [25], this is seen in East Asian countries such as Japan and Taiwan, but less so in China. In South Korea, a number of cultural variables play a role. In less affluent and more rural countries in the Far East, such as Cambodia, Vietnam, the Philippines, and Malaysia, a protracted adolescence is less often seen. Across many of these countries, the trajectory of girls' transition into adulthood is much more complicated than that of boys. The concept, noted by Erickson, of a "psychological moratorium" has been particularly notable in many societies over the past 20–30 years, with delays in joining the workforce or living independently from parents.

Other Theories

While the above theories are related to mandatory progressive stages with critical time periods, other theories have been developed without such constraints:

Schenker's heuristic model of religiosity is comprised of three primary elements: (1) religious judgment, an individual's cognitive framework of interpreting the world through a theological lens; (2) personality characteristics/personal religion; and (3) salience and depth of such beliefs/practice [26].

Religious judgment was a theory developed by Oser and later expanded upon in partnership with Gmünder. His definition was the following: "Religious judgment is the way in which an individual reconstructs his or her experience from the point of view of a personal relationship with an Ultimate (God). Religious development is concerned with the age-related, meaning-making qualities of this reconstruction" [27] (Table 3.2).

Oser's and Gmünder's theory of religious judgment (RJ) [28] is similar in certain aspects to Erikson's psychosocial theory of development in its use of polarities. In RJ theory, polar pairs include sacred vs. profane, transcendent vs. immanent, freedom vs. dependency, hope vs. absurdity, trust vs. anxiety, eternity vs. ephemerality, functional transparency vs. opaqueness, and

Table 3.2 Oser and Gmünder's stages of religious judgment

Stage		
Stage 1	Deus ex machina	The Ultimate Being (God) acts, humans react
Stage 2	Do ut des	The ultimate being can be influenced by prayers, offerings, the following of religious rules, etc.
Stage 3	Deism	The individual assumes responsibility for his or her own life, and for matters of the world. The ultimate being is apart. He has his own field of action; we have ours
Stage 4	Divine plan	Now an indirect, mediated relationship with an ultimate being has come into existence. The ultimate being becomes the condition for the possibility of human freedom, independence, etc., via the divine plan
Stage 5	Universal solidarity	The ultimate being appears in every human commitment yet transcends it at the same time. Transcendence and immanence interact completely. This total integration renders possible universal solidarity with all human beings

what is given vs. what is self-produced. Numerous Eastern religion researchers have found validity in this theory. Included in these were Dick's studies of Hindus, Jains, and Buddhists in India [29].

Adulthood

Also featured in Oser's and Gmünder's developmental theory is the concept that as one ages, one develops a transcendent mind-set. The Swedish gerontologist Lars Tornstam coined the term "gerotranscendence." However, in a study by Bruyneel et al. [30], the core concept of a transcendent connection (subscale of the gerotranscendence scale) was only weakly related to age. In Wink and Dillon's study of spirituality across the lifespan [31], spirituality increased at a more rapid pace among women than men, and the time of most robust increase was between late-middle and older adulthood. Villani et al. [32] reported that spirituality was positively correlated with an individual's subjective sense of well-being, independent of religious status. Wink and Dillon noted that in later life, while well-being could be derived from both spirituality and religiousness (importance of tradition-centered religious beliefs and practices), it occurred associated with the latter via relationships/connectedness/service.

Social/Cultural Aspects

To expand research that had primarily been done within Western, Judeo-Christian settings, McClintock et al. surveyed 5500 individuals. In their study, "Phenotypic Dimensions of Spirituality: Implications for Mental Health in China, India, and the United States" [33], the following participant religious affiliations were noted: 20% Buddhist, 21% Christian, 11% Hindu, 2% Muslim, 26% nonreligious, and 9% other. Their findings supported the concept of spirituality as a universal phenomenon. Shahaeien et al. [34] reviewed culture in the context of theory of mind development. They found that in contrast to Australian and US children aged 3–6 years, Iranian children showed a sequencing in the stages of theory of mind similar to Chinese children in that they understood knowledge access earlier than opinion diversity. The authors felt that this was attributable to areas of similar cultural importance, such as "filial respect, dispute avoidance, and acquiring knowledge."

Personality

Granqvist and Kirkpatrick [35] theorized that attachment styles predict relationships to both parents and religious deities. Secure attachments were seen as healthy, correlating with the philosopher and psychologist William James' concept of the "healthy-minded" individual. In James's lectures on "the sick soul" [36], he described the dilemma of a pluralistic view of theism. He labeled as "healthy minded" those individuals who subscribed to the concept of God as not responsible for the existence of evil. In such a theory, individuals with insecure styles of attachment may be expected to distance themselves from religious figures. However, a counter theory explained the seeking of a robust relationship with God as a stress-related, coping response. Granqvist and Kirkpatrick saw this as correlating with James' description of "the sick soul."

Regarding one's identity, Eastern philosophies describe particular personality types [37]. Within Buddhism, the Arhat personality (all "healthy factors") is attained through mindfulness.

In Hinduism, the aspect of one's personality is determined by the combination of three characteristics, or gunas: the Sattvic, or guna of spiritual quality; the Rajasic, or guna of active quality; and the Tamasic, or guna of material quality. The determination of personality within the Upanishads is known as "swabhaava." This term is also used in Buddhism, although there is discrepancy within the sutras as to a link to personhood.

Sufism is considered an Islamic mysticism. Ruh, or the spirit/true self of an individual with Allah, contends with overcoming man's primal nature, manifested in seven levels of nafs. Progressing through the influence of nafs in stages is accomplished by awareness, the intellect (aql).

In the Jain religion, karma is a significant driver, and individual action is necessary to reach nirvana, overcoming the life/death cycle. As in other Eastern religions, there are guidelines for living correctly: Right Faith (Samyak Darshan), Right Knowledge (Samyak Jnana), and Right Conduct (Samyak Charitra).

Self, Group, and Universality

Dimkov [38] notes that with minor exceptions, the concept of "self" within Eastern and Western philosophies is in opposition. Per Dimkov and others, in the East, self as an essence does not exist; it is illusory. The group, not the individual, is the priority. In the West, self exists as separate from others, and the individual is prioritized.

In Confucianism, sense of self is strongly tied to the social/cultural environment. In Taoism,

self is a manifestation of the cosmos, and ultimately "selfless." In Hinduism, the self again is relational—the human soul, Atman, as part of the divine spiritual truth, Brahman ("That art Thou").

In Buddhism, Atman or atta is the concept of self/soul. However, it is not an unchanging self; selfhood is an illusion. Buddhism is concerned with altruistic, ethical conduct, as noted in the Four Noble Truths and Eightfold Path. While many have used the term "suffering" as the primary focus in Buddhism, others have interpreted the term dukkha as "dissatisfaction."

East and West

From a religious/spiritual standpoint, in the West, the cognitive dissonance of the concept of evil is externalized, projected outward, whereas in the East, it is dealt with internally. Commonalities between "East and West," however, include mysticism and, as noted above, the frequent developmental progression of self/group/universality. In tying Eastern religion and spirituality to Western psychological developmental theories, perhaps the best example is Jayaram's clever analogy [39] noted in Figs. 3.1 and 3.2, between Maslow's "Hierarchy of Needs," swabhaava, and the Four Aims (Purusharthas) of Hindu life:

Experiences and Change

Many posit that cognitive development is a requirement for "higher" religious stages, though arguments against this are the well-known "abrupt conversion" experiences, where individuals have a significant precipitous change in their religious outlook. These can occur during stressful times, related to life events, pilgrimages, etc. A common occurrence (in the West, in particular) is that of an individual in the throes of addiction turning his or her life over to a higher power. The story of Bill W., one of the founders of Alcoholics Anonymous, is a prime example [40]. More rare phenomena related to pilgrimages are (usually) temporary psychological conditions such as the "India syndrome" and

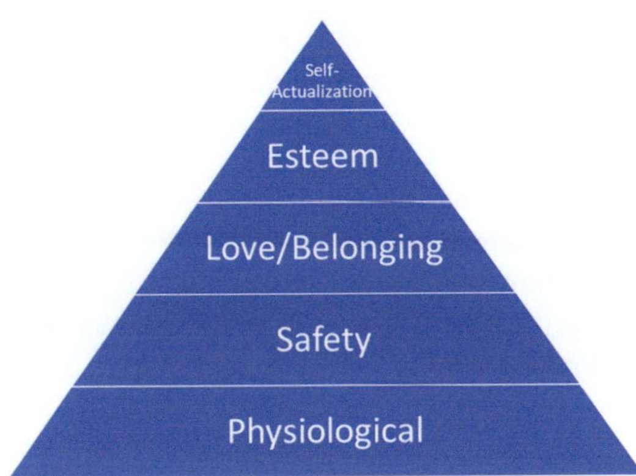

Fig. 3.1 Maslow's Hierarchy of Needs

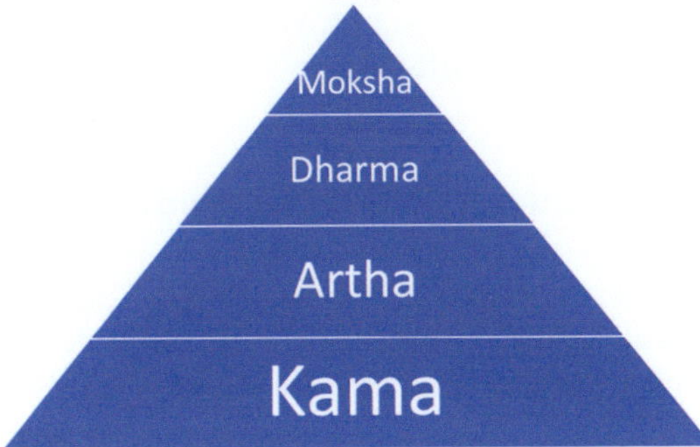

Fig. 3.2 Four Aims. Kama: desire; artha: wealth; dharma: righteousness; moksha: liberation

"Jerusalem syndrome" [41]. In these episodes, individuals experience profound religious obsessions and beliefs, often delusional. Typically, the symptoms dissipate upon return to the home country. Theories related to the etiology of these events abound.

Hallucinogens and Religious Experiences

Another type of seminal experience potentially impacting spirituality is the use of hallucinogenic drugs. For many, these are used within a foundation of culture, and psychedelic drugs have been associated with religious practices for millennia. Indigenous populations, especially in the Americas, have utilized these (particularly mescaline, psilocybin, and ayahuasca) in religious rites.

Vedic hymns, Hindu works over 3500 years old, mention the use of soma in divine rituals, although there remains debate as to the specific properties. Cannabis and *Datura* are also noted. Such uses are much less likely in other Eastern religions [42].

Whether we are talking about a particular brief "syndrome," an experience from hallucinogen ingestion, or a mental illness episode with religious manifestations, even temporary events can leave long-lasting impacts on one's spiritual and religious life.

Nature (Genetics)

David Sloan Wilson (Darwin's Cathedral) [43] and others have argued that religions are biological adaptations which, from an evolutionary standpoint, allow groups to function as single units.

Spector [44] comments on UK studies as well on those in the United States, Netherlands, and Australia, the findings of which pointed to a 40–50% heritability of spirituality/religiosity. In non-adopted twins raised by biological parents, no significant genetic influences were found from parents' practices until the young adults emancipated. D'Onofrio et al. [45] have also noted the link between the family environment and religious affiliations in their genetic studies of twins.

Neurology, Neuroimaging, Religion, and Spirituality

In literature, there are many instances of ties between particular types of seizures and spirituality. Perhaps, best known is the work of the Russian author Dostoevsky, who himself had epilepsy and had incorporated this malady into a number of his characters. He had described to family members one episode that he experienced: "I felt that heaven was going down upon the earth and that it had engulfed me. I have really touched God. He came into me myself, yes God exists I cried, and I don't remember anything else" [46].

Rim and colleagues [47] undertook a systematic literature review of neurobiological correlates of religion and spirituality (R/S), focusing on 25 studies. Tools frequently utilized in these studies included MRI, fMRI, PET, and EEG. Religious groups included Christians, Muslims, and Buddhists. Their findings showed potential associations between R/S and multiple brain regions, including the medial frontal cortex, orbitofrontal cortex, precuneus, posterior cingulate cortex, default mode network, and caudate.

Zhu et al. [48] looked at neuroimaging in relation to the psychological self-structural differences noted between East Asian (interdependent) and Western (independent) subjects. In an fMRI study measuring brain activity judging personal trait adjectives regarding self, mother, or a public person, they found that "Chinese individuals use the medial prefrontal cortex (MPFC) to represent both the self and the mother, whereas Westerners use MPFC to represent exclusively the self, providing neuroimaging evidence that culture shapes the functional anatomy of self-representation."

Han and Ma [49] reviewed self-referential processing through fMRI and noted that both Chinese Buddhists and Christians had increased activity in the dorsal medial prefrontal cortex (DMPFC) (vs. increase in the ventral medial prefrontal cortex (VMPFC) in Chinese nonreligious). In addition, Buddhists had decreased functional connectivity between the DMPFC and posterior parietal cortex. The above findings led the authors to assume that there was a relationship between such neural activity and the Buddhist doctrine of "no-self." They also found that "East Asian cultures are associated with increased neural activity in the brain regions related to inference of others' mind and emotion regulation, whereas Western cultures are associated with enhanced neural activity in the brain areas related to self-relevance encoding and emotional responses during social cognitive/affective processes." Wu et al. [50] studied neural activity in subjects of two Chinese ethnic groups (Han and Tibetan) to review the potential role of religion in self-representation. (An assumption within this study was that all Tibetans were Buddhists.) The findings led the researchers to the conclusion that a difference in neural activity was due to the nominal sense of "I-ness" among the Tibetans.

Gupta and colleagues [51] described a controlled study involving spiritual practice such as meditation and prayer, and spiritual transformation experiences. fMRI results showed increased network as well as increased frontal lobe perfusion and improved mood compared to controls.

Numerous studies utilizing EEG, MRI, and fMRI have pointed toward the inferior parietal lobe (IPL) in perceptual processes related to spirituality [52]. In particular, the left IPL may be involved in the sense of a visuospatial presence outside of one's self [53].

Case Study: A Convert to Hinduism

His mother was a practicing Roman Catholic, and his father a nonpracticing Anglican. After his First Communion at age 11, George Harrison (who would later become known as "the quiet Beatle") decided that he would not go on to receive the next rite, that of Confirmation. "I thought, 'I'm not going to bother with that, I'll just confirm it later myself'" [54]. While he appreciated the impact of his church attendance on his senses—the stained-glass windows, the images of Christ, and the smell of incense—he was skeptical of the authoritarianism of the church and sensed hypocrisy. Some individuals raised similarly find their way to remain in the church through the social justice movements often developed outside of such authority— George ventured "outside" and found such companionship, purpose, and enlightenment through Hinduism. He later said, "I came to understand what Christ really was through Hinduism" [55].

As noted, parental religious belief and foundation have a strong influence on the spiritual and religious development of their children, and a key Eriksonian "counterplayer" is the mother. Despite her religious and cultural background, George's mother appreciated others' cultures and perhaps unknowingly fostered her son's interest as well.

While in utero, he was bathed in Indian music from his mother's Sunday listening to the Radio India program [56]. Even at the height of the Beatles' popularity, George was writing to his mother about spiritual matters and his search for self-realization and God. He appreciated the presence of the feminine and masculine in Krishna/Radha. George remained close to his mother and soothed her on her deathbed with readings from the Bhagavad Gita.

Episodes

George described episodes beginning in childhood where he would have odd vibratory sensations, feeling extremely small and then expanding at rapid speed and "coming out of it," fearfully. He later learned to induce these episodes [57]. Whether they were neurologic (doubtful, due to the ability to induce) or psychological (derealization/depersonalization, though there was no history of psychological trauma) is uncertain. There is no mention of a particular relationship between these experiences and spirituality.

As mentioned earlier in this chapter, adolescence is a time for experimentation, trying new and exciting things, beginning the search for "finding yourself." George was still a minor when he joined the Beatles and began playing in Germany, exposed to many worldly matters earlier than most. In terms of the Four Aims of the Hindu life (pyramid above), he experienced artha (wealth) quite quickly.

The first club the band was scheduled to perform in was, ironically, called the Indra, named for the primary god of the Rig Veda who defeats evil and deception. Within a few years, a particular event would launch him toward his new religion.

The term psychedelic, Greek for "showing the soul," was originated by the psychiatrist Humphry Osmond [58]. In his early 20s, George had his first experience with LSD, slipped to him and others while at a friend's house. Though initially frightening, he was quoted as saying, "I had such an overwhelming feeling of well-being, that there was a God, and I could see him in every blade of grass. It was like gaining hundreds of years of experience within twelve hours. It changed me, and there was no way back to what I was before" [59]. Around this time, he and his friends more frequently utilized LSD; he and his bandmates developed a formally shared interest in Eastern religion, philosophy, and music, although George was the only member whose interest led to a life of devotion. After becoming acquainted with the sitar, he was introduced to Ravi Shankar, who provided him with teachings of Hinduism. He also met Maharishi Mahesh Yogi and the founder of the global Hare Krishna movement, Swami Prabhupada. He stopped utilizing LSD as he became more serious about his religious practice, believing that while the drug had initially been quite useful, it no longer served a purpose for him. In addition to traditional Hindu texts, he frequently read the I Ching and Yogananda's Autobiography of a Yogi. George believed that you must practice your religion and experience it—meditation and transcendence. He often mentioned that he was seeking the face of God. The Hare Krishna form of Hinduism was a good fit due to his appreciation of both individual and communal music in the form of chanting. He felt that music, along with meditation, was one of the vehicles to obtain enlightenment. "Through Hinduism, I feel a better person. I just get happier and happier. I now feel that I am unlimited, and I am more in control ..." [60].

George was uncomfortable with celebrity, and when he found like-minded people within the Hare Krishna movement, he felt unburdened. As a youth, he had not advanced in school and had been an electrician's apprentice and the son of a bus driver, and the people who knew him best felt that he was a very humble individual. He had a long-standing empathy for others, particularly those who were suffering, and for the underdog and the common person. He would go on to establish the template for benefit concerts with The Concert for Bangladesh, not only helping hundreds of thousands of people, but also enlightening others about Asian countries and Eastern religions.

Case Summary

George was raised by a religious mother and set out at an early age in search of meaning. In the material world, he faced human challenges. While Paul McCartney, in an interview a few years ago [61], indicated that the Beatles worked through their mental health issues with their songs, there is no indication that George suffered from a mental disorder. He and his friends certainly used drugs (an occupational hazard of rock stars), and ex-wife Pattie Boyd noted that for George, cocaine was particularly negative for him during their marriage [62]. However, drug use seemed to significantly wane, and it is clear that he found a sense of well-being and happiness as a result of his spiritual journey. He was able to find his group or "tribe" in the Hare Krishna tradition of Hinduism and clearly developed a universal mind-set as he grew older. "We have the same qualities as God, just as a drop of the ocean has the same qualities as the entire sea …" [63]. He felt that his body was simply a vessel for this life, and his hope was, as with all Hindus, to have freedom from samsara (rebirth) and arrive at moksha (liberation). George Harrison, a bridge between West and East, died with family and friends surrounding him, as verses were chanted from the Bhagavad Gita. His ashes were scattered in the holy Ganges.

Conclusion

The entirety of this book is dedicated to the connection between mental health and Eastern religions/spirituality. As one can see, if and where one lands in terms of one's spirituality can be influenced by many factors. There can be a fostered, religious upbringing; there can be active searching for spirituality; and at times, there can be an abrupt and unintended meeting with it. While there continues to be support for religious/spiritual developmental theories across the lifespan, particularly in correlation with psychological theories, science also has shown us the importance of "nature" as well as selective, experiential events impacting one's religious/spiritual journey.

References

1. Medina J. The epistemology of resistance: gender and racial oppression, epistemic injustice, and resistant imagination. Oxford: Oxford University Press; 2013.
2. van Uden MHF. Religion in the crisis of mourning: an explorative study by in-depth interviews. Dekker & Van de Vegt: Nijmegen; 1985.
3. Sinnott JD. The development of logic in adulthood: postformal thought and its applications. New York: Plenum; 1998.
4. Monod S, Brennan M, Rochat E, Martin E, Rochat S, Büla CJ. Instruments measuring spirituality in clinical research: a systematic review. J Gen Intern Med. 2011;26:1345–57.
5. Koenig HG, Kvale JN, Ferrel C. Religion and Well-being in later life. Gerontologist. 1988;28:18–28.
6. Elkind D. Age changes in the meaning of religious identity. Rev Relig Res. 1964;6(1):36–40.
7. King PE, Boyatzis CJ. Religious and spiritual development. In: Handbook of psychology and developmental science, vol. 3. Wiley; 2015. p. 975–1014.
8. Bergin AE. Values and religious issues in psychotherapy and mental health. Am Psychol. 1991;46:394–403.
9. Woyciechowski D. The relationship between intrinsic/extrinsic religiosity and meaning in life. Rowan-Theses and Dissertations. 2007. p. 884.
10. DeHaan LG, Yonker JE, Affholter C. More than enjoying the sunset: conceptualization and measurement of religiosity for adolescents and emerging adults and its implications for developmental inquiry. J Psychol Christian. 2011;30:184–95.
11. Erikson EH. The life cycle completed. New York: W.W. Norton & Company; 1982.
12. Smith C, Adamczyk A. Handing down the faith: how parents pass their religion to the next generation. Sociol Relig. 2022;83(4):536–8.
13. Bornstein MH, Putnick DL, Lansford JE, Al-Hassan SM, Bacchini D, Bombi AS, Chang L, Deater-Deckard K, Di Giunta L, Dodge KA, Malone PS, Oburu P, Pastorelli C, Skinner AT, Sorbring E, Steinberg L, Tapanya S, Tirado LMU, Zelli A, Alampay LP. 'Mixed blessings': parental religiousness, parenting, and child adjustment in global perspective. J Child Psychol Psychiatry. 2017 Aug;58(8):880–92.
14. Piaget J. Cognitive development in children development and learning. J Res Sci Teach. 1964;2:176–86.
15. Schenker D, Reich KH. Oser/Gmünder's developmental theory of religious judgement: status and outlook. In: Archive for the psychology of religion, vol. 25. London: Sage; 2003. p. 180–94.
16. Cartwright KB. Cognitive developmental theory and spiritual development. J Adult Dev. 2001;8(4):213–20.
17. Haidt J. The happiness hypothesis. New York: Basic Books; 2006.
18. Kohlberg L. The psychology of moral development: the nature and validity of moral stages (essays on moral development, volume 2). Harper & Row; 1984.

19. Rizzuto AM. The birth of the living god: a psychoanalytic study. University of Chicago Press. 1979;
20. Fowler JW. Stages of faith. New York: Harper & Row; 1981.
21. Barry CT, Sidoti CL, Briggs SM, Reiter SR, Lindsey RA. Adolescent social media use and mental health from adolescent and parent perspectives. J Adolesc. 2017;61:1–11.
22. Good M, Willoughby T. Adolescence as a sensitive period for spiritual development. Child Dev Perspect. 2008;2(1):32–7.
23. Spilka B, Hood RW Jr, Hunsberger B, Gorsuch R. The psychology of religion: an empirical approach. 3rd ed. New York: Guilford; 2003.
24. ChildTrends. Religiosity among youth. 2013. http://www.childtrends.org/?indicators=religiosity-among-youth.
25. Yi CC. Adolescents and transition to adulthood in Asia. In: Quah S, editor. Routledge handbook of families in Asia, vol. 13. New York, NY: Routledge; 2015. p. 1–20.
26. Shenker D. The influence of religiosity on coping with existential issues in young and young adults. Unpublished Lizentiatsarbeit, School of Education, University of Fribourg, Schweiz; 1996.
27. Oser F. Stages of religious judgment. In: Brusselmans C, O'Donohoe JA, editors. Toward moral and religious maturity. Morristown, NJ: Burdett; 1980. p. 277–315.
28. Oser F, Gmünder P. Religious judgement. A developmental approach. (Trans. By Norbert F. Hahn, 1991). Birmingham, AL: Religious Education Press; 1984.
29. Dick A. Drei transkulturelle Erhebungen des religiösen Urteils. Eine Pilotstudie. Unpublished Lizentiatsarbeit, School of Education, University of Fribourg; 1982.
30. Bruyneel S, Marcoen A, Soenens B. Gerotranscendence: components and spiritual roots in the second half of life. Psychology. 2005.
31. Wink P, Dillon M. Religiousness, spirituality, and psychosocial functioning in late adulthood: findings from a longitudinal study. Psychol Aging. 2003;18(4):916–24.
32. Villani D, Sorgente A, Ianello P, Antonietti A. The role of spirituality and religiosity in subjective well-being of individuals with different religious status. Front Psychol. 2019 July;10:1–11.
33. McClintock CH, Lau E, Miller L. Phenotypic dimensions of spirituality: implications for mental health in China, India, and the United States. Front Psychol. 2016;27(7):1600.
34. Shahaeian A, Peterson CC, Slaughter V, Wellman HM. Culture and the sequence of steps in theory of mind development. Dev Psychol. 2011;47(5):1239–47.
35. Granqvist P, Kirkpatrick LA. Attachment and religious representations and behavior. In: Cassidy J, Shaver PR, editors. Handbook of attachment: theory, research, and clinical applications. The Guilford Press: New York; 2008. p. 906–33.
36. James W. The varieties of religious experience: a study in human nature. Modern Library N Y. 1902;6:7.
37. Mohanty A, Ravi A, Girish D, Gumber M, Chaudhary V. Eastern traditions: perspectives on psychology of personality and motivation. Indian Transp Psychol. 2019.
38. Dimkov PR. The concept of self in eastern and western philosophy. In: 5th international e-conference on studies in humanities and social sciences, Belgrade; 2020. p. 197–204.
39. Jayaram V. Maslow's hierarchy of needs and purusharthas of Hinduism. https://www.hinduwebsite.com/hinduism/essays/maslow-and-hinduism.asp.
40. Thomsen R. Bill W: the absorbing and deeply moving life story of bill Wilson, co-founder of alcoholics anonymous. New York: Harper & Row; 1975.
41. Bar-El Y, Durst R, Katz G, Zislin J, Strauss Z, Knobler HY. Jerusalem Syndrome. Br J Psychiatry. 2000;176:86–90.
42. https://en.wikipedia.org/wiki/Religion_and_drugs. Accessed 22 June 2023.
43. Wilson DS. Darwin's cathedral: evolution, religion, and the nature of society. University of Chicago Press; 2003.
44. Spector T. Identically different: why we can change our genes. New York: The Overlook Press; 2013.
45. D'Onofrio BM, Eaves LJ, Murrelle L, Maes HH, Spilka B. Understanding biological and social influences on religious affiliation, attitudes, and behaviors: a behavior genetic perspective. J Pers. 1999 Dec;67(6):953–84.
46. Mayne EC. (Trans.) Letters of Fyodor Mikhailovich Dostoevsky to his family and friends. New York: Horizon Press; 1961.
47. Rim JI, Ojeda JC, Svob C, Kayser J, Drews E. Current understanding of religion, spirituality, and their neurobiological correlates. Harv Rev Psychiatry. 2019;27(5):303–16.
48. Zhu Y, Zhang L, Fan J, Han S. Neural basis of cultural influence on self-representation. NeuroImage. 2007;34(3):1310–6.
49. Han S, Ma Y. Cultural differences in human brain activity: a quantitative meta-analysis. NeuroImage. 2014;99:293–300.
50. Wu Y, Wang C, He X, Mao L, Zhang L. Religious beliefs influence neural substrates of self-reflection in Tibetans. Soc Cogn Affect Neurosci. 2010;5(2–3):324–31.
51. Gupta SS, Maheshwari SM, Shah UR, Bharath RD, Dawra NS, Mahajan MS, Desai A, Prajapati A, Ghodke M. Imaging & neuropsychological changes in brain with spiritual practice: a pilot study. Indian J Med Res. 2018;148(2):190–9.
52. Miller L, Balodis IM, McClintock CH, Xu J, Lacadie CM, Sinha R, Potenza MN. Neural correlates of personalized spiritual experiences. Cereb Cortex. 2019;29(6):2331–8.
53. Farrer C, Frith CD. Experiencing oneself vs another person as being the cause of an action: the neural

correlates of the experience of agency. NeuroImage. 2002;15:596–603.

54. The Beatles. The Beatles anthology. San Francisco: Chronicle Books; 2000. p. 25–6.

55. Shankar R. Raga mala: the autobiography of Ravi Shankar, vol. 230. New York: Welcome Rain Publishers; 1999.

56. Greene JM. Here comes the sun: the spiritual and musical journey of George Harrison. Hoboken, NJ: Wiley Publishing; 2007. p. 2.

57. Tillery G. Working class mystic: a spiritual biography of George Harrison. Wheaton, IL: Quest Books; 2011. p. 17.

58. Tanne JH. Humphrey Osmond. BMJ. 2004;328(7441):713.

59. The Editors of Rolling Stone. Harrison. New York: Simon and Schuster; 2002. p. 145.

60. Harry B. The George Harrison encyclopedia. London: Virgin Books; 2003. p. 321.

61. Reilly N. Interview with Paul McCartney, NME. 2020. https://www.nme.com/news/music/paul-mccartney-says-the-beatles-suffered-from-mental-health-issues-there-were-a-lot-of-things-we-had-to-work-through-2833462. Accessed 12 June 2023.

62. Boyd P. Wonderful tonight. George Harrison, Eric Clapton, and me. New York: Three Rivers Press; 2007.

63. Belmo. George Harrison: his words, wit and wisdom. Fort Mitchell, KY: Belmo Publishing; 2002. p. 36.

Eastern Religions and Their Influence on Parenting

4

Aradhana Bela Sood, Sarah Arshad, and Jayaprabha LaFontaine

Introduction

"Children are the narcissistic extension of an Indian parent's identity" …. These words echoed in my mind as I sat nursing the subtle hurt that grew in me.

A colleague of 20 years, whom I respect, articulated his observation while I had been musing over my children's academic progress. I had immigrated to the United States in 1982 and had three children who in the early 2000s were in the formative stages of establishing their "second separation individuation" by choosing a college and a career. In retrospect, I am not sure to what extent I was fully aligned with the traditional dictum "be successful or else" from my South Asian ancestry. However, the fact that it hurt made me ponder and think.

I would argue that children are, by and large, considered their parents' creation and thus a reflection of them. In varying degrees, my colleague's observation could be universally applied to anyone from Eastern or Western hemisphere.

A. B. Sood (✉)
Virginia Commonwealth University, Richmond, VA, USA
e-mail: bela.sood@vcuhealth.org

S. Arshad
DCAPBS, Philadelphia, PA, USA
e-mail: Arshads@chop.edu

J. LaFontaine
Nixa, MO, USA

However, there are easy-to-spot differences based on our backgrounds: these values are emphasized in our role as parents and which we do not consider to be the fulcrum around which we formulate our mores and actions as parents.

So, to what is this variance attributable? Is it religion that defines what one turns to at the birth of our first child or is it the prevailing culture that surrounds us when we were children ourselves? What molds our sensibilities as parents? Is parenting a skill that is taught or is it passively imbibed through exposure to behavior? How much of it changes with the ever-expanding influence of life experiences, new information that comes from observation of others, education, travel, migration, and especially intermarriage or cross-pollination of religion, race, and ethnicity in couples?

The objective of this chapter is to discuss Eastern parenting with consideration given to spirituality and religion. The writing is not meant to be an exhaustive or critical review of religions but a broad overview of their influence on parenting.

The term East refers to a large and diverse area [1], which has several religious traditions. If we include the Middle East, we have religions like Christianity, Judaism, and Islam that all had their origins in that area. However, the conscious decision to tailor the discussion and to focus on the regions that are geographically in the East was made to (a) work within boundaries to maintain a focus for the topic and to (b) specifically examine the influence of geographical proximity and cultural similarities on the religions included. Islam will be included in the discussion as it has wide representation in the Eastern hemisphere, e.g., Pakistan, India, and Indonesia, to name a few countries, whereas Christianity and Judaism, both Abrahamic religions like Islam, have mostly populated the Western hemisphere and the Middle East, respectively, with relatively marginal representation in the East.

Spirituality and religion are often understood as separate concepts [2] in which religion is a specific set of organized beliefs and practices shared by a community or a group, while spirituality is an individual's private/personal relationship to something larger that can lead one to experience peace, purpose, meaning in life, and connection with others. It could be argued that one's religious beliefs help the development of one's spiritual life. Although a person may move away from the rituals of one's religion, growing up surrounded by a belief system validated by the majority culture could influence the imbibing of thematic values and mores that the religion has created as a structure for itself. This may be an important part of an individual's spiritual life. Hence, operating from the broad assumption that spirituality is connected to values that spring from a culture and to some extent the religion of a geographic area, we will discuss parenting in relation to the religions of the East.

The Eastern religions that arose in Greater India including Hinduism, Buddhism, Jainism, and Sikhism loosely share the concepts of Dharma (one's duty), Karma (one's actions), and reincarnation (the soul will be reborn), while East Asian religions that are followed in Korea, Japan, and China make use of the concept of Tao (natural order of the universe) and include Confucianism (focuses on filial piety, humaneness, and rituals), Shintoism (respect of nature), and Shamanism (spirit healing) [3]. These religions are generally considered polytheistic (unlike those in the West such as Christianity that tend to be monotheistic) and derive from philosophical teachings with a representation of folk traditions that guide daily living. The values of

Islam, a monotheistic Abrahamic religion represented in many parts of the Eastern hemisphere including the Indian subcontinent, strongly guide parenting.

Before we venture into the impact of Eastern religion and spirituality on parenting styles, let us review the traditional scaffolding of how parenting is characterized in the literature and then attempt to extrapolate what we learn from those descriptors to cultural and religious influences on parenting.

Types of Parenting

Parenting styles are described broadly as authoritarian, authoritative, permissive [4], or uninvolved. Each refers to the degree of involvement parents have with the child and the nature of the overarching philosophy they use in giving children core values, a way of living, and their place in the community and home. A qualifier before we discuss this is that none of these descriptors are always rigid. They could exist as a combination in a person and find expression when certain triggers occur or could be the predominant style in their parenting. Some of these styles may be consistent with the cultural and social background of the family and rationalized through religious teachings or rituals that were passed down intergenerationally. As there is a broadening of life experiences and exposure to other cultures, these styles may alter based on the psychological malleability of the parent and receptivity to change. Conclusions expressed regarding outcomes of each parenting style do not have a rigorous research base but are accepted in psychological formulations of character and personality development.

Parenting Styles

In authoritarian parenting, an overinvolved parent believes that the child is important but does not have agency to make decisions on their own, that they should follow the parents' directions in day-to-day living, and that their aspirations and goals both immediate and long term should be determined by the parent. Obedience rather than negotiated rule setting is the norm with little if any input from the child as rules are enforced. Disagreeing with the parent can lead to negative consequences on a psychological and a physical level. The focus on discipline for stepping out of line rather than teaching children to make better choices may cause guilt and fear in the child. Research suggests that children raised by authoritarian parents are at risk for poor self-esteem, harbor aggression and anger, and are less capable of forging an independent path for themselves as adults.

In authoritative parenting, the parent may be overinvolved and directive, but decisions are discussed with the child and made collaboratively, i.e., reasoning is prominent, and a sense of give and take exists. Rules are enforced but not without explaining the reason for the rule. The emphasis on creating a positive relationship with the child includes validating the child's feelings or perceptions. Praise and rewards are embedded in the discipline style. There is consensus that authoritarian parenting is perhaps the best fit for raising confident and self-assured children who are more adept at making decisions as adults and assessing safety risks in adulthood.

At the other end of the spectrum, permissive parenting is marked by loose boundaries regarding rules for the child. If there are rules, they are rarely applied consistently. The parent assumes the role of a "friend" to their child. Although communication is encouraged, they do not help the child avoid bad choices or correct bad behavior. Leniency with expectations and the idea that the child will learn best on their own is a value held by permissive parents. Children growing in permissive environments are known to be at risk for academic underachievement, sadness, and health problems because of a paucity of supervision over nutrition and exercise choices. They may be at higher risk for behavior problems as they do not like being held to rules [5].

In uninvolved parenting, the parent does not see the need to be available to the child on a day-to-day basis. This could be because they believe that the child will raise themselves or their own

life circumstances such as economic hardships keep them away from home. Occasionally, depression or substance abuse or a lack of knowledge of child development can lead to uninvolved parenting. Uninvolved parents have a cursory idea of their child's whereabouts and rarely supervise their homework or see to their day-to-day needs. Such children are at risk for underachievement in multiple arenas as adults. They are likely to struggle with sadness and poor self-esteem.

Let us examine and explore Eastern religions, with a special focus on the Indian subcontinent and minor allusions to the Far East that includes China, Korea, Japan, and Vietnam. This will be followed by short narratives from two adults who grew up under the influence of Hindu and Muslim traditions, in countries that are geographically insular from the country in which their parents grew up. We will also explore whether those principles travel with them upon migration and remain operative even when those values are not validated by the majority culture of the country where they make a new home. To what extent did religion and spirituality drive parenting styles or was it the culture/environment and societal beliefs that defined parenting philosophy? The conclusions can be complex and nuanced.

Keeping the four parenting styles as the scaffolding around which most parents hover, we will now explore what influence the predominant religions of the East have on individuals who grow up there.

Eastern cultures are similar in their values yet broad in their traditions and cultural perspectives. These cultural influences have a unique influence on parenting, which is expressed explicitly in their religious or spiritual reference texts. In review, are they different or just so in their external trappings?

Let us examine the similarities that influence parenting, then the differences, and how those differences can be explained. Can these be explained through religious/spiritual beliefs or the culture or the individual interpretation of the religion? The broad-brush strokes approach presented in the following section as reflective of Eastern parenting practices is qualified in that there are significant variations in these values. In this century, due to globalization, Western exposure, urbanization, and generational difference, the interpretation of religious practices continues to change.

1. Collectivism (rather than individualism) [6]: The family or community takes precedence over the individual. Hence, there will be harmony, cooperation, and teaching of children the importance of considering how their actions reflect on the family and not just on themselves. Decisions both good and bad are thus given strong weight to be thought through and deliberated upon before enactment due to the potential impact on the family honor. As a result of this tolerance for collectivism, raising an individual within a "joint family" is encouraged and leads to strong connections to their family tree. Childcare is seen as a collective venture.

2. Filial piety [7] and with it respect and obedience of elders: Parents and ancestors are revered, and this core value leads to an almost irrefutable assumption that the elders are to be respected by children and cared for as they age.

   Ancestral worship is a vital part of the rituals in some Eastern cultures. Remembering the deceased parent through peace prayers a year after their passing (Shraddha ceremony for Hindus) is an example of a social and religious event underscoring the respect of elders and ancestors. Obedience to parents and seeking their guidance on important matters are an expectation.

3. Regarding children, the values that appear common and strongly emphasized by parents are (1) academic achievement: Education is valued; parents will often measure the child's success based on academic achievement. Parents will put pressure on their children to succeed academically, and hard work is highly valued (2). What follows then is a strong push for perseverance and hard work. Parents will encourage their children to work hard and strive for excellence (3). Discipline and structure: Parents set a clear structure and expectation for their child's behavior that is validated by the broad culture within which they live. This is reinforced by following prescribed rules, being consistent in respecting adult opinion, and being responsible and predictable in behavior as reflected in adequate self-control (4). Being humble and self-effacing about achievements are qualities that are culturally rewarded. Others might praise you, but doing so yourself is crass. Being pompous or self-aggrandizing is discouraged. Emotional expression is thus also muted, particularly when negative or where there is conflict or disagreement. Emotional restraint and respect of those who are senior in age trump any independent contrary views that may be foundationally accurate.

4. Religious traditions are concretized in rituals which often are the backbone of rites of passage passed down through generations where each age or stage of child's life is marked by a ceremony/blessing that is a harbinger of the next phase. As an example, the Upanayanam, the first step to the knowledge of oneself, is a Hindu Brahmin ceremony that marks puberty for the male child. Parents also see themselves as the decision makers of marriages. This thinking can be traced to several underlying assumptions including that age confers wisdom to parents who will therefore choose the most appropriate match. This match will lead to a strengthened family system and support cultural traditions.

5. Gender roles vary across different cultures in the East, but expectations of male and female children are distinctly set. Parenting is strongly influenced by these roles in relation to how male and female children are raised. Historically, countries dependent on agrarian economies preferred the male child as physical labor was necessary to support the family livelihood [8]. As more labor markets have opened for the female, the value of the girl child is also changing.

After a brief comment on the Far East, our major focus will be on the Indian subcontinent and the major related religions of that area.

China (and the Far East)

Though we only discuss China and its religions here, in relationship to parenting, similar themes permeate child raising in other Far East countries such as Korea and Japan. Religion in China is a complex topic today as the People's Republic of China is officially an atheist state. However, it would be fair to say that the government recognizes five religions, which include Buddhism (10–16%), Taoism (10%), Christianity (2.5%), and Islam (0.83%), but 80% of the population practice folk religion [9]. Most of the population believes in the natural order of the universe and a proper path for existence. In the past two decades, there has been a revival of Confucianism and Chinese folk religion. A common theme in Chinese religious philosophy is that this is a way of life rather than a single, rigid system of belief. Within this construct, the Chinese believe strongly in respect for elders and ancestor worship.

Children are raised with a very strong awareness of how their behavior could impact the fate of their ancestors. Children are taught the value of the extended family and never to bring shame to the family/ancestors [10]. Another major theme is a focus on success in life as traditionally there are few spots in the hierarchical structure of society and competition to succeed is intense. To "make it" and be the best of the best is the goal, thereby being a credit to the family and ancestors. Children are often pressured to work extraordinarily hard. Parental success is measured by the success of their children. The role of the mother is emphasized in the raising of children. Academic success opens doors to a better future, and that success leads not only to one's personal betterment but also to a sense of pride for the family and the ancestors. The usual conclusion drawn about failure is that it is "the parents' fault." Parents are willing to pay an incredible personal price in giving up their leisure time to push their children to excellence by supervising and providing resources to reach the goals set for them.

In summary and briefly, the Chinese child is raised with expectations of academic and job excellence, which will define whether they have suc-ceeded. Responsibility for upholding the family name and dedication to "getting ahead" but putting in a lot of hard work to do so are common in Chinese children growing up today. There is a strong sense of appreciation for family and ancestors, and any behavior, negative or positive, has an impact on the immediate family and the ancestors.

Related Religions of the Indian Subcontinent That Inform Parenting

For the purpose of this discussion, the authors will qualify that the following is neither an exhaustive list nor an in-depth description of all Eastern religions but rather a representative overview.

Hinduism

Hinduism is the predominant religion practiced in India (79.8%). Other religions of the subcontinent include Islam (14.2%), while Jains, Sikhs, Buddhists, Christians, and Zoroastrians make up the rest of the 6%.

As in any religion, parenting practices informed by a Hindu religious tradition can differ by regional traditions, by the caste or sect to which one belongs, and by personal beliefs of orthodox versus liberal versus a middle road view in the interpretation of those teachings. Hinduism is a polytheistic religion that is the world's third largest, followed by 1.3 billion people and perhaps one of the oldest ones traced back to 500 BCE [11]. It is practiced not only in India but also in Bali, Nepal, Mauritius, and Indonesia and in many countries where Hindus migrated.

Many Hindus describe Hindu traditions as being a "way of life" derived from comprehensive written and spoken texts that are complex conglomerations of schools of philosophy, the Vedas, Upanishads, and Puranas.

The practice of Hindus may vary from ritualistic to spiritual based on what the familial traditions are. Since Hinduism is most often considered a way of living, one cannot be ostracized for not following the core beliefs [12].

It could be argued that the socialization of the Hindu to differences in the practice of their own religion and tolerance of this pluralism produces an acceptance of other religions and their tenets with more ease than would be expected.

Hindus worship in temples with their children, as part of their religious journey, where children are exposed to Hindu texts such as the Bhagavad Gita and the Ramayana, but this exposure to religious studies could occur at home as well. These texts aim to instill ethical values and guide children to make virtuous choices emulating the lives of multiple deities of this polytheistic religion. Festivals mark the calendar year reminding devotees of their deities.

The term Karma, an important concept in Hinduism, means the law of cause and effect. One's actions always have consequences. Children are taught by parents to think before engaging in action. Hence, virtuous living is emphasized; otherwise, penance in this or other lives is a given. Following this idea is the notion that loss, pain, and misery result from one's own actions in this or a past life [13]. Despite the fatalism in this notion of "destiny" ("this was meant to be and was in my fate") versus the Judaic, Protestant, and Catholic Western tradition of "free will" (the power to act without the constraint of necessity or fate), this principle could lead to thoughtfulness in one's actions. Rather than an external focus of cause and effect, it encourages the finding of explanations through the examination of one's own willful behavior.

Yoga and meditation for physical and mental well-being and the promotion of respect for nature are encouraged. Vegetarianism has the goal of promoting harmony with the environment.

In keeping with this is the notion of ahimsa or nonviolence in day-to-day living or resorting to nonviolence even in conflict. Parents teach children to treat all living creatures with kindness and compassion. There is a strong emphasis on teachers being considered as important as God ("Gurudevo bhava"). Children are taught to treat all adults and formal educators with unconditional respect.

The balance between material and spiritual pursuits is also emphasized by appreciating academic and employment success but maintaining a sense of detachment from material wealth.

The value of family (nuclear and more importantly the extended) is emphasized—particularly bonds with cousins and grandparents. Respect for elders includes not abandoning older people as they age.

There is strong emphasis on teaching the child their duties in various roles, i.e., family member, student, friend, and a citizen of the country.

In summary, parenting influences in Hinduism are strongly driven by the values outlined in the shared beliefs of Eastern religions.

Sikhism

Unlike Hinduism, Sikhism is a monotheistic religion that started in the Punjab region of undivided India in the fifteenth century, influenced by Sufism and Hinduism. Many Sikhs today live in the state of Punjab. The devotee prays to a single God who is formless, and the Sikh believes in "seva" or selfless service, social justice, and equality of all. These tenets are imparted to children daily for their ethical and spiritual growth. "Ik Onkar" or "There is one creator" are the first words in the holy scripture of the Sikhs, "The Guru Granth Sahib." Just as in Islam, Sikhs believe in a single God which is not deified as an idol [14, 15].

Sikhs have the highest rate of formal religious teaching of Eastern religions of their children through the Gurudwara, their place of worship.

Just as with other religions, there is an emphasis on honesty and integrity. Parents model and encourage humility, contentment, and gratitude with what one has. Meditation, remembrance of God (Naam Simran), and mindfulness are expected to lead to inner peace and spiritual connection to the divine, a process to which parents introduce children early in life and continue to support regularly through "paath" and Gurbani (recitation of the Granth Sahib through communal singing). Scripture provides children with lessons regarding ethics and spirituality. Teachers are regarded as the ultimate repository of knowledge, able to show a path to God. Communal praying, called a sangat (community gathering), emphasizes the importance that Sikhs give to treasuring community networking, making connections and friendships within their religious community. Sikhs are known for the free community kitchens (langar) where anyone from any faith, caste, and creed can be fed and have a place to stay. The Golden Temple of Amritsar in India is known to serve 100,000 meals a day. Sikhs and others serve in such places as a part of "Seva" or service and pass on these values to the children. This has extended to creating langars in places of need such as places hit by natural disasters or war.

The Sikh child wears his hair long (kesh) and when a youth dons the adult turban along with four other symbols of Sikhism: a comb (Kangha to comb the long hair), a small sword (Kirpan), a bracelet (Kada), and Kacha (underwear). These are the five Ks that personify the Khalsa or "the pure." Adhering to these external elements of dress demonstrates a Sikh's adherence to Sikh rehni (or the Sikh way of life). Female Sikh children likewise never cut their hair.

The tenets of Sikh living that permeate into parenting are the following:

Oneness and equality of the whole human race connected through God, such that everyone is equal, and everyone is respect/compassion worthy, regardless of their race, gender, or social status

"Seva" or selfless service of others by way of acts of kindness to help those in need and the larger society wherever there is a need for help

Honesty and integrity and standing up for what is right

Sikh parents pass these values, along with personal discipline, hard work, and service to others, on to their children in their day-to-day religious instruction. They are both monotheistic and socially committed.

Islam

Islam is an Abrahamic monotheistic religion which follows the teachings of the Quran (the holy book of Islam) and the sayings and actions of Prophet Muhammad (the Hadith). Muslims or adherents of Islam are two billion globally, second only to Christianity in the world. Islam teaches that God or Allah is the one and only God, and Prophet Muhammad is the last prophet (preceded by Prophets such as Jesus and Moses, among others) [16].

Parenting by followers of Islam is influenced by the teachings in the Quran and the Hadith, following these principles:

Tawahid (monotheism): The idea that Allah is the only God, and his teachings and qualities should be imbibed by children.

Parents deserve respect, obedience, kindness, and care.

Children should learn from the Quran and the Hadith honesty, humility, and compassion.

They should also better themselves through religious and secular education.

Formal religious practice includes daily prayers (five times a day, called Salat or Namaz) that have the goals of developing a strong connection with Allah and of explaining the reasoning for Islamic rituals and act as Dua or supplication to God for guidance and help in whatever stage a person is. This provides the child fortitude to work through any stress.

Ramadan is a period of fasting intended to promote the development of restraint and self-control so that wrongful desires and bad habits can be overcome. The singular focus on God during the month of fasting enhances the spiritual focus of the child and reduces desires to usurp the rights of others ("If I give up what is rightfully mine, why would I look at anything that belongs to others?").

Charity and generosity (Zakat), particularly during the holy period of fasting, are also inculcated in children.

Modesty of attire and behavior are considered an expression of pious behavior. So are patience (Sabr) and perseverance in the face of challenges that children face. These attributes are modeled and taught in formal or informal ways, including by reference to historical figures who lived exemplary and moderate lives.

Family bonding through shared mealtimes and community activities provides the communal context that is the hallmark of Eastern cultures.

Jainism

Although culturally and regionally connected to the religions of Buddhism and Hinduism in the Indian subcontinent, Jainism is distinct. It is believed to have begun in the seventh and fifth century BCE in the Eastern Gangetic Plain contemporaneously with Buddhism. Its first practitioners did so with the idea of moving away from ritualistic Brahmin traditions of the Hindu faith, particularly valuing ascetic living and abandonment of worldly concerns. Spiritual leaders (but not God) are called Tirthankara; the last or 24th Tirthankara was Mahavira. Although a large number of Jains do not believe in praying to an idol when they do pray to a physical form, Mahavira is traditionally the form they worship [17].

The main tenet of the Jain faith is the "conquering of base passions" by ancient renunciants/monks/nuns to achieve enlightenment. Those who achieved enlightenment were called Jina and their lay followers the Jainas, with their communities called "Sangha." There are six million Jains in the world with the majority living both in North and South India. With globalization, Jain emigration to North America and the UK has been on the ascendency.

Although the Jain Monks follow a strict ascetic way of life, Jain followers apply the following five Anuvratas (partial rejection of sinful activities) on a day-to-day basis and transmit these to Jain children from a young age. These are the following:

1. Ahimsa or nonviolence: Vegetarianism is a practical example of this, along with eating early/before dark (so as not to swallow a flying insect that may not be readily visible in the night).
2. Satya or truthfulness: Like other religions, Jains value honesty.
3. Being nonacquisitive or not desiring anyone else's material possessions: "Do not steal" is a dictum emphasized by parents.
4. Celibacy: Any carnal activity is perceived as sinful, but the Jain religion acknowledges that this applies to those not married and that there is a period of "sansarik sambandh," i.e., earthly connections/obligations when that dictum is put on hold.
5. Aparigraha or non-possessiveness of material possessions.

In addition, Jain children are taught to value resources and not to waste. Practical examples might be not letting water run while brushing teeth, serving more than one can eat, or throwing away food.

Children are taught to develop strong control of their senses with the idea of keeping desires in check.

Tapasya or meditation is emphasized as a way to learn how to further control desires. Meditative practices emphasize the control over the mind (Mana), words (Vachan), and body (Kaya).

Paryushan Vrata is an 8-day period of fasting during which children along with parents practice control of their taste buds. Fasting allows them to experience hunger. They are encouraged to eat less or give up their favorite food, eat before sunset, etc., and they are rewarded for that by parents in nonmaterial appreciation.

Another important value taught is "Kshamapana" or forgiveness. Children learn to ask for forgiveness for any sins they may have committed and are taught to forgive others. Humility and self-effacement are well regarded, culturally sanctioned, and validated.

Jainism is distinct in its leanings toward an ascetic and explicitly stated value system of nonviolence and self-sacrifice. Children of Jain ancestry have strong communal ties and depend on each other, a common thread in many contextual cultures and religions explored in this chapter.

Buddhism

Buddhism developed in the Gangetic Plain of India around the fifth century BCE as an offshoot of Hinduism and is based on the teachings of Buddha, a Hindu prince who gave up all worldly possessions in search of liberation from the grief of repeated cycles of life and death. To achieve liberation from this suffering, he went on a journey of self-exploration and achieved enlightenment, and then Moksha or absolution from the cycle of life. During his period of meditation and self-discovery, he came upon the middle way, a path for spiritual salvation which became the basis of his teachings that could be applied to the ordinary man's life and included the eight jewels and threefold path. Buddhism spread from India far and wide over the centuries to the South Asian countries of Sri Lanka, Thailand, Nepal, Tibet, China, Vietnam, Taiwan, Korea, Japan, Burma, Laos and Cambodia, Mongolia, and Russian Kalmykia [18].

The tenets of Buddhism include the three jewels that purify and uplift the spirit through seeking the Buddha, seeking the Dhamma (upholding the centered self and natural order of the universe) and Sangha (community). Buddhism also teaches Sila or the ethics for living through right speech, right speech, and right living. Meditation, mindfulness, restraint over the senses, not stealing, not lying, abstaining from non-proscribed sensual pleasures, not using alcohol or drugs, and ahimsa or nonviolence are some of the precepts of Buddhism.

Parenting in Buddhism differs from that in other Eastern religions in that rather than inculcating various virtues such as honesty and compassion, Buddhists encourage the acceptance of the child in whatever form they are. They try to recognize and accept life's imperfections, eliminate desires and unrealistic expectations of children, and also parent with the rightness of belief, a right resolve, right speech, right conduct, right livelihood, right effort, right mindfulness, and right meditative awareness. In these ways, Buddhism can be described as a way of life.

Christianity will not be discussed here as it is not an Eastern religion. Cultural influences support blending in with the majority culture in parenting styles.

Zoroastrian

Zoroastrians are also called Parsis ("Persians"). Most live in the Indian subcontinent and number about 60,000. They originally migrated from Iran to India in ~600 CE, as they were persecuted by Muslim invaders there. Their God of wisdom is Ahura Mazda, whose teachings Prophet Zoroaster spread across the land [19]. They tend to marry within their faith. Since their parenting style is marked by a philosophy of living life to the fullest and radiating happiness toward others, the Parsi child is encouraged to grow up with a sense of being charitable and philanthropic.

Summary

Despite the distinctive worship styles, beliefs held, and the historical evolution of each tradition, one can appreciate several common themes that permeate parenting within Eastern religions:

1. Children are raised in environments with strong community and contextual connections.
2. Parenting is an active process for parents from Eastern religions, with moderate to intense involvement of the parent with the child's upbringing.
3. Developmental milestones are marked by rituals that acknowledge these transitions.
4. Religious education occurs predominantly within the home and community through modeled behavior and (infrequently for most) in places of worship.
5. Religion is often a way of living typically marked by values of obedience, dependability, and nonviolence.
6. Teachers and family or community elders are to be respected. The assumption is that age confers wisdom and advice/instructions from elders must be followed.
7. Many values are shared with Western religious teachings, such as the importance of honesty and moral behavior.

How is this broad range of values common to Eastern religious traditions reflected in the way individuals perform the tasks of life? The answer must of course be qualified by the pluralistic influences of family culture, geography, temperamental differences, tolerance for deviation from the norm, etc.

The following two self-portraits of two practicing child psychiatrists who have been highly influenced by their Eastern ethnic and religious backgrounds shed light on how these influences can impact the lives of children and youth as they negotiate developmental tasks.

"My Journey: The Good Muslim Daughter or the ABCD": Sarah Arshad

I was born in the Bronx, NY, to immigrant parents. They were both born and raised in Pakistan, from upper middle-class families that emphasized education and religion. My dad settled in the United States as a teenager after his older brothers had also moved to the United States, and my mother joined him after their arranged marriage (they were introduced by their parents and had exchanged letters and pictures but met in person for the first time the week of their wedding), waiting to finish medical school in Pakistan before moving to the United States. My dad had an African American colleague, who, along with his wife, "adopted" my parents and became my "American grandma and grandpa" to help them navigate American culture and society. My parents had three children and parented their children with the values with which they grew up in a country very different from the one in which they were raised.

As an adult, I can only imagine what they were dealing with, as I start to appreciate their difficulties in raising three children, all born in the United States, and how difficult it must have been for them to adapt to a new country and culture while also adjusting to married life, navigating their professional lives, having children, and raising a family. But as a child and then as an adolescent, I often felt confused, and I identified as an "ABCD," or American-Born Confused Desi as an adolescent. It felt as though I was being held to standards and expectations that were literally foreign to me and inconsistent with the culture in which I was born and raised. Reflecting, I recall times of authoritarian parenting especially in regard to our Pakistani heritage that I did not inherently understand and often struggled with.

As a child and as a teenager, I felt a heavy sense of not belonging. I did not feel "American enough" for my friends whose parents had also been born in the United States, I did not feel "Pakistani enough" for our South Asian family friends, and I was also confused about my Muslim identity and why some of our practices differed from Muslim families we knew from other cultural backgrounds. Religion and culture were often conflated, such that I was not sure what traditions were Pakistani and which were Muslim, making it more difficult for me to navigate my intersectional beliefs.

In elementary school, I remember feeling like "the other" when at lunchtime, my meal looked so different from that of my peers, and I confessed that I had no idea what a "baloney" sandwich was. After I learned, I did not know how other children could eat pork when it was "haraam" for me. I also felt isolated when I did not celebrate the same holidays and remember always being frustrated during the winter when our art and music activities revolved around Christmas and Hanukkah, but I never got to celebrate Eid ul Fitr or Eid ul Adha in school. My parents were unable to help me navigate my frustration and sadness at singing songs and painting pictures for other people's holidays in school, but never being able to celebrate or even acknowledge my own with my peers or teachers. Similarly, around South Asian or Muslim children, I also felt different—I spoke Urdu more hesitantly and with a clear American accent, and I discovered that even Muslim families can have different practices. My parents were not able to help me with this identity confusion, let alone help me shape my identity going forward, and did their best to raise me to belong in both cultures, not realizing that I felt lost in the chasm between them.

My parents were likely plagued with their own worries about how their children would grow up, faced with how to teach them the values they held dear when in a culture that was so different from what they knew (1970s/1980s

Pakistan). There was a strong desire to raise their children as religious Muslims, but less ability to help their children navigate how to do that when they were of a minority religious belief, and "haraam" behaviors (such as eating pork, drinking alcohol, or having sex before marriage) were socially acceptable. To some degree, they likely reinforced the way they were parented—with authoritarian styles, dictating that parents knew best, and kids should not question. We were instructed that these behaviors were impermissible because we were Muslim, but not taught about why they were not impermissible to others or given guidance for how to fit in in such a different social atmosphere. In the third grade, I decided that I was no longer going to wear shorts because it was not modest, but I was not sure how to respond when other kids or teachers would ask me if I was hot in the summer. As a teen, I was very conscious about watching the TV shows my peers were watching (What if my parents found out there were kids drinking alcohol? Or that teenagers were in physical relationships?) and what my parents would think, or whether it made me a bad Muslim.

That said, my parents were relatively lax (compared to some other families I knew)—they would ask and encourage us to engage in religious activities (the five daily prayers, reading Quran, fasting, etc.) but did not force us and, as I grew up, became more authoritative, engaging with me in intellectual discussions about religion. And they made exceptions for school—they did not expect us to comply with the five daily prayers during schooltime but would ask us to make these prayers up when we came home. They also encouraged us not to fast during the holy month of Ramadan if we had exams. They encouraged the rituals without force so that we could grow and connect to God, and to the religion, which for me ultimately provided a source for hope. When good or bad things happened, we were instructed to always remember God, say "Alhumdulillah," and pray earnestly. Over time, this reminded me that for Muslims, everything happens for a reason, and we rely on the fact that God is All Knowing and has a plan for us all. In my adulthood, this connection to, belief in, and reliance on a higher power had utterly grounded me when otherwise my world would be spinning around me.

Once I got to college, I connected more with my faith, separately from my cultural heritage, and drew many values from Islam. My intellectual growth also allowed me to (respectfully!) engage in more discussions on the deeper values of religion with my parents, who were then more authoritative in their styles of discussion; they would still state what was right or wrong but were engaging in the discussion as to "why," perhaps because it was clear that I was attempting to gain knowledge. I feel as though my parents' introduction to Islam grew into a curiosity to learn more about the religion and the values underlying the practices. In college, I found a community, helping solidify my Muslim identity. I kept up with their earlier expectations of avoiding "haraam" due in part to their parenting, but also to their openness and my own discovery of my religious identity and being able to choose that life for myself as a semi-independent young woman. While it did mean avoiding certain social gatherings and parties in college, I was also able to find a community of others (Muslim and non-Muslim) who also chose to avoid those settings. I was finally able to find a collection of peers with similar values while still engaging in social activities and connecting with those around me. And while I appreciated Pakistani culture—the food, the clothes, and the music—I also struggled with and rebelled against aspects of Pakistani culture, especially when I found it contrasting with the Islamic values I was coming to better understanding.

When my parents grew up in Pakistan, there was a strong expectation of respecting and obeying one's parents, and they expected this of their children. Values of respect were often conveyed with authoritarian styles, with little room for discussion. Their ideals may also have been stuck in the past from when they left, and it would feel like I was compared to historical children in Pakistan as opposed to the current generation. In addition, they may not have prepared me for the questioning attitude American society and culture also seemed to emphasize—including with your parents, which may have felt to them as though their children were "talking back" or "questioning their authority" when instead this was how I was taught to learn more. Immigrant parents often also value privacy less and so can feel entitled to know about their children's lives, including information that many American teens may tell their parents is "none of your business." Moreover, this can continue past adolescence into adulthood, even when their children are married and become parents themselves.

Pakistani culture is also more collectivist; for example, parenting is not the job of the parents alone, as family members and community members can also teach, comment, advise, and lecture. Some aspects of this can be useful—the "village" can help raise the children, and there can be huge amounts of community support. We were always taught to respect the community and always encouraged to be generous (charity is also one of the five pillars of Islam) and listen to the advice of elders. However, this brings with it concern about the respect of the community and worry about straying from norms due to "log kya kahenge" or "what will people think." This can lead some parents to discourage their children from standing out due to concern for censure or possible damage to their reputation. This concern can also lead to the hiding of troubling (and, in fact, "haraam") behavior within a home for the sake of a family's external reputation—including abuse (between partners, or of in-laws, in cases where a woman's in-laws expect her to not only move into their house but also serve them and the family), mental health concerns, and other behaviors that would lead to stigma—which in turn can result in the propagation of intergenerational trauma.

In families privileged with higher socioeconomic status, Pakistani parents often emphasize the importance of education. As siblings, we were often compared to each other or to other family friends' children, which felt frustrating at the time, if likely intended to be motivational. Pakistani parents are very involved and often help their children, including sometimes minimizing expectations of household chores if their kids are studying or helping them with assignments to prioritize academic achievement. I have strong memories of doing math worksheets with my dad (to be honest, I asked him for these for fun) as well as science assignments and projects with my mom. The child's achievement can, in part, also become the parent's achievement and can be a status symbol (e.g., if they go to the Ivy League, get into medical school, accomplish another milestone the community would respect). These life milestones also carry expectations from the family, in part due to expectations held by the community—what the most reputed professions were (doctor, engineer, etc.), when people should get married, etc. And within my family, there was a fine line between getting high achievements and thanking God for them, but also not announcing them publicly for fear of "nazar" or the evil eye, and concern that other people may consciously or subconsciously wish you ill due to your success.

Family involvement has its perks; for example, there was more family support (academic, social, financial) than I saw with my American peers, especially those with permissive or uninvolved parents—I never worried about being expected to leave the house at 18 to live on my own, and in fact, my parents provided full financial support for my undergraduate education, as well as some support for my housing during graduate school. For some families, the support is expected in reverse after the child completes their education and starts earning an income—parents may expect to live with their children and be fully supported (emotionally, socially, financially) by them, as often occurs in South Asia.

My parents demonstrated significant pride when I accomplished the professional milestones expected. And yet, there was also tremendous anxiety in my household as I grew older, without a husband in sight. I often felt like a failure for not being able to check off this life achievement and was forced by social norms to politely provide a nonresponse when community members would ask me "when will you give us good news?" (I was not allowed to respond snarkily, asking why my professional news and good health were not "good news" enough) or even when community members instructed me to lose weight, take off my hijab, or in some way make myself more physically attractive in order to attract a husband.

It was not clear to me why our strong faith did not relieve the anxiety—after all, God has a plan and everything happens for a reason. Alhumdulillah. And I also found myself struggling with how to find a husband, because I was not sure how to do so. Luckily, my parents were more open-minded in that they hoped I would find a Muslim husband, but did not care about his race or ethnicity, unlike many other South Asian parents I knew who had more stringent criteria. But they also could not rely on their experience, as finding a spouse in 1980s Pakistan held no similarity to getting married in modern-day America, and I had to navigate my unique path to finding a life partner. And I was raised with religious values, including that dating was impermissible, and never saw my parents engage in any physical affection as that is not culturally acceptable. I was not taught how to talk to someone for the sake of marriage or how to assess compatibility, in part because my parents did not know—their parents had arranged it for them. My ideals of dating resembled the Victorian novels I read to merge a conservative belief system with my own romantic ideals of love and affection. And yet when the community saw me, I knew that there was talk of how I was getting older, and what a shame that I was not married, because I could not possibly be happy.

In Pakistani culture, there are social expectations for politeness. As an American-born person, part of the expectations, perhaps due to it being a "guess culture" vs. an "ask culture," felt passive. I was not allowed to express how I felt in the tone or language I wanted to but had to engage in social niceties for the sake of others. I always felt "othered" in my South Asian community by traits sometimes viewed differently by my American-born community—I was an extrovert, sometimes loud, more independent, and often more defiant and questioning. And Heaven forbid that I accept the offer of something—food, a gift, etc.—without showing some "takalluf," or politely declining two to three times first. Growing up, I felt very confused as to why it was expected that I

decline a desired offering, but I also felt like I was not allowed to question it as it would only further point out my cultural naivete. Fitting into the ideal—a demure young woman who carried herself well and followed the unstated rules with poise—always felt wrong and like I it was shameful to fully be myself. And I found historical Muslim women who were models for being leaders (intelligent, well-spoken, confident)—and wondered why that was not the expected ideal.

I often wonder how much of this was colored by my gender. Within Pakistani culture, values align with traditional gender roles—women are often in charge of household tasks such as cooking and cleaning, for example, even if they are as well or better educated than their husbands and work full-time jobs. My parents defied the norm in teaching all of their children (regardless of gender) these household chores, and equally encouraging us to pursue education, including if it meant moving away for school (which some families allow their sons to do, but not their daughters). That said, there were also expectations for me to "carry myself" a certain way: to be demure, soft spoken, and offer more help at home, especially when I was old enough to be married and we were around families with appropriately aged, marriageable sons. Again, I questioned how these aligned with Muslim values, in which there are some gender roles but also examples of women with impressive professional accomplishments and men playing an active role in raising children and taking care of household tasks.

Now that I am older and more experienced, I am better able to understand the difficulties my parents faced and how the racism and microaggressions they must have faced likely affected how they tried to get us to belong in this culture as well as their own. They faced the same challenges as any parents, but on top of this, the challenges of their own immigration and acculturation. They parented their children with the hopes that they would carry on the traditions, culture, and religion they valued while also trying to prime them for success in the United States. And they likely used the models and styles their parents had used before them—largely authoritarian, though with time they became more authoritative, allowing for more discussion from their children to understand their values on a deeper level. And I struggled through my adolescence to find myself while often feeling like I had to pretend to fit norms I did not quite understand. But after much introspection and examining my values through multiple lenses, whether cultural or religious, I have found myself. And I am no longer "confused," but a proud Muslim American and an "American-born desi."

Echoes of So Many Pasts: "I Carry All of You Within Me": Jaya Nair

I was born in India and raised by an atheist mother from a Kerala Christian family and a Hindu father. We immigrated to the United Arab Emirates shortly after my birth and lived there till I was 11 years of age. By way of this immigration and choices my parents made regarding my education, I have enjoyed describing myself in those early years as a "Hindu child attending a Catholic school in a Muslim country." Every morning, I woke up to hearing the ringing of the bells and chanting of a Sanskrit prayer by my father, who would utter these words wearing nothing but a sarong or towel in supplication to the Gods, while the Imam would sing Quranic verses over the loudspeakers. This is perhaps why I would stop to pray at Mother Mary's shrine every day at St. Joseph's school, even while most of my Christian friends walked on.

Religious syncretism is prevalent in Kerala, India, where according to the census, Hinduism is followed by 54.7% of the population, Islam by 26.6%, and Christianity by 18.4%. While Kerala has seen bouts of religious violence since the early nineteenth century, the state has enjoyed long periods of harmony between the different groups in contrast to several other states in India.

One experience in life which brought home to my awareness Kerala's intrinsic and interwoven nature of worship took place when my mother and I enlisted the help of a Muslim girl to learn the proper rituals to perform at a Hindu temple preceding my brother's wedding. While life outside the home was diverse and inclusive, life within the home was a singular and strict path.

My father was the quintessential Southern Kerala Nair man. The Nairs are a warrior clan-like culture of Kerala whose social intra-caste hierarchy preceded Brahminism. They had a feudal society with powerful landlords who possessed their own cavalries and engaged in territorial wars with each other until the early 1700s. In south Kerala, nobles from eight ruling houses attempted to subvert the rightful ascension of the late King's nephew Marthanda Varma to the Travancore throne but were defeated by the prince who quelled their revolution, acquired their lands, and consolidated their power. My father's ancestral family served that court in the nineteenth century. Nair society is one of only two matrilineal ones in India. Among the Nairs, men were born into the cavalry and women were regarded as the future mothers and property owners. The men were trained from birth for the purpose of righteous service to the Kingdom. The Nairs upheld honor, duty, and piety above all else. To die in battle was the greatest of honors. Every Nair home of substance held its armory as its most sacred room. For young men to fall in service to his King was not atypical, after which the family continued with their wives, mothers, and daughters at the helm. There, the women held much power and sway in matters as they were sure to outlive most of the men in the home. These traditions were strongly rooted in my father, who saw fortitude in life and service as the most important characteristics of a person. Members of his family served in both World Wars in the British Indian Army; his grandfather returned from WWI to be appointed by the King as "in-charge" of the police in his district, having served during the Malabar rebellion of 1921. My father's uncle died as a POW in a German concentration camp during WWII. I remember seeing my great uncle's portrait on the wall of the main hall in my ancestral home as a child. He was a young man still in his teens when he enlisted. I remember listening to how devastating the loss had been for my great grandmother who lost her only son. My father credited his own strict upbringing as having given him the strength to survive the numerous deaths in his family, including his father's when he was 21 years of age. Thrust into the role of patriarch, he faced severe economic constraints and social pressures of settling his siblings into their lives and providing for his family; he shouldered this burden while pursuing and attaining an engineering degree without a promise of employment as India suffered a devastating economic depression from drought and wars at its borders in the mid-1960s into the 1970s.

Perhaps, it was due to this history and tradition of pain and trauma that my father directed his fatherly duty toward us with a sense of unyielding purpose. His task was threefold—to instill in his children not just the tenets of Hinduism, but our cultural Nair heritage, as well as bestow upon us the grit to overcome unimaginable odds in an increasingly unpredictable world. Within this construct, ritual was important in the home, as was a strict adherence to time. We woke up at the same time every day, ate at the same time, and slept at the same time, and there was to be no changes in this. My brother, seen as the bearer of my father's name, was raised in much harsher conditions than I; he was rarely afforded the luxury of failure or misbehavior. Conversely, achievement was met with quiet acceptance. Celebration for what he was "supposed to do" was seen as unnecessarily emotive. While I enjoyed much more freedom within the home, possessing more of my father's warmth and affection, I was held to similar standards of behavior and achievement once I entered middle school. He was authoritarian in his parenting style, and this fit perfectly within his Nair identity. For his part, my father saw himself to be much more engaged with the family than his own father. He spoke to us about important matters of the world and heard our take on the issues.

My mother in contrast came from an affluent and influential Christian family who were intimately involved in the Indian revolution. Her uncle was a philanthropist who served closely with the revolutionaries who founded modern India. She too experienced the prioritization of service, duty, and education within her family, having been supported by her father to obtain her

engineering degree. In raising us, therefore, she settled comfortably into the Nair lifestyle of my home, adamant about keeping to our father's mission. She became an extension of his will even in his absence.

My family was isolative in the early years of our immigration to America. We first landed in Houston and then came to make our home in New Orleans, Louisiana. My parents created a microcosm of Hindu Nair principles and lifestyle amidst a completely alien Western culture. While there was much diversity in religious practices in Kerala, and subsequently the Keralite communities in the Middle East where all identified as either Keralite or more broadly Indian, this was no longer the case in the United States.

I suddenly found myself thrust into a sixth-grade public school classroom with Latinx, African American, and White students. My brother and I were aware of the differences in our family life when compared to my Indian friends, many of whom, while being Hindu and from India, did not have the extent of discipline in the home as I did. It was hard to be the only student in my middle-school marching band who had to sit out from performing with the group on Bourbon Street for Mardi Gras as my parents did not want me to be exposed to the debauchery that is typical of the festival. Perhaps due to my family's isolative nature, I felt more urgency to establish clearly what I believed in and who I identified myself to be.

Through the years, my brother and I became very close, as he served the function of second father and best friend. Perhaps, the strictness of our home enabled us to overcome sibling strife. He was brilliant and a voracious reader, eager to share his thoughts and what he learned with me. Being five and a half years younger, I remember following him around like a little shadow. His interests became my interests. And like him, I found a passion in Vedic literature. Through this, along with my father's encouragement in the study of South Indian classical music, I settled more fully into a Hindu identity rather than simply an Indian one. Where I did not have much socialization outside the home, these activities, discussions around the dinner table with my brother and father, and absorbing stories my brother told me helped me find release and freedom. These activities remain my outlets to this day.

As I matured, I inevitably adopted several American virtues as my own. Eastern communal behaviors and ideals are in stark contrast to the adventurous individualistic American ideal. This contrast can often result in internal and external conflicts for first- and second-generation Indian immigrants for whom the term "ABCD" or "American-Born Confused Desi" was coined. I remember first encountering that term when I was a college student at the University of New Orleans and deciding that whatever I identified as, I would not accept confusion as part of my identity. In retrospect, this rejection of uncertainty within myself was perhaps in unconscious adherence to my Nair upbringing. As I embark on the most important work of my life, as a mother to my 2-month-old daughter and wife to my Southern Cajun White husband, I am reminded of my own childhood and understand the richness of what I have gained as well as the pain of what I suffered.

I watch my father now with my daughter, and with his two other grandchildren from my brother, freely expressing his joy and love, relishing his closeness to their minds and hearts. In the grandfather, I see glimpses of the father I had always wanted. It inspires me in my approach toward my daughter—while I want her to know her Nair heritage, and how it informs the Hindu traditions that my family practiced, I hold her with warmth and allow her some liberties in knowing the community she is a part of and engaging in more activities than with her peers. Meanwhile, I also want her to know the path of her ancestors, without feeling stifled or constricted in being who she is. I would like to follow in my father's footsteps in nurturing her mind, and I also would celebrate her heart. I would want her to have both my genuine deep interest in a Hindu lifestyle with an understanding of Hindu spiritual ideals while being able to appreciate and welcome the exploration of other religions and cultures as well. I would not push rituals on her. Rather, as my father did on so many occasions around that dinner table, I would

weave the stories, the ancient tales that teach the importance of having compassion for herself and others, of the importance of righteousness and honesty, of love and faith. Most importantly, I would want her to see herself in all who cross her path.

Summative Comments

Coming full circle, in superimposing what we have learned about Eastern values in parenting and the "parenting style" scaffolding alluded to at the beginning of the chapter, we encourage asking whether a parent is authoritarian or authoritative, and how these values translate into day-to-day living and development.

These vignettes provide a rich and real-life context for understanding the advantages and possible drawbacks of what have been described in the previous section as core values of Eastern religions and parenting primarily in the greater Indian subcontinent.

Table 4.1 summarizes these dilemmas with their nuanced and complex implications:

- The positive elements could be broadly summarized as follows:
- Strong involvement of parents and family that allows generational transmission of values and traditions
- Strong family and community support for counsel, role modeling, and help in times of distress
- Strong emphasis on education and life skills to succeed in the material and spiritual world; industriousness and perseverance emphasized at a young age that sets a strong foundation for a desire to succeed
- Respect for elders, their opinions, and appreciating the wisdom synonymous with age
- High degree of supervision that prevents exposure to developmentally inappropriate trauma

However, the other side of the coin is that if these values and resulting parenting styles are rigidly enforced without psychological space for the

Table 4.1 Positive and negative trajectories conferred by parenting informed by Eastern religious and cultural traditions

Value conferred by religion and culture	Pros	Cons	Comments
Religious emphasis	Solidification of identity, belongingness Pride in origins	Isolation within society if rigid adherence and rejection of that which is not "me"	Secular culture may protect against a belief system that does not tolerate differences
Emphasis on education	Tools to succeed are acquired as a minimum expectation. Transition into adulthood easier Sets standards for industriousness and perseverance. Quality-pervaded approach to any task at hand = success	Development focused on academic instruction and achievement at the cost of a well-rounded education that includes fine arts, sports, or exploration of unique interests a child may have	Comparison with others: siblings, neighbors, other kin who are relatively more accomplished = self-esteem impacted Subliminal gossip in extended family, community regarding lack of achievement = rejection of community
Emphasis on family	Strong network of support Dependability of and for people The "auntie" and "uncle" culture that connotes closeness and dependability Strong relationships can trump even kinship "Takes a village to raise a child"	Intrusion into the psychological space of another is culturally supported Dependence on the opinion of others Reputation of family paramount Actions may be dictated by "what will 'X' say/think?" Dishonor to the family name avoided at any cost	Parents expect children will remain an "open book" and all their information should be shared openly even as adults Psychological closeness but at the cost of "not allowed to grow independently" or make mistakes Being a "daily witness to one's life" can buffer the fear of being alone
Obedience to adults and respect of elders	Open to instruction from others Willing to accept parents' "wisdom" and values that are passed down from "elders" Maintains familial peace and connections Collective wisdom from the millennia retained and maintained Built-in consultation on complex topics available	Children should not "talk back" or question parents/adults and accept that adults "know the best" No reasoning provided leading children to be resentful/angry Acquiescing due to guilt leads to resentment/anger. Rejection, pushback, or rebellion Religion is used as reason for why "rules" exist	Adults and children may benefit if reasoning for "rules" explained rationally The relationship may benefit from a give and take of rationales, viewpoints, and willingness to compromise without abandoning core values

(continued)

Table 4.1 (continued)

Value conferred by religion and culture	Pros	Cons	Comments
Gender roles	Clear expectations set for males and females In theory, women are to be protected and seen as mother figures Rarely are they objectified in literature or in religion Many important deities in the Hindu tradition are women gods with attributes of strength, courage, wealth, etc.	The role delineation may not be equitable Women will marry and "belong" to the husband's home and follow the proscribed rules of that role Prescribed roles for the girl child: household chores Modesty in clothes and demeanor Stricter rules or choices regarding career, education, social interactions, i.e., curfew, freedom to make independent choices or friends or nontraditional activities	Often a source of conflict and resentment As women's interaction with the outside world is increasing through education and careers, women are aspirational to achieve more and have more choices in their life
Unconditional support of parents for their children	It is an expectation for parents to financially and emotionally support children till they complete their education or marry. Reciprocal dependence on child as parents age	Parents use guilt to persuade children to accept "rules," i.e., "sacrifices" made to raise the child Significant familial upheaval when there is imbalance in this equation, not only on an individual level but also loss of face within the larger religious or social community	Recognition of the phases of life and how cultural and contextual changes have accelerated the wisdom of "pay it forward," i.e., parents give to their children and their children give to theirs: rarely does it come back. This is the cycle of life Respect must be commanded and not demanded
Expression of emotions	Expressions of love: strong representation in literature, poetry, and arts Lack of demonstrated physical affection between couples in public Affection and love are acknowledged as important feeling states but are implicit rather than explicit and often are relationship and commitment based	Could provide stability in a committed relationship; less likely to disintegrate under stress But young adults in the twenty-first century envision love as essential to a long-term relationship and reject such alliances	Arranged marriages are acceptable although on the wane The work-around is to allow interaction between individuals to assess compatibility Families still play an important part in the vetting and approval process of a mate Connects to obeying the advice of elders

Table 4.1 (continued)

Value conferred by religion and culture	Pros	Cons	Comments
Migration	The impact of migration is multifold and can depend on whether the family has assimilated vs. acculturated vs. isolating or integrated with the majority culture It tests inherent resilience, perseverance, and psychological sophistication of the family matriarchs and patriarchs	Parents and therefore families may be "frozen in time" to the point of migration. Their ethnic, cultural, and religious values mimic those of the time they left their country Cultural bereavement must be negotiated. It can put significant stress on a system	Children in families are also "stuck in time" and are often surprised by the vision of the real vs. imagined home country when they do visit. A sense of not belonging in either place with a resulting rejection of their ethnic religious and cultural identity can ensue
Mental health and eastern religions	Familial support serves as a safety net against normal everyday stressors Eastern religions and culture support the notion of community support	Strong stigma against diagnosis of mental illness (MI) Somatic expression of MI: headaches/stomach aches Poorly acknowledged "What is there to be depressed about, you have everything!"	Intergenerational trauma reenacted and could be potentiated without professional intervention

child-parent dyad to understand the reasoning behind dictates, allowance for missteps, and evolution of the relationship in which parents are able to individuate from the child at appropriate phases of their development, then the same values that were positive influences in childhood can become stifling and curb psychological growth in the young adult. Following are few examples of the downsides of Eastern family values:

- Being adult centric in relation to power within the family
- Parental agenda for life choices given primacy
- Potential to support conformity and stifle individual thought and creativity
- Limited tolerance for mistakes
- Appropriate and powerful supervisory role in childhood but unable to give up control in young adulthood impacting problem-solving, independent thinking, etc.

Conclusion

The understanding of parenting and its connection to family values and change is nuanced and complex. Although deliberately simplified in this chapter, the wise will appreciate that culture, imbided through traditions, rituals, and values, is ever evolving with geographic migration of groups, adaptation of parents through education, and psychological malleability to embrace novel ideas while keeping core values that allow them to be the best version of a parent they can be. Most parents want the best for the next generation. To that point, it would be fair to categorize religions from the East as conferring authoritarian or authoritative parenting styles. Conversely, permissive and uninvolved parenting styles, if present, stand out. They are noticed as aberrant and are generally rare and inconsistent with the core values that spring from an upbringing rooted in Eastern traditions.

References

1. Coogan MD, Narayanan V. Eastern religions: origins, beliefs, practices, holy texts. Sacred Places: Oxford University Press; 2005. ISBN: 0195221907.
2. de Blot P. Religion and spirituality. In: Bouckaert L, Zsolnai L, editors. Handbook of spirituality and business. London: Palgrave Macmillan; 2011. https://doi.org/10.1057/9780230321458_2.
3. Coward HG, Neumaier-Dargyay EK, Neufeldt R, editors. Readings in eastern religions. Wilfrid Laurier University Press; 1988. p. 1. ISBN: 0889209553.
4. Oxtoby WG. World religions: eastern traditions, vol. 2. ISBN: Oxford University Press; 1996. p. 0195407504.
5. Robinson CC, Mandleco B, Olsen SF, Hart CH. Authoritative, authoritarian, and permissive parenting practices: development of a new measure. Psychol Rep. 1995;77(3):819–30. https://doi.org/10.2466/pr0.1995.77.3.819.
6. Rezai Niaraki F, Rahimi H. The impact of authoritative, permissive and authoritarian behavior of parents on self-concept, psychological health and life quality. Eur Online J Nat Soc Sci. 2013;2(1):78–85. https://european-science.com/eojnss/article/view/24.
7. Triandis H. Collectivism v. individualism: a reconceptualisation of a basic concept in cross-cultural social psychology. In: Cross-cultural studies of personality, attitudes and cognition. London: Palgrave Macmillan UK; 1988. p. 60–95.
8. Dai YT, Dimond MF. Filial piety. J Gerontol Nurs. 1998;24(3):13–8.
9. Hansen CW, Jensen PS, Skovsgaard CV. Modern gender roles and agricultural history: the Neolithic inheritance. J Econ Growth. 2015;20:365–404.
10. de Groot JJ. The religion of the Chinese: English version. 1–142: CreateSpace Independent Publishing Platform; 2016.
11. Lakos W. Chinese ancestor worship: a practice and ritual oriented approach to understanding Chinese culture. Cambridge Scholars Publishing; 2010.
12. Tarakeshwar N. What does it mean to be a Hindu? A review of common Hindu beliefs and practices and their implications for health. In: Pargament KI, Exline JJ, Jones JW, editors. APA handbook of psychology, religion, and spirituality (Vol. 1): Context, theory, and research. American Psychological Association; 2013. p. 653–64. https://doi.org/10.1037/14045-036.
13. https://www.pewresearch.org/religion/2021/06/29/diversity-and-pluralism/.
14. https://reddit.com/submit?url=https://www.hinduismtoday.com/hindu-basics/karma-and-reincarnation/&title=Karma%20and%20Reincarnation.
15. Kalsi SS. Sikhism. Religions of the world. Philadelphia: Chelsea House Publishers; 2005. p. 41–50. ISBN 0-7910-8098-6.
16. Cole WO, Sambhi PS. The Sikhs: their religious beliefs and practices. Sussex Academic Press; 1995. p. 200.
17. Rahman F, Mahdi MS, Schimmel A. Islam. Encyclopedia Britannica; 2023. https://www.britannica.com/topic/Islam.
18. Strohl GR, Dundas P, Shah UP. Jainism. Encyclopedia Britannica; 2023. https://www.britannica.com/topic/Jainism.
19. Harvey P. An introduction to Buddhism: teachings, history and practices. Cambridge University Press. 2012; https://www.worldhistory.org/zo.

Learning About Death and Dying in the Eastern Traditions

5

H. Steven Moffic

There are more things in Heaven and Earth, Horatio, than are dreamt of in your philosophy—Hamlet.

In Shakespeare's famous play, Hamlet, Hamlet and his good friend Horatio are discussing a belief in ghosts, which in this situation would be the ghost of Hamlet's murdered father. More generally and to date, it questions what we still do not know about any afterlife hundreds of years later. For example, not long ago, on December 1, 2022, my best friend of 70 years died. We had talked much in recent years of our impending deaths and what might happen in the afterlife, if indeed there was something after life. Our conversation might go something like this:

He: Maf (loving contraction of Moffic), what do you think happens after we die?

Me: Don't know, Kucs (loving contraction of Marcus), but hope there is something good. You know I've had all these serendipities happening to me, almost every day, over the past few years. Makes me wonder if something is guiding me from beyond. An ER physician colleague said my writings are "a vessel of the divine." But even a Rabbi said it might just be chance.

He: You know I've been Buddhist, too, and there is a belief in a reincarnated afterlife, but I'm not so sure of that. I guess we won't know until after we die.

Me: Probably my big fear is that even if there is something, it will be separate from my loved ones: Rusti, you, ancestors. Made me even intrigued with the Mormon belief that married couples stay together in the afterlife forever.

Kucs: Interestingly, but terrifying at the same time.

We had hoped to get together in the summer of 2023 when we would both be 77. In the meanwhile, I had even written a chapter on the social psychiatric aspects of death and dying for a new textbook [1].

It was not meant to be.

Knowing his cardiac problems, I was not caught by surprise and, in fact, my wife and I had visited him from afar in October of 2022, just to be sure. That might have been divinely inspired too. Unexpectedly, the Canadian border opened to pre-pandemic status on October 1, 2022, and we had a chance to fly to Victoria Island from Toronto, and did so, just in case. Actually, that was also due to my own health concerns, having needed a pacemaker a year prior, with some continuing related problems afterwards. After I had the pacemaker put in, with the need discovered by apparent chance, I asked my cardiologist, who was Indian and Christian, why she thought the deadly problem was discovered. She said that, along with her own recovery from breast cancer, we were both still needed in this world. Such an unusual spiritual response from a cardiologist! How did she know?

H. S. Moffic (✉)
Milwaukee, WI, USA

While I cannot imagine that my best friend was still not needed, especially by his wife, children, grandchildren, and creative communities, I at least had no regrets about not seeing him. He died suddenly in the hospital, probably from an embolism. His wife thought maybe he was giving up on getting better. I wondered: Did he have any last thoughts about dying as he passed away? More importantly, will we ever meet again? I do still act and think as if he is still alive; he readily comes to mind.

But what did surprise me was his funeral. Interestingly, we had not discussed that. I guess I thought we would both be buried in a casket. That is the general Jewish way, in large part due to the sanctity of the body.

Studying Other Religious and Spiritual Ideas About Death and Dying

In contrast to the specific afterlife of a Heaven (or Hell) in Christianity and Islam, Judaism generally is not specific about an afterlife, instead emphasizing the importance of doing good things in this life, in the Tikkun Olam of making this world a better place. However, an intermediate place called Sheol for the transition of the soul is mentioned, as well as the possible further development of the soul in its relationship to our monotheistic God.

Even so, in the Jewish mysticism tradition of the Kabbalah, there is a concept called gilgul, where souls are reincarnated. The goal is a perfect state of reintegration with the divine. One's actions in life will influence subsequent reincarnations, for good or ill. Great souls in each generation can lead and model other souls on their journey.

Such beliefs are matters of faith, though studies about near-death experiences attempt to lend some scientific explanation to the dying process. A new study suggests the possibility of a covert consciousness during what seems to be an unconscious time of dying [2].

I wondered, given that this book was in process at the same time as my best friend's death

and reading this new study, how did other religious and spiritual traditions from the East view death and dying? To begin to learn more, it seemed obvious that I should learn from my co-editors, and being an academic, to explore some of the literature. Let us see what I found.

Starting with the long-standing imminent dying process, I found that science may be substantiating some of the faith. Clearly, my learning is still in flux, and it is likely that I will misinterpret or oversimplify along the way. Please forgive that.

For instance, in Tibetan Buddhism, there seems to be a related dying process called tukdam that posits mental conditions beyond what is known and accepted in psychiatry. It pertains to meditators who die in meditative equipoise. Apparently, their bodies do not decompose as usual, but much more slowly over even weeks after clinical death. They can remain sitting upright in meditation posture and seem lifelike. This particular process is being researched scientifically, as presented in a 2022 documentary film Tukdam: Between Worlds. Initiated by the Dalai Lama, the multidisciplinary Tukdam Project connects the Center for Healthy Minds at the University of Wisconsin, headed by the neuropsychologist Richard Davidson, with Tibetan collaborators in Dharamshala, as well as with Russian and Indian scientific collaborators. Though the results are still unclear, for the Tibetan Buddhists, there exists a presence, called mind, at least in this intermediate period of death.

What has not been common at all in Judaism until recent years is cremation of the body. That so many Jewish bodies were burned up in the concentration camps in World War II only intensified a negative associated with cremation for many. My best friend was cremated. Forbidden in Islam, I did know that cremation was more common in Eastern religions and spirituality.

Psychiatry, Death, and Dying

My son is a reform rabbi, and we have sometimes joked about the aftermath of a congregant or patient who has died. Generally, the eulogy that a rabbi or other Western clergy provides at a funeral is a solely positive one about the deceased. We psychiatrists know that when there is more ambivalence or negativity about the deceased, and that is omitted from the eulogy, loved ones may need some psychotherapy to process the loss afterwards.

Psychiatry has also paid much attention to the grieving process for the loved ones of the deceased. Kübler-Ross developed some varying stages of normal grief—denial, bargaining, anger, depression, and acceptance—while after her death, her colleague added a last one called finding meaning [3]. However, it is important to note that this process was actually studied with those dying, not those who were grieving after the deaths of loved ones.

Now, when grief does not dissipate, we have in psychiatry a new formal classification of prolonged grief for DSM-5, along with some specific therapeutic techniques.

Besides trying to prevent suicide or homicide in our patients, death and dying may come up for various reasons in treatment, and need to be discussed and processed, as existentially oriented psychiatrists like Yalom have done in depth [4]. In his clinical work, he often found that fear of death was the unconscious basis of much undue anxiety and needed to be brought out for discussing and processing. Paradoxically and unexpectedly, Yalom was faced with his own denial of death and dying when his wife Marilyn developed a terminal aggressive cancer. With her encouragement and involvement, they together wrote a book about how she gradually released from life and helped him to release her [5]. Though both were Jewish, this turned out to be a place of ultimate Buddhist-like suffering for a newly wounded-again healer. Yalom concludes that the basic living lesson he learned is that life is lived meaningfully and happily through the creative pursuit of learning in order to end up with as regret-free as possible [6].

In clinical work, Yalom's work suggests that we just have to be as sure as possible not to let our own countertransference concerns about death and dying intrude upon the patient. From both sides of the clinician and patient relationship, knowledge of cultural, religious, and spiritual values is essential to guide the processing. Some of that knowledge may be already known, but each can also teach the other, which individualizes the beliefs and overcomes translation problems from an original language one does not know. Here is how a Christian friend and colleague described to me about how he was still processing his wife's death, which occurred a couple of years ago, after hearing of this chapter:

Him: I occasionally sense the presence of my late wife Pam, like throughout today.

Me: That's so interesting and usually reassuring, whether you are imagining it or her presence is really there.

Him: "Steve, I appreciate your reaction to my sensing Pam. Here are some recent examples:

- Last month, in the evening, I was unusually lonely; I cried out her name and then, mysteriously, I felt her kiss me on the lips.
- This past week, however, I seem to have merely felt her presence.
- And recently, I heard her laugh, hearty laugh that I hadn't heard in years.

My therapist said that it was not unusual in that there is, apparently, an energy that must be omnipresent. These occurrences don't freak me out, Steve, rather, I find them a source of fascination."

Me: Fascinating examples, Chuck, and I like your therapist's openness.

Him: Thanks again, Steve, for all that you have done for me and my spiritual growth.

In the supportive psychiatry realm, there are now death doulas, sort of peer counselors, who help people who are preparing to die. Those dying may be unaffiliated religiously or isolated. An important process, when possible, is the talk with the dying about what has given their life meaning, purpose, and joy, a sort of counter to the existential agony of approaching death.

Certainly, all health and mental health staff who work in a hospice have opportunities to process upcoming death with patients and to help make them more comfortable.

Finding Out About the Eastern Traditions

Given that all humans evolved out of Africa, at least according to anthropologists and historians, it would be expected that beliefs about death and dying would have some similarities and differences. The similarities would come from basic human nature and common ancestral practices, while the differences would come from long periods of geographical separation and ignorance of Eastern or Western practices. None of the religions and spiritual traditions around the world seem to deny the reality of death, though there have always been pockets of people who quest for immortality.

Nevertheless, most traditions believe that the benefit of death is to make life more meaningful. This contrast, between a desired meaningful life and a death that seems to end that, results in a challenging psychological dialectic for us all.

I probably understand Buddhist spirituality best due to the beliefs of my best friend; I discussed some of that in my other book chapter. Some Buddhist traditions meditate on death daily. The Tibetan Book of the Dead, otherwise known as the Bardo Thodol, is a sacred cornerstone of Buddhist thought, and the Western world has come to recognize its psychological insights into the processes of death and dying [7]. Tibetan Buddhists call the interstitial period the bardo. Composed in the eighth century CE, the book claims to clearly show the various manifestations of the mind in the manifestations of entities in the mind of the deceased right after death. Psychiatry refers to this mechanism as a Freudian projection process. This unconscious uncovering of manifestations of one's own mind can be comforting or frightening. Prayers and explanations are also communicated.

The deceased in this immediate postmortem period may very well fit the possibility of a covert consciousness that was brought up as a possibility in recent medical research [2]. The purpose is "to rest the soul of the dead" and to ready the person to return to earth as another reincarnated human being. The psychiatrist Carl Jung advocates for the psychological benefits of convincing ourselves of the soul's immortality.

One of my older main sources for understanding more about the Eastern traditions has been the Rubin Museum in New York. Besides its various artistic and educational exhibits, it publishes a periodic magazine called Spiral. The first edition of 2023 was called "Life After" and examined the concept of life after, aka death, through stories, art, and studies.

One of the articles was by Dzigar Kongtrul Rinpoche. His brief bio reads that he "was recognized by his root guru, Kyabje Dilgo Khyentse Rinpoche and the Sixteenth Gyalwa Karma, as a reincarnation of Jamgon Kongtrul Lord Thaye." His article is entitled "Death, the Bardo, and Rebirth in Tibetan Buddhism" [8]. He describes two bardo phases. First, your consciousness struggles to understand that you have left your body and died. You find you cannot do the same things anymore. Tremendous grief can arise. It is said that you can read the minds of loved ones who are alive and perceive their emotional states. You try to comfort them.

In the second phase, you perceive flashes of where you will be reincarnated. If it is in the human realm, you look for an entry way. If you are to be born as a boy, there are usually aggressive feelings toward the father, while for a girl, there is the opposite. These dynamics can continue in life. This sounds to me like the basics of the Freudian Oedipal conflict, does it not? It is also an explanation of why traditional Tibetan Buddhism starts counting age at the presumed point of conception. At best, you are on the journey toward unconditional love and care for all living beings.

Like Buddhism, it seems to me that Hinduism emphasizes the importance of preparing for the soul's afterlife and reincarnation after death. Karma is the principle of receiving what is deserved by one's actions, the dharma of right duties and practices. For those who have done especially bad, there are hellish realms.

I cannot say that I have never had any wondering or belief about reincarnation. Somehow, that seems to fit "love at first sight," as if the spirit of the person was somehow familiar. Such is the case with my first sight of my wife. Later, I was to learn that most anything about the Holocaust was too painful for her to think about. Could she have been reincarnated from the Holocaust? She was born soon after World War II ended, perhaps a soul who knew how important it was to bring sunshine to the world, especially those in need.

For me, I have always felt more connected to the psychiatrist Viktor Frankl, rather than Freud, as far as the Holocaust goes. Frankl found meaning even in the concentration camps [9]; Freud escaped the camps, but just about left too late in his underestimation of the Nazi's genocidal goals for Jews. Later in my life, my connection with the Holocaust intensified. I was asked to discuss a movie about Hitler's children. These were not his children, of course, as he did not have any, but the children of the top Nazis. Maybe half went on to redress the harm done by the Nazis, while the other half continued to support Nazi ideology. The thunderbolt that struck me, as if it was a Shofar blast from the past, was that, among the infinite number of variables that account for one's birth, for me the Holocaust was one of them. My father joined the war effort late as a lawyer and met my mother at an Armed Forces mixer, and then I was conceived, even though my mother was medically not supposed to have children. From then on, addressing the intergenerational transmission of trauma from the Holocaust became a professional priority, as well as doing anything I could to reduce antisemitism [10].

Also as for Buddhists, there is a Hindu preparatory practice in approaching imminent death, with the afflicted repeating the monosyllable Om, which concentrates the mind and refers to the creator, Brahman. Death apparently best occurs on the ground, not in bed.

It is common for Hindus to try to cremate the deceased's body within 24 h of death, though such practices vary with location and sect. It is often conceived as an offering to the god of fire, allowing the soul (atman) to pass out through the head openings. In some places, it seems to be thought that the souls of the really wicked depart through the rectum. Children under 2 years are often buried, not cremated, as the child is thought to have had troubled prior lives. The Ganges River is a sacred place for the funeral pyre and ashes.

After death, the soul is usually reincarnated in another body or form, on a journey of spiritual development and final emancipation. I found it fascinating that it is thought that sometimes a group of souls will sequentially incarnate into an expected family, so that a grandchild may be the returned soul of a grandparent.

For Confucianism, a spiritual tradition in which there is no deity, life and death are inseparable. After death, the spiritual essence is thought to return to a Heaven, but that Heaven can be considered transcendence rather than a place as in Christianity. For dying patients with those beliefs, it is best to involve the family [11].

A unique mourning process can be found with the isolated Sora Indigenous people in the highlands of Odisha in eastern India. They routinely talk with their dead through the mouths of shamans in trance [12].

Tentative Conclusions

So far, with these selected examples and sources, my journey of trying to add the Eastern traditions to those of the West in addressing death and dying brings some tentative conclusions. It is a subject that has some clinical and personal relevance for all patients and people, religious, spiritual, atheist, or agnostic. All of us have some degree of death anxiety, conscious or unconscious.

There is so much to still learn. Keep in mind that any generalities of major religions are subject to variations depending on geography, local culture, subgroups, and the individual person.

For all, community involvement and support are psychologically helpful. There seems to be a looser religious and spiritual structure in the East, resulting in more individual practices. In general, the Western religions seem to deny death more during life than the East, especially in the United States.

Imminent death, other than, say, an immediate one from an accident, offers the opportunity to say farewell to life and prepare for death. There are Western religious traditions for the transition, though many of the Eastern ones seem more elaborate. In Eastern traditions like Hinduism, Buddhism, and Jainism, this period of spiritual death (Sallekhana) has certain common rules and rituals, including:

- Giving up material aspirations
- Obtaining and giving forgiveness
- Meeting with a spiritual guru
- Meditating on the innermost self of the true "I"

In the Eastern traditions, cremations are used much more than the burial practices of the West, though cremation seems to be increasing in the West.

There is an important intermediate period after death in many of the Eastern traditions, though there is some belief of that in Judaism. Probably the biggest differences are with the ensuing period of the afterlife. The Hindus and Buddhists believe in reincarnation of the soul until it reaches perfection, in Buddhism called Nirvana.

Christianity emphasizes eternal life in Heaven or Hell. I recall that when we lived in Alabama in the rural South, usually the first question the natives would ask us is: What church do you belong to? When they found out we were Jewish, they often tried to persuade us to take Jesus as our Savior, so that we would be saved in the afterlife. Telling them that Jesus was born and raised Jewish did not change their recommendation. Judaism is more vague about the afterlife, though both Judaism and Christianity look forward to a future messianic age of peace and the gathering of souls.

With all these apparent similarities, differences, and overlaps, it appears that the means may be somewhat different, but the end goals similar. The end goal seems to be an emphasis of having a good life for the soul of a person. Do what is right. Show care. Be sincere. Appreciate the impermanence of existence. Perhaps, this goal should put to rest the terms Western and Eastern, as they are artificial geographical differences of the northern hemisphere in a circular globe.

A limiting factor is not only my developing knowledge, but that there are so many sects and a range of practices within these religions and spir-

itual practices. Tying us all tighter is mortality. That we all die can potentially unify us toward peace and love or, on the other hand, conflict and hate. We are hardwired to be fearful about perceived differences, but our cognitive capabilities can overcome that.

Dialectical Resolutions

So, I am left with the dialectic between how I live life and the uncertainties of the afterlife.

My Judaism seems to have its own internal dialectic, a mainstream view that continues to emphasize doing morally good while alive and a mystical view that has similarities to many Eastern traditions, such as karma and reincarnation. Judaism's external dialectic with other Western religions and spiritual approaches tends to provide various specific views of the afterlife, like the Christian and Muslim heavens. Most of these belief systems connect having a good life with a good afterlife. So, in a way, perhaps the death and dying beliefs of Judaism may be a bridge or connection between so-called Western and Eastern religious and spiritual traditions.

Those who quest for immortality will potentially lose the meaning of death, let alone solving the need for more resources. Perhaps, then, all are searching for the perfect and beautiful world imagined in the afterlife to be present in this life. It is where psychiatry overlaps with spirituality. I will keep searching for how we can each find that psychological space "somewhere over the rainbow" together. It is the "eternal now" as one of our chapter writers told me. Or, as guru Ram Das, originally a psychologist, said many times: "Be here now!"

Kucs, are you out there somewhere? I sure hope so.

References

1. Moffic HS. Death and dying. In: Gogineni RR, et al., editors. The WASP textbook on social psychiatry: historical, developmental, cultural, and clinical perspectives. Oxford University Press; 2023.

2. Xu G, et al. Surge of neurophysiological coupling and connectivity of gamma oscillations in the dying human brain. Proc Natl Acad Sci. 2023;120:e2216268120. https://doi.org/10.1073/pnas.2216268120.

3. Kessler D. Finding meaning: the sixth stage of grief. Scribner; 2020.

4. Yalom I. Staring at the sun: overcoming the terror of death. Jossey-Bass; 2009.

5. Yalom I, Yalom M. A matter of death and life: love, loss and what matters most in the end. Platkus; 2021.

6. Moffic HS. Disclosing ourselves: a review of 4 psychiatrist memoirs. Psychiatric Times. 2020.

7. Sambhava P (Compiler), Thurman R (Translator). The Tibetan book of the dead: the great book of natural liberation through understanding in the between. Bantam, 1993. Scr Theol. 2020.

8. Rinpoche D. Death, the Bardo, and rebirth in Tibetan Buddhism. Spiral; 2023. p. 26–7.

9. Frankl V. Man's search for meaning. Beacon Press; 2006.

10. Moffic HS, et al., editors. Anti-Semitism and psychiatry. Springer International; 2019.

11. Lee S. East Asian attitudes toward death—a search for the ways to help east Asian elderly dying in contemporary America. Perm J. 2009;13(3):55–60.

12. Vitebsky P. This spiritual tradition could be the most poetic bereavement therapy ever documented. Sci Am. 2023.

Emily Diamond

Practice and Faith in the Eastern Traditions

I grew up in a house with an altar. *Butsudan* is what it is called in Japanese, and versions of these home Buddhist altars exist in families in Hong Kong, Vietnam, mainland China, Taiwan, and other places. When I was growing up, the first cup of tea of the day went to this small altar, along with the burning of some incense. We would be in the kitchen drinking coffee, but my mother's parents and grandparents who died when she was young got green tea. If there were big exams coming up, or occasionally on my birthday, my mother would ask me to put a fresh cup of tea at the Butsudan and light some incense and tell her parents and grandparents the news or ask them to help me to do well. Over the years, they got flourless chocolate cake, perhaps pieces of pecan pie, foods they never tasted in their lives. I have asked her if her parents liked things like cake, and she would say, *of course.*

How was it when my mother was a child? It was WWII, and fruits or occasional sweets were rarer when there was not always enough to go around. She and the other children waited patiently for the adults to give the signal to the children that the spirits have had their fill of the treats, and the treats could come down from the altar and be eaten.

Here in our home in the USA, my mother got a gift of a sculpture we think depicts Quan Yin, so she is part of the butsudan. Almost always there is a small vase of flowers from the garden there too. Losing both her parents at a relatively young age and coming to the USA in 1960, I think the incense, the prayers, and the conveying of news of her children kept a connection to her own mother as she raised her own in a different country, in a different language, and in a different time.

In the Thai culture, there are Spirit Houses that one can see in homes, gardens, and businesses, with offerings to the protective spirits of the place, so they might stay and congregate, warding off the more troublesome ones. I learned about Spirit Houses long ago, and though not exactly a part of a tradition I grew up with, it is near enough to something I do know, to feel natural. Syncretism of different traditions, some spiritual and some philosophical, makes spirituality in East Asia and throughout Asia harder to parse apart. It also allows them a rootedness in everyday life. What you place at the altar, a flower from your new native land or a new treat you happen to like, these may change, while the practice itself is ancient.

To see someone pray often leads me to think about what is being prayed for; it is one part of knowing who people are and what they care about. Something else hard to understand is exactly what we mean by belief. I think a lot

E. Diamond (✉)
The Wright Institute, Berkeley, CA, USA
e-mail: ediamond@wi.edu

H. S. Moffic et al. (eds.), *Eastern Religions, Spirituality, and Psychiatry*,
https://doi.org/10.1007/978-3-031-56744-5_6

about this because so much in the Eastern traditions is about seeing the duality in things, but language, perhaps the English language especially so, pushes on those grey zones in an effort at precision, so we see people write things like the inelegant, "*both/and.*" This story may get to some of that.

In 2011, an earthquake so large that it altered the axis of the Earth hit Fukushima, Japan, also causing the meltdown of three nuclear reactors. Triggered by the earthquake, a tsunami formed in the Pacific that in some places made a wall of water 133 feet tall. As it moved onto the shore, not only did it destroy whole towns, but also thousands of people were swept away when the waters retreated, never to be seen again. In all, about 20,000 people died [1]. In the minutes, hours, and days after the event, people frantically called the phones of their children, spouses, parents, grandparents, and others, hoping that they were alive. There is now a telephone in the town of Otsuchi, Japan, called the *Phone of the Wind* [2]. It is a phone booth in the midst of a garden, unconnected to any phone lines. Tens of thousands of people have visited it, calling the phone numbers their fingers will never forget, and speaking about how much the other is missed, how children or grandchildren are doing, and how they are doing. It is a moment to feel through the act of speaking, a connection. It also allows one to perhaps feel the textures and weight of one's own grief and hopes. This may have originated in Japan, but other countries now have Wind Phones too; some are attached to majestic trees, and there is one on the Appalachian Trail. There are Wind Phones in Wisconsin, Texas, British Columbia, and Washington State. There are Wind Phones in Australia, Poland, Denmark, Lithuania, Italy, and Germany.

What has this to do with the modern practice of Buddhism? At the bottom is a practice of connection. In part, this is why even when the communists rose to power in China, they did not demolish temples or stamp out altars to family members who died, because for so many, this was the realm of cultural practice. Practices that strengthen the notion of family, bridging those living with those who have gone before. Practices that ran much deeper because they are interwoven with Confucianism and Taoism, and the pre-Buddhist spirituality of China.

Syncretism in East Asia

Buddhism, Taoism, and Confucianism have become over time a syncretic set of beliefs, so where one starts and ends are often hard to tell. Each arose in the fourth century BCE, so the East Asian countries have more than 2000 years with these ideas overlaying their native belief systems. What is more, both Confucianism and Taoism arose from thinkers who were reaching back in time to earlier thinkers in order to develop their own thinking. These ideas have to do with not only how people should relate to one another but also how one relates to those who came before.

Many years ago, when I was a graduate student, I interviewed for a training clinic where my supervisor was originally from India. He took each prospective student out to dinner to get to know them, and I remember we talked about many things, and this included my parents and grandparents. My grandmother was a clinical psychologist who started one of the first schools for children with developmental disabilities in California, and he wondered if he had ever met her. It was nice to start off the year with that connection. A year or two later, at a different training site, I went to my first hour of supervision with a psychiatrist. He asked me to tell him about myself. I began by telling him that both my grandparents were clinical psychologists, my grandfather trained in Germany before WWII, and my father was a pediatrician, and that had something to do with my interests. I remember how he told me that the convention in the USA is when someone asks you to tell them about yourself, that this means—just you.

All these years later, I supervise research students from different states and different countries. Many meetings start with asking about how the student is and sometimes asking after their family. It has been an honor to try and shoulder some of the concerns they have when an illness strikes or, in our era, floods, fires, hurricanes, and pandemics. It has been a rich experience to learn of family members from generations back and feel the wonder of how that great-grandchild came to be my student or came to enter our field. I will never forget my student's parents from Appalachia who took me out to dinner during a visit to California where I teach. Just as we were about to part ways, my student's father said, *"Take good care of her, she is the most important thing in the world to me."* I assured him I knew that. I still ask how her parents are doing, and they still ask after me and my parents. This is familiar to me. It reminds me of how some of my own professors in Japan were towards me, or the Japanese professors I had here were. One such person was a tremendous inspiration to me because it was an education that reached far beyond the syllabi, lectures, and the weeks of the course. She was a mentor, she invited students to her home, and eventually, she became a family friend.

The Beginnings of Buddhism

What were the beginnings of Buddhism, a tradition at once philosophical and spiritual?

About 400 years before the Common Era, Buddhism, Confucianism, and Taoism each came into being. Perhaps more amazing is that these ideas and thoughts would traverse countries, branch into differing schools, spread within contexts of preexisting native spiritual practices, and take root. What is more, they persisted culturally through war and revolution and came with immigrants to their new countries. Of all the countries of Asia, there is only one that no longer has a sizable Buddhist population, and that is the Philippines. Here, the island archipelago's native spirituality and Buddhism were diminished when they became a Spanish colony in 1565 [3].

The date is uncertain, but scholars think that it was somewhere between 563 and 483 BCE, in a region we currently know as Nepal, where a boy of princely background was born named Siddhartha Gautama into a world of many deities [4]. As a young man, much to the unhappiness of his parents, he left his wealthy family to think about the pain, suffering, and poverty he saw. His questions were about release from suffering, freedom from ignorance, being released from being driven by desire, and the cycle of birth, death, and rebirth. To do this, he put himself in the crucible of those factors and became an ascetic, with a life focused on wandering, meditation, contemplation, and begging for his sustenance.

Leaving the Himalayas behind, he traveled down to the vast fertile North Indian River Plain, which is 172 million acres that rests like a raised brow across the top of present-day India, with Pakistan on one side and Bangladesh on the other. Siddhartha Gautama is thought to have achieved enlightenment in Bodh Gaya, which is about 225 miles away from his place of birth, in present-day India. Eventually, he developed a monastic order of his own. In this context, enlightenment means that he is released from a cycle of life, death, and rebirth and is now Nirvana bound. His name became Buddha, meaning *the Enlightened One*, and his teachings were passed down for centuries in an oral tradition that helped spread Buddhism further West into Pakistan, Afghanistan, as far as Iran. Buddhism also spread eastward and south to Korea, Thailand, Japan, Vietnam, Cambodia, Indonesia, the Philippines, and Malaysia. In time, there would be other Buddhas.

What is known is that Siddhartha Gautama developed the idea of the *Eightfold Path* [5]. It involves having the *Right View* or *Right Understanding*, which means that the person sees the nature of reality clearly. The person should have *Right Intentions*, which is an unselfish motivation for wanting to pursue enlightenment. *Right Speech* means that people should use speech compassionately. *Right Action* is ethical and compassionate conduct. *Right Livelihood* is about an ethical occupation that is not destructive or harmful. *Right Effort* is about having good and ethical motivations. *Right Mindfulness* is working towards full awareness which includes mind-body awareness. *Right Meditation* is about having a dedicated and focused practice of some kind.

Where did I learn of the Eightfold Path? My father, a humanistic retired physician who was born in New York to parents whose families came from Europe. Does my mother, born in Japan, know it? I do not think so. Where did I learn about the hand gestures of Buddha and bodhisattvas, and what these gestures mean? His parents, both of them with a love of art and art history. I also learned about them because for a short while, I was a bookseller, and our collections included rare books on all topics, including *mudra*, the gestures.

As Buddhism does not have an origin story about how the world came about, and because centuries of Buddhists have had their altars in their homes, there are families in which some members see Buddhism more as a philosophy, and perhaps others see it more as a religion. Perhaps their feelings change as events in their lives unfold, dipping into feeling faith or philosophy as their needs prescribe. There is a story that is told where someone asked the Buddha if he was a god. The Buddha said that he was not. The person asked: What are you? The Buddha, not wanting to define himself through that duality of human and god, replied, "*I am awake.*"

In this context, what is Nirvana, so often translated as Heaven? In Buddhism, there are what is known as the three poisons: greed, hatred (anger), and delusion (ignorance) [6]. How does one escape the interwoven and insidious nature of these? Through generosity, loving kindness, and wisdom. On an average day, at the family altar or a visit to a temple, how often in the silent prayers do these thoughts come to mind? Of course, one cannot know this. I know that I tend to always wish for the health of my family, and often I wish for a more peaceful world and for far less suffering in the world. I do not recall wishing for good grades or a raise, but surely that happens too. I know that in English, *wishes*, *hopes*, and *prayers* mean different things and imply different relationships to spirituality and can be charged with implications that I do not see in Japanese.

The Bodhisattvas of Buddhism

For centuries, people learned about Buddhism orally. Sometime during these years, the bodhisattvas arose, exactly when we do not know.

They are also enlightened ones. Travelers from different regions, some merchants, some philosophers, and those keen to learn about Buddhism carried the name of Buddha and the bodhisattvas back to their own countries. Here, the Buddha and the bodhisattvas would eventually take on names that would better fit the native language. In Japanese, Buddhism became *Bukyo* and the word bodhisattva became *bosatsu*. In Korean, a bodhisattva is *bosal*, and in Vietnamese, they are *Bồ Tát*.

One such bodhisattva is Quan Yin. Knowledge of her came to China through a seventh-century Chinese monk, Xuanzang [7], who journeyed West to India and still farther to Afghanistan to further his knowledge of Buddhism. His travelogue includes seeing the enormous Buddha carved into the mountainside in Bamiyan, Afghanistan, which was destroyed in 2001. When he did return to China, he had brought back knowledge of Quan Yin. She is known as *Kannon* in Japanese, and when Jesuits in China in the sixteenth century saw statues of her in temples, they called her the Goddess of Mercy. Her lore is that when she became fully enlightened, she was invited to enter Nirvana. As she made her way there, she heard the cries of the multitude of anguished here on Earth. She turned back to Earth, deciding she would not enter until all on Earth could enter with her. I have a few small sculptures of her in my home. The first one I got came during graduate school when I was working with my community's elders, all of them medically fragile, mostly alone in the world, and suicidal. I choose the sculpture because her face looks like my mother's face.

Quan Yin is Quan'Am in Vietnam and Kanin in Indonesia. Not only did her name change, but sometimes the bodhisattvas changed gender. Quan Yin is female in many East Asian countries, but not so in India where he is known as Avalokiteśvara. Further north, in Tibetan Buddhism, the successors of Dalai Lama are thought to be incarnations of Avalokiteśvara. So this bodhisattva is a placeholder for a being that listens with compassion.

I remember once talking with my mother about a particularly beautiful sculpture of a bodhisattva I saw, and she told me gently and with a laugh not to compare the beauty of sculptures, because maybe they are listening, so it's best to say they are all beautiful.

Very likely the first Jesuit missionary to learn Chinese was the Italian, Matteo Ricci, who lived in China in the sixteenth century [8]. It likely helped his missionary endeavors to make sense of Quan Yin as being like Mary, and in making that connection, the West would come to use words like deity, or Goddess of Mercy, and in that, this compassionate being changed once again. Belief systems change through having to flow through the available words of the cultures they become a part of. So a tradition that works against entrapment of duality has to find its way into a worldview where there is a tradition of mind-body dualism, one which has made an artificial line on the continent of Eurasia to separate Asia from Europe or believer from nonbeliever or wish from prayer.

I have struggled with this a bit because it feels like the Western world is pulling for dualities that I am often not seeing or perhaps resisting. As a high schooler, I learned about debate clubs where there would be winners and losers. I could not fathom why teachers would want to teach their students to take positions they did not believe in and win through rhetorical device. I did not understand why teachers would not be interested in teaching strategies to get beyond division. I slowly realized that I had a different culture, and this realization I mostly kept to myself.

Years ago, on a day I should have been working on my dissertation, I learned of another bodhisattva. I had decided to drive out to the coast. I would often listen to Corelli's Op 6 as it seemed to help me organize my thoughts as it unfurled notes to create worlds I like to contemplate and doing so with an inventiveness that I found astounding. Partway there, I came to a shop of knickknacks and found a small sculpture. On the bottom was taped an explanation; it was a name I had never heard, with a face that I did not recognize, and at first I was not sure if the sculpture was Hindu or Buddhist. The tag on the bottom said that he was the bodhisattva of wisdom, Manjushri. It did not matter what tradition he was

from; it was an easy decision to bring him home. I remember telling my parents about it, and after some discussion, we realized that he is who the Japanese call *Monju*, the *bosatsu* or bodhisattva of wisdom and education.

My Manjushri, depicted in an Indian manner, remains on my desk. My choice to bring Manjushri home happened before I knew much at all, only that I should have been home writing my dissertation and could use any bit of help I could get. So while I never wished or prayed for jobs or grades, with Manjushri, I hoped that the sword he carries, which is supposed to cut through the veil of ignorance and duality would work for me. Let us not forget that he carries a scroll too, a scroll that this graduate student could not resist. While in his right hand, he carries a sword, in the other hand, he carries a lotus blossom and a scroll that contains the *Perfection of Wisdom*.

From the Tang dynasty onward (A.D. 618–907), he is occasionally depicted astride a lion. Visiting the temple of Monju before a big exam is common. This association is strong, so when Japan began building nuclear reactors to meet its energy needs, and there was the need to win public approval on this earthquake-prone archipelago, the powers that be named one of them, *Monju* [9].

Another very popular bodhisattva in Asia is in Sanskrit, *Ksitigarbha*. He is often depicted with a shaved head of a monk and is called *Dìzàng* in Chinese, *Jizō* in Japanese, *Jijang in Korean, Địa Tạng* in Vietnamese, and *Sa yi snying po* in Tibetan. He is known to try and save those in the lower realms, realms that in the West we would think of as hell. Like Quan Yin, he made a vow to remain a bodhisattva until all those trapped in the lower realms were free.

In Japan, sometimes the *Jizo* is a small sculpture often about 2 ft tall, and he is thought of as the protector of children and the guardian of the souls of children who have died (Fig. 6.1). *Jizo* is also a protector of travelers. Sometimes, one can see small stone *Jizo* sculptures with bright caps to keep their head warm and red bibs around their necks. Occasionally, people leave candy and small toys for them, and when I see this, I feel a deep sadness that this was perhaps left by some-

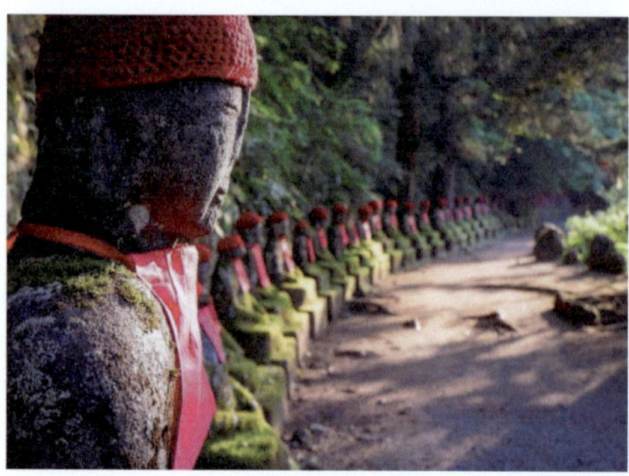

Fig. 6.1 Photo by Susann Schuster, Unsplash

one who lost a child. In paintings, the *Jizo* is often carrying an orb, and that symbolizes wisdom. The Jizo, Quan Yin, Buddha, and sometimes the laughing Buddha are also sculptures I see frequently in gardens where I live in California.

The Rise of Confucianism

We do not know the date of Buddha's birth in Nepal, but we know that farther East, in China, in about 551 BCE, the person the West would come to know as Confucius was born, in what is now Shandong Province [10]. He was educated in music, archery, charioteering, writing, and arithmetic, but in the hierarchy of the time, it was not enough to rise into the ruling class, the positions held by hereditary aristocrats. *Kǒng Fūzǐ (Master Kong)* is his name, and Kong is the clan or family he came from, and his given name was Qiu. His era was one marred by the violence of warring states. He reached back in time to learn from earlier periods of the Zhou Dynasty (1100 BCE to 256 BCE) to understand philosophical and societal factors that he felt would lead to more stability.

He was born at a time that would later give rise to three philosophies that would deeply impact China, the rest of East Asia, and parts of Southeast Asia to varying degrees: Confucianism, Taoism, and Legalism. The latter would draw upon Confucianism and Taoism and lay down the

administrative methods that would support a growing bureaucracy for a more unified China under the Han, one with deepening foreign relationships. This era is known as the Golden Age of Chinese Philosophy or Hundred Schools of Thought.

Confucius is known as *Kōshi* in Japan and *Khong Tu* in Vietnam. There is no single book more important to understanding Confucianism than The Analects of Confucius, called *Lunyu* in Chinese. This is where some of the most important thoughts of Confucius and his students were compiled in a series of brief sayings and later memorized by centuries of students.

Taken together, the sayings build on the idea that if every unit starting with the family abides by rules of deference in their relationships with each other, and this system was allowed to organize all relationships within society, then the whole would be more stable. So there is a proper way for a younger brother to relate to the older brother, wife to husband, student to teacher, younger person to elder, and friend to friend. In so doing, the family, village, municipalities, and regional governments would be more stable too. The translated word in English is often *harmonious*.

It is more than a system of propriety and deference. There is great importance put on learning and the relationship between student and teacher. It comes through in this phrase: "*A teacher for a day is a father for life.*" As I write these words, I remember meeting the brother of a college classmate in the USA. He asked me what I wanted to do after college. I said that I was thinking of being a teacher. He replied, "*You know what they say, those who can't do, teach.*" It was the first time I had heard it, and it was so alien that I never forgot it.

Here, after a doctor's appointment or a class, a person is asked to grade or rank their teacher, and this also goes for nearly every purchase or service. Sometimes, I know that things have gone well when there is growing trust over time, not how an interaction went over a moment or a course. One of my past students is now a professor. When his father passed away recently, I offered to teach his courses for a week. It was wonderful meeting his students, and I told them that if they felt I might be able to answer a question for them, now or in the future, they should reach out to me and I would do my best for them. I was not inspired by The Analects; I think I had learned that from my favorite professor from Japan, and she perhaps learned it from hers; it is a part of more than 2000 years of cultural practice.

There is not only great importance on cultivating characteristics that would keep stability in the family and society, but also a great emphasis on developing *wisdom*, and these two work together. You can see it in this phrase, *"The nobleman who studies culture extensively and disciplines himself with propriety can keep from error."* Other key passages discuss *righteousness*, and the importance of cultivating a profound idea of *benevolence*, and *trustworthiness*.

China is the first known country to have a written civil service exam; the very first of these began in 581 [11]. Chinese classics and in particular The Analects had a central role in it. It transformed a society of inherited positions, which had earlier shut Confucius out of the higher ranks, into exploring meritocracy, for sons. If you could afford the books and the time to study, how you did was ranked, with each rank corresponding to a particular animal that would be embroidered across the front of your uniform for all to see [12]. Over the various dynasties, the focus on Confucianism could change, but it remained central to the education of civil servants for centuries. Analogous systems arose in the Ryukyu Islands, Japan; Korea; and Vietnam.

One day, after I had taught a class on the history of testing and measurement, a student told me how one of her ancestors did on that exam. This is to say that what may appear to be a scholarly tradition is more than that, and after 1500 years, it is not quite a religion, nor is it simply a set of ideas.

This is a portrait of a young official done by Weng Pu, who got the rank of 7 on the exam, and you can see that rank reflected in the Mandarin duck embroidered on his official outer coat (Fig. 6.2).

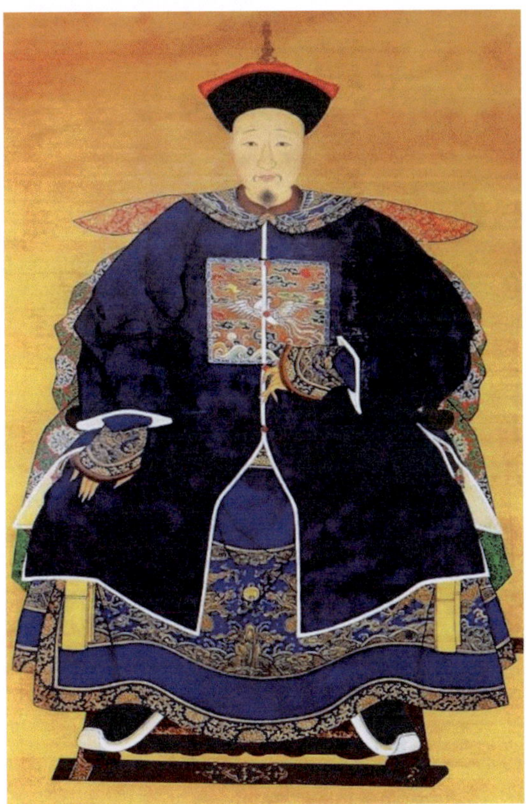

Fig. 6.2 Portrait of Weng Pu, Wikicommons, public domain image

Harmony and Statecraft in Confucianism

There are passages in The Analects where it is clear that what Confucius and his students were hoping to achieve was bigger than stability in the household.

One can see this in these passages of The Analects [13]:

1.2 "It is rare for a person who is filial to his parents and respectful to his elders to be inclined to transgress against his superiors. And it has never happened that a person who is not inclined to transgress against his superiors is inclined to create chaos. A gentleman looks after the roots. With the roots firmly established, a moral way will grow. Is it not true then that being filial to one's parents and being respectful to one's elders are the roots of one's humanity [ren]?"

More on governing is in this passage:

2.3 "If you guide the people with ordinances and statutes and keep them in line with [threats of] punishment, they will try to stay out of trouble but will have no sense of shame. If you guide them with exemplary virtue [de] and keep them in line with the practice of the rites [li], they will have a sense of shame and will know to reform themselves."

I was in college when I first read The Analects, and it was then that I could better see how my own mother, born in the 1930s, had been raised. These were years of Japan's gearing up for WWII and imperialistic expansion throughout Asia, in part aided by a resurgence of Confucianism. She describes how people were expected to cheer and send off young men called up for the military. She tells me how the military came door to door asking for valuables to support the war effort. She remembers her mother handing over her engagement ring, and with that, every tangible thing from her father was gone, because he passed away when she was 2 years old. One did not have to know The Analects or be scholarly at all to have its norms shape expected behavior.

This history of Japanese imperialism is something I talk about with my students. From Western eyes, it may be that there is a group called Asians, and with time, the preferred words and geographic boundaries of newer terms change. To ourselves, and to the student whose ancestry is in Korea, the Philippines, China, or any place Japan sought to dominate, it is important to show I know that painful history and show how I feel about it.

When I think about how ideas come through culture, often this story comes to mind. After a car accident many years ago, I was left with some shoulder pain and wanted to know why and what to do. My doctor, a Chinese person, showed me a page from his textbook, a page of illustrations of shoulders and tendons. Mine matched a picture of one where the tendon was torn, but not all the way through. I thanked him for showing me his textbook, and he said, "*A doctor is a teacher to one person at a time.*" In the many years that have passed, I sometimes tell that story to my own students to see how that feels to them. How does that fit in a world where patients are clients? How do these worlds collide for them?

The Rise of Taoism

Another major cultural, philosophical, and spiritual development, also going back to around the fourth century BCE, is Taoism, sometimes called Daoism. The character in both Chinese and Japanese is the character for *path* or *way*, so one can see it written sometimes as *The Way of Tao*. Some of the ideas arose out of ideas of the *School of Naturalists* of which philosopher Zou Yan was a guiding member (305–240 BCE) [14]. This organized the world broadly into *yin* and *yang*. The *yin* is associated with the negative, dark, cold, and female, as opposed to *yang* which is associated with the positive, light, hot, and male. There are also *five elements*: water, fire, wood, metal, and earth [15]. In this cosmology, the cause of disease and poor well-being is that the *qi*, or life force, is out of balance, very often between the forces of *yin* and *yang*. These ideas may have traveled by way of the Silk Road and be the origins of the Greek and Roman humoral tradition. Regardless of how far these ideas may have traveled, they have penetrated deeply where they began. It is the 2000-year-old tradition on which Chinese traditional medicine is built. There are now practitioners across the world, and sales of these treatments bring in $50 billion in annual revenue for China's economy [16]. In places where contemporary medication may be prohibitively expensive, or for other reasons, one can see that traditional Chinese medicine has taken a foothold. This was in part facilitated by the Chinese government advocating for traditional Chinese medicine to have a dedicated chapter in the ICD-11. It is also why when I teach students about how to do a comprehensive intake, no matter the patient's ancestry, I make sure that they ask about all things people are taking to try and solve their problems.

If we can imagine a time in life when we might want fervently for everything to go right, it is pregnancy. In this cosmology, if you are pregnant, the mother is *yin*, and pregnancy is believed to increase *yin*. So the mother-to-be might be encouraged to avoid cool foods, which would increase *yin* even more. Behaviorally, emotions like anger and fear might be very bad for one's *qi*, because they add yet more *yin*, potentially causing more imbalance and leading to a state of unhealthy disharmony.

Similar to Confucian's focus on keeping harmony, in this cosmology, the body, the family, and other tiers of society can be healthy if all the building blocks also remain in harmony. For the body, this means that things that make up our world, our emotions, foods, beverages, temperature of things, and behaviors, can upset this balance and may need to be adjusted or corrected.

As with Confucians, there is an aspect of Taoism that is about statecraft. One can see it in the *Tao Te Ching*, written about 400 BCE and credited to Lao Tzu [17]. This is from the section called *Keeping People Quiet*. It is about the power of governing with what is called *non-assertion*. The idea is that if you put something into the world for people to know, envy, or covet, you will create problems in keeping your power:

Not boasting of one's worth forestalls people's envy.
Not prizing treasures difficult to obtain keeps people from committing theft.
Not contemplating what kindles desire keeps the heart unconfused.
Therefore the holy man when he governs empties the people's hearts but fills their stomachs. He weakens their ambition but strengthens their bones. Always he keeps the people unsophisticated and without desire. He causes that the crafty do not dare to act. When he acts with non-assertion there is nothing ungoverned [18].

I remember a year of college spent in Japan, and the ever-present sounds of life in one of the world's megacities, Tokyo. I remember being introduced to Taoist poetry and being taken with themes of simplicity and nature and the idea of freedom from the cares of the world. No system that was all about deference, propriety, and ultimately cultivation of docility could likely survive without some counterforces too. You can see it in this poem by Tao Yuanming who was born in about 365 in what is now Jiangxi Province, China. His great-grandfather, grandfather, and father were all in government, as was he. He wrote *Returning to the Fields*, translated from the Chinese by Arthur Waley [19]. The last line I liked then, and still do:

When I was young, I was out of tune with the herd:
My only love was for the hills and mountains.
Unwitting I fell into the Web of the World's dust
And was not free until my thirtieth year.
The migrant bird longs for the old wood:
The fish in the tank thinks of its native pool.
I had rescued from wildness a patch of the Southern Moor
And, still rustic, I returned to field and garden.
My ground covers no more than ten acres:
My thatched cottage has eight or nine rooms.
Elms and willows cluster by the eaves:
Peach trees and plum trees grow before the hall.
Hazy, hazy the distant hamlets of men.
Steady the smoke of the half-deserted village,
A dog barks somewhere in the deep lanes,
A cock crows at the top of the mulberry tree.
At gate and courtyard—no murmur of the World's dust:
In the empty rooms—leisure and deep stillness.
Long I lived checked by the bars of a cage:
Now I have turned again to Nature and Freedom.

The Three Teachings, Buddhism, Confucianism, and Taoism Together

Together, Buddhism, Taoism, and Confucianism make up what are known as *the Three Teachings*. Here, Confucius is handing the baby Buddha to Lao Tzu (Fig. 6.3).

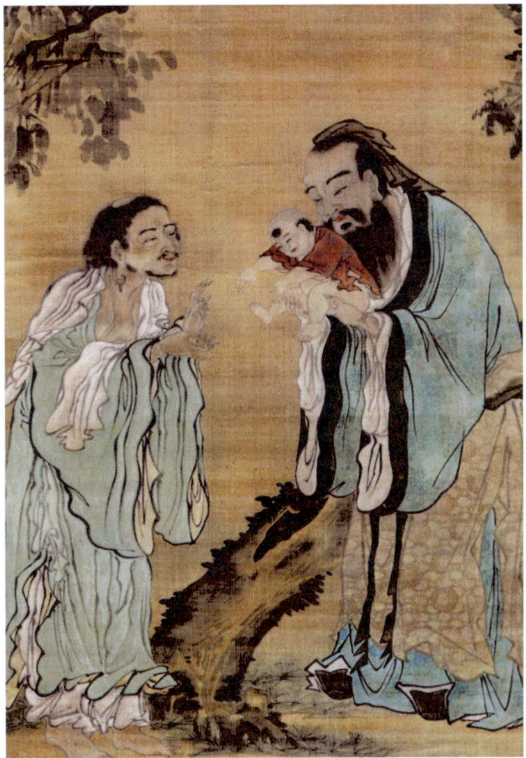

Fig. 6.3 *The Three Teachings*, Wikicommons, public domain image

They are together again in this sixteenth-century Japanese painting, called the *Vinegar Tasters* (Fig. 6.4). It is Confucius, Lao Tzu, and Buddha from left to right, each tasting vinegar and discussing it. There are other paintings in this genre, with Buddha likely to have thought that life was largely bitter and full of suffering, Confucius believing that the nature of existence is more sour with a need to build mechanisms to correct the sour ways of people, and Lao Tzu able to taste elements of sweet amidst the tart acidity.

Buddhism, Confucianism, and Taoism did not arise in a monotheistic tradition, and they also spread to countries with native spiritualities and religions to which they became an additional layer.

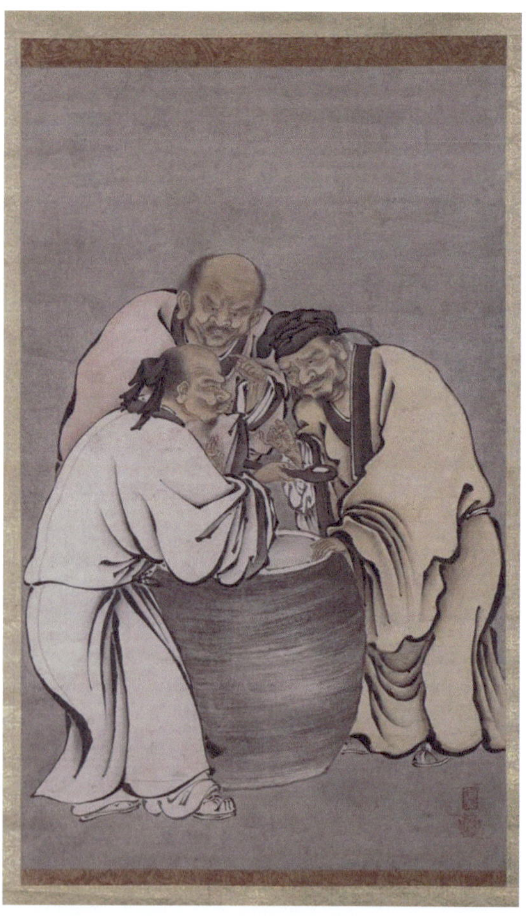

Fig. 6.4 *The Vinegar Tasters*, Wikicommons, public domain image

The Three Teachings Make Their Way Among the Native Spirituality of Asia

You can see the esteemed place of the dragon in much of Asia, the Fu Dogs of China, the 12 animals of the Lunar Zodiac, and the myriad *kami* (divine beings) in the native Japanese tradition that beyond these teachings is also a world of another spirituality. In pre-Buddhist times, Korea had a native religion where trees, mountains, and other elements of life were animated with spirits [20]. Particular mountains might have unseen spirits, and animals too could have scared spirits in them. The Philippine islands had their deities and spirituality too, with differences between their 2000 inhabited islands on their archipelago of more than 7000 islands [21]. Vietnam too has a native religion, with local deities.

In Japan, the native religion is Shinto. In Shinto, the Japanese islands were formed by the sun goddess Amaterasu Ōmikami. Up until the end of WWII, it was said that the royal family was descended from the Shinto gods, a story that the emperor was forced to formally retract as part of Japan's surrender at the end of the war [22].

You can sometimes come across Shinto shrines in nature; they are noticeable because they will have been garlanded by rope, giving the spirit its place and letting others know that there is a *kami* there. It is the same *kami* as in *Kamikaze*, the pilots of *"divine wind"* who flew suicide missions in WWII. So if the making of modern Asia is profoundly sculpted by Confucianism, Taoism, and Buddhism, the native spiritual beliefs were also used as part of statecraft.

This is a shrine, called the Meoto Iwa, or Husband and Wife Rocks (Fig. 6.5). The shrine gate is faintly visible on the larger rock.

In the Shinto traditions, these deities have days on which they are feted; these festivals are called *matsuri* [23]. *Matsuri* are when the community comes together, and the main street leading up to the shrine has special stalls of foods and goods, and there will be an evening of folk music, dancing, plays, and fireworks on the shrine's grounds. I remember this, and the charm of it has stayed with me all my years.

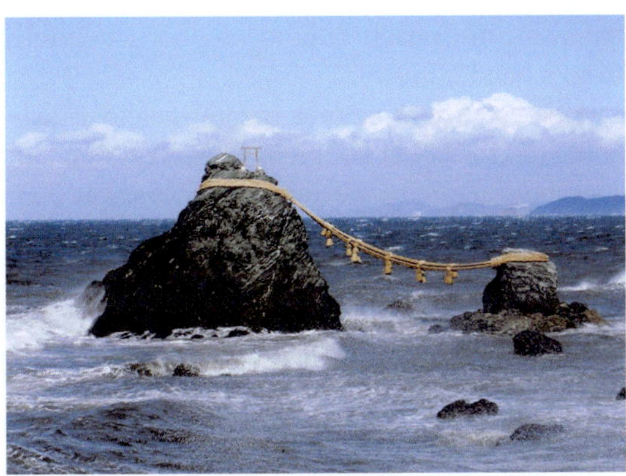

Fig. 6.5 Shinto Shrine, *Meoto Iwa*. Public domain image

In this system of local deities and main deities, there is the ability to call on different ones depending on the circumstance and situation. On the other side of Eurasian continent, the Romans did this too. As their empire expanded, they learned of new Greek deities and others from other lands, they left offerings and prayers, and made many of them their own. One that they had which the Greeks did not have was *Vesta*, the god of the doorway, from which we have the word, *vestibule*. In Chinese folk religion, door or gate gods are called *Menshen*, and I have seen these guardians of thresholds put up at Lunar New Years and as guardian sculptures at temples in Japan [24].

This comparison matters because it is difficult to explain a world populated by so many spirits and beings, some with no form and some with human form. It is easy to feel that this is a uniquely Asian phenomenon, exotic even, but it was not throughout the Eurasian continent in the time before the Common Era began. It is even difficult to explain what it means to believe as one looks out from a skyrise onto the canyons of concrete that can be modern Asia. Even still, every prefecture in Japan has a temple and some have more than a dozen. There are tens of thousands of Shinto shrines across the islands, some very small and local, and some are grand and bring in visitors and tourists from far away.

I remember the shrines to the fox deities that were near our house in Japan, and I recently gave my mother a little carving of a fox in carnelian because I thought maybe she missed them. They were part of the aesthetic world we lived in.

For me, it was a world animated and charming, one where there are fourteenth-century temples of Buddha or a bodhisattva and, not so distant, a shrine to a deity, perhaps in a rock, tree, human, or fox. Then, there is a temple for an old scholar and his students. There is also the altar in the home and the smell of incense that is as familiar as a friend. All of these are connections to emotional, aesthetic, philosophical, and spiritual worlds and difficult to recreate far from Asia.

I remember one professor said during a lecture that Asian people were not very introspective. I did not know what she meant. I did know that to be introspective in the Western sense is often to be in the foyer of conversations about one's family. I like to think that what she meant was that it is not in general a culture where people will freely complain, accuse, or blame their parents or other family members. In immigrant families, the first generation here has had to struggle to learn a new language and raise their children with the values they care about, but also new ones they are less familiar with. They hope that it will help them fit into a culture that they are themselves learning, much of it from their own children. I think that there may be a special reticence to say things that sound like accusations, failures, and complaints because you can see that your parents feared untethering you from cultural posts they know, into a world they were only just learning, with everyone holding out the hope that this new chapter of the family will be safe and successful.

Around the time I heard Asians are not very introspective, I remember finding a book on Morita therapy. Shōma Morita was a Japanese psychiatrist born in 1874, and he focused his career on people who were anxious, worried, and deeply self-conscious and many who had depression. Though his treatment style would later be taken up by clinics throughout Japan and be based in hospitals, initially patients went to his home. They were for a time part of his family. Treatment started by giving the person space to rest from their sleeplessness and exhaustion from wrestling with their thoughts and feelings. He himself had firsthand experience with wrestling with grief, as he and his wife experienced the young death of their only child [25]. His home clinic included a contemplative garden, which was central to treatment. In some descriptions, it is a Zen garden, a place to contemplate such things as seasons, stillness, imperfection, and the negative space that lies between elements in the garden. People who went there spent the first days calibrating their sleep and wakefulness to the day, by waking up with the sunrise and listening to birds, watching the light as it moved across the garden, and going to sleep when it got dark. Morita let them experience and hopefully come to understand that their thoughts were natural and not something they could control, much as one cannot control the light, the birds, the sounds of the cicadas, or the seasons in the garden. Through the garden, he hoped to extend their awareness outside of themselves, and to understand that they are a part of nature and to let their consciousness extend outward to it. He gave this kind of consciousness the name *mushojushin*, peripheral consciousness. When they were ready, they were urged to observe life in the garden more closely, noticing and writing about things they saw, like how an insect walks the length of a blade of grass [26]. Slowly and over the course of weeks, they could begin to reengage with life, starting with small tasks and getting stronger over the course of treatment. Sometimes, they wrote haiku and did other Zen-related activities like calligraphy; other times, they worked in the garden itself, until ultimately they were ready to rejoin their lives at home. The things they did and what they noticed and wrote about were not because Morita asked it of them. He felt that lasting changes would be because they felt pulled by nature itself to do it, because their awareness was now less inward and now outward. As someone who has written poems for a lifetime, I resonated with this.

For me, it has been a long road of learning. In the USA, you can go into interviews and you can present yourself as though you have no family at all, as though all that you have done or achieved comes entirely from you alone. It reminds me of one of my favorite stories my mother used to read to me. It was called *Momotaro*, an ancient Japanese folk hero who sprang fully formed from the inside of a peach, later to save his community from a band of ogres.

Here is where getting mental health can be about talking about your family in ways that I am sure must not feel easy for people who grew up in a different way, with different values, and with different parts of life sacred and meaningful. I had known one of my students for several years when one day at lunch she told me that when she was little, a parent had been mentally ill and was abusive at that time. She took her time, she waited for a moment there was confidence in me, and she told the story in a very compassionate way. How does this bode for our world of time-limited sessions? How does it bode for a world where you do not even realize the kind of confidence the other person needs to have in you?

When a painful disclosure is about a family member, how does it feel when there is not a firm line between what is your life and the lives of your parents? If you know a little about the history of psychology, you might worry that you will be trapped in an eddy where you discuss individuation and independence and might seem a failure by a metric you do not fully understand. You may worry that your doctor may have read, as I have, that the religion is about ancestor worship, and so you do not want to talk about your spiritual life because while those words do not fit, more fitting words do not easily come, like *homage* or respect, or simply connection. It might be difficult to lay open your mind and thoughts only to find yourself using the time in explanation, or perhaps a defense of things you hold dear. Maybe you feel like your doctor should be more like a teacher for one, and you wonder why you are doing most of the talking and the silence is alienating. When you do talk, maybe you feel the language pulling for one either/or after another. Maybe the therapy you get for your English-speaking self does not quite work for the part of you that is thinking and feeling in another language.

I have heard people say that there is only one god but with different faces around the world. I think it is an attempt, often well-intentioned, to make a bridge. In recognizing that impulse, I tend not to say anything. Study these layered traditions a while, and see and feel if that interpretation continues to feel right.

Were it possible to follow a thread in time, it would go back to the time before written history. The newest additions come from the fourth century BCE. What it is, is the world before monotheism. What it is, is a world where a spirit or deity could belong to the woods behind your town, where a person could have their favorite among the deities. It is a world where there was a person whom people came to call Buddha, and there is a temple to pay respects to an old philosopher and his students. It is not at odds with the modern cities that have sprung up around these places. In the world of many gods, they have been there, used, and misused, but holding their space for contemplation of what might be sacred. They have been there as places to voice one's smallest and biggest hopes. All the while, the newest iterations of society have grown up and been replaced in a cycle going back thousands of years.

In writing this, I am reminded that like musicians, we are often playing someone else's repertoire from another place or time. The thinkers in this essay confronted the inequality, turbulence, and violence of their times and tried to meet it by thinking about such things as how much the *self* matters, the meaning of life, and the varieties of virtue. Some like Confucius borrowed social mores from earlier times. Clinically, someone like Morita saw the rising colonial wave that eventually took his own brother's life in Manchuria, and his son's death from disease, and he met that grief by helping people to see that thoughts and feelings will rise and subside and that we must find a way to keep on going, our gaze turned out to the small elegances and meaningful pauses and spaces in the landscape. On the best of days, perhaps these could be turned into haiku or beautiful calligraphic art, observations to share with family and friends. At about the same time, in Austria, a medical doctor named Freud, saw the rising fascism closing in on his country, and he responded to his times by turning the perspective inward, hoping to help free people from their various troubles by going back into

their pasts. We know from the last photographs taken of his office, days before he was allowed to leave for England, that Nazi flags draped the buildings along Berggasse, the street on which he lived. In his office was a collection of dozens of archeological artifacts from all over the world. His tray of pens lay at the base of a sculpture of an old Chinese scholar he was said to have greeted every morning [27].

We now confront challenges of a different order, a climate that is destabilizing, the growth of vast inequalities, temperatures that are not easily survivable, rivers gone dry, and a rise in violence, physical and emotional. It is a desecration. As the physical world ails, so too do we, in ways we can see and define and in ways that we do not yet have words for. For some, depending on where you live, you can write and speak about it, for others not. Wherever you are, I think it is not so much a matter of whether our attentions are turned outward or in, or even to the past or the lightly outlined future. We need the freedoms of these thinkers. Those freedoms allow us to take what works for us and let go of what does not. What is more, we will need that freedom so that we can revisit, revise, and at times resist. I write this on days that are thought to be the hottest in the last 125,000 years. We will need to learn how to meet this heat and fire with freedom and fluidity. We are musicians having learned a repertoire, maybe more than one. It is not so much which to like better, allegiances, or how to rectify the differences, but the freedom and strength to compose pieces of meaning, resilience, and tenacity for ourselves and our loved ones to get us through these times.

In writing this, a phrase my grandfather kept on his desk comes to mind from Terence, the playwright born a slave in North Africa around 195 BCE, who died a celebrated writer in Greece. My father showed it to me when his father passed away, and I was about to enter graduate school and getting ready to be a listener to stories I worried might be unlike any I was familiar with; the note on my grandfather's desk read: *Homo sum, humani nihil a me alienum puto.* I am a human being, nothing human is alien to me.

References

1. Nakahara S, Ichikawa M. Mortality in the 2011 tsunami in Japan. J Epidemiol. 2013;23(1):70–3. https://doi.org/10.2188/jea.je20120114.
2. Howard K. Dealing with grief: japanese phonebooth connects the living and the dead. 2017. https://allthatsinteresting.com/phone-of-the-wind. Accessed 3 Nov 2023.
3. Barrow D. A history of the Philippines. New York, Cincinnati, Chicago: American Book Company; 1905. p. 126–56.
4. Thomas EJ. The life of Buddha: as legend and history. New York: Kegan Paul, Trench, Trubner; 1931. p. 126–56. https://archive.org/details/in.gov.ignca.7358/page/n55/mode/2up.
5. Bodhi B. The noble eightfold path the way to the end of suffering. Buddhist Publication Society. Kandy, Sri Lanka. The Wheel Publication No. 308–311; 1998.
6. Nyanatiloka. The Word of the Buddha: an outline of the teachings of the Buddha in the words of the Pali Canon. Kandy, Ceylon, Buddhist Publication Society; 1907. p. 31. Electronic version Accessed 11 Mar 2023.
7. Wriggins S. The silk road journey with Xuanzang. Basic Books; 2004.
8. Spence JD. The memory palace of Matteo Ricci. New York, NY: Penguin Books; 1983.
9. Johnson E. Nuclear cash cow Monju now a liability for residents as plant faces ax. The Japan Times. 2016. https://www.japantimes.co.jp/news/2016/10/04/national/nuclear-cash-cow-monju-now-liability-residents-plant-faces-ax/.
10. Huang Y. Confucius: a guide for the perplexed. London: Bloomsbury Press; 2013. p. 1.
11. Wang R. The Chinese Imperial examination system: an annotated bibliography. Scarecrow Press; 2013.
12. Breedlove B, Fung IC-H. Auspicious symbols of rank and status. Emerg Infect Dis. 2020;26(5):1056–7.
13. Confucius. The Analects: Lunyu. (Chin, A. trans.). Penguin Books; 2014. p. 77.
14. Ronan CA, Needham J. The shorter science and civilisation in China: volume 1. Cambridge University Press; 1978. p. 153.
15. Ronan CA, Needham J. The shorter science and civilisation in China: volume 1. Cambridge University Press; 1978. p. 144, 153–5.
16. Editors. The World Health Organization gives the nod to traditional Chinese medicine. Bad Idea Scientific American; 2019. https://www.scientificamerican.com/article/the-world-health-organization-gives-the-nod-to-traditional-chinese-medicine-bad-idea/.
17. Laozi. The speculations on metaphysics, polity and morality, of "the old philosopher" (Chalmers, J. trans.). London, Trübner and Co. (Date of original work unknown); 1868. p. viii.
18. Tze L. The canon of reason and virtue: Lao-tze's Tao Teh King. (Suzuki, T.D., and Caras, P. trans.). La Salle, Illinois, Open Court. (Date of original work unknown). 1913. https://www.sacred-texts.com/tao/crv/crv009.htm.
19. Bai J. A hundred and seventy Chinese poems. United States: A. A. Knopf. (Waley, A. trans.). New York: Alfred Knopf; 1919. p. 113.
20. Koehler R. Religion in Korea: harmony and coexistence. Seoul Selection; 2012.
21. Hislop SK. Anitism: a survey of religious beliefs native to The Philippines. Asian Stud. 1971;9(2):144–56.
22. Emperor, Imperial Rescript denying his Divinity (professing his humanity). 国立国会図書館—National Diet Library. (n.d.). https://www.ndl.go.jp/constitution/e/shiryo/03/056shoshi.html. Accessed 13 Mar 2023.
23. Festivals (Matsuri). 2022. https://www.japan-guide.com/e/e2063.html.
24. Pregadio F. The encyclopedia of Taoism: 2-volume set. Routledge; 2013. p. 744.
25. LeVine P. Classic Morita therapy: consciousness, Zen, Justice and Trauma. 2017. https://openlibrary.org/books/OL27412229M/Classic_Morita_Therapy.
26. LeVine P. Morita therapy according to Morita: dwelling in the tension between hardy and fragile life. Int J Ecopsychol. 2020;1:8.
27. Engleman E. Sigmund Freud's home and offices, Vienna 1938, the photographs of Edmund Engelman. Chicago: The University of Chicago Press; 1976.

Spirituality: Relationship with Religion, Health, Wisdom, and Positive Psychiatry

Bruno Paz Mosqueiro, Alexander Moreira-Almeida, H. Steven Moffic, and Dilip V. Jeste

Spirituality has been known and valued since the beginning of the human culture. However, empirical scientific research on this topic has been a phenomenon of the last few decades. Yet, even today, many clinicians and scientists dismiss constructs such as spirituality and wisdom which they view as fuzzy, despite a robust body of research on these topics. It is worth noting that many entities that were considered fuzzy and unscientific for centuries are now accepted as critical scientific entities. Examples include consciousness, stress, emotions, cognition, and resilience. Most researchers today agree that these entities are not only real ones, but they also have neurobiological correlates. The static and compartmentalized separation of human characteristics into psychological, social, and biological categories is wrong and anti-science. Fortunately, the field of health and health care is broadening, and rigid conceptualizations are gradually being replaced with more open-minded ones, focusing on the overall well-being of the individuals and the communities. Over the past three decades, a substantial number of high-quality scientific studies have been published on the association of spiritual beliefs, experiences, and practices with different clinical outcomes related to health and well-being.

In this chapter, we will primarily discuss the emerging science of spirituality in terms of its relationship with religion, health, wisdom, and positive psychiatry and its implications for mental health care. There is even a new focus on spiritual intelligence, as spirituality seems to be gaining more followers as participation in many formal religions decreases. We will also discuss similarities and differences between Eastern and Western religious and spiritual traditions and practices. We will consider how religiosity/spirituality (R/S) impacts health and how clinicians can address it.

B. P. Mosqueiro
Psychiatry Department, School of Medicine at Universidade Federal do Rio Grande do Sul,
Psychiatrist at Grupo Hospitalar Conceição,
Porto Alegre, Brazil

A. Moreira-Almeida
School of Medicine, Federal University of Juiz de Fora (UFJF), Juiz de Fora, Brazil
e-mail: alex.ma@medicina.ufjf.br

H. S. Moffic
Milwaukee, WI, USA

D. V. Jeste (✉)
Social Determinants of Health Network,
La Jolla, CA, USA

Definition of Spirituality for Research and Clinical Practice

There is no single consensual definition of spirituality in medical sciences and psychology. However, for academic purposes, a more specific definition is certainly necessary. A comprehensive review of different scientific publications and theoretical backgrounds suggested that *"the distinctive aspect of spirituality is the relationship or contact with a transcendent realm of reality that is considered sacred, the ultimate truth or reality"* [1].

A more broadened and useful working concept of spirituality has been proposed as part of a palliative care consensus conference and panel discussions about the integration of spirituality into health care and development of strategies to create more compassionate systems of care (*Improving the Spiritual Dimension of Whole Person Care: Reaching National and International Consensus*). This definition seeks to highlight the amplitude and connection of spirituality to multiple dimensions of people's lives and in clinical care and states: *"Spirituality is the aspect of humanity that refers to the way individuals seek and express meaning and purpose and the way they experience their connectedness to the moment, to self, to others, to nature, and to the significant or sacred"* [2].

Religion, which will be interweaved into this focus on spirituality, is generally defined somewhat differently. Among the usual definitions is an institutionalized system of beliefs in a superhuman power like a god or gods. Spirituality is usually more personal than institutional, though there can be overlap between religiosity and spirituality. Atheists, who do not believe in a god or formal religion, can have spiritual beliefs, and follow some of the moral principles of religions. Agnostics are uncertain about formal religious beliefs, but can also pursue spiritual ones. A recent movement called "New Age" is sort of a catch-all of a variety of cultural phenomena, which draws upon ancient pre-Christian traditions, questioning science and organized religions.

Spirituality as an Essential Component of Health

In ancient times, health was considered to be largely under the influence of religiosity/spirituality (R/S). Illnesses were often attributed to the wishes of demons and supernatural forces, and these had to be appeased to achieve cure.

Therefore, religious practices such as praying and sacrificing to the gods were thought to be necessary to achieve health [3]. Around the fifth century BCE, Hippocrates, considered the "Father of Modern Medicine," became the first authority to separate medicine from magical and religious beliefs and to consider diseases to be a result of the effects of environmental and personal factors. To be fair, Hippocrates was not irreligious, but emphasized the need of searching for natural causes [4]. Increasingly, especially during the twentieth century, Western medicine tended to view R/S as being mostly peripheral, irrelevant, or even harmful to physical and even mental health, and thus, the original pendulum has swung to the opposite end.

During the last few decades, there has been a move to expand the field of medicine from diseases and disabilities to overall well-being. In 1948, the World Health Organization (WHO) defined health as *"a state of complete physical, mental, and social well-being, not merely the absence of infirmity or disease."* There has been an ongoing debate about adding a spiritual component to the WHO definition of health [5]. The relevance of spirituality as a key dimension of quality of life across different cultures is reinforced by the World Health Organization, WHOQOL spirituality, religiousness, and personal beliefs (SRPB) instrument, a helpful research tool developed to evaluate how spirituality, religiosity, and personal beliefs (SRPB) are related to quality of life in health and health care. Currently, different international health organizations recognize the importance of integrating R/S issues in clinical care, including the American Psychiatric Association (APA), the Royal College of Psychiatrists, the German Psychiatric Association, and the Brazilian Psychiatric Association [6–8]. The World Psychiatric Association, for instance, published a Position Statement recommending the assessment and integration of R/S in clinical care, teaching, and research, as part of culturally sensitive and compassionate care in psychiatry [9] (Box 7.1). It is now available in seven languages.[1]

---

[1] https://religionandpsychiatry.org/main/wpa-position-statement-on-spirituality-and-religion-in-psychiatry/.

Box 7.1 World Psychiatric Association Position Statement on Spirituality and Religion in Psychiatry

WPA proposes that:

1. A tactful consideration of patients' religious beliefs and practices as well as their spirituality should routinely be considered and will sometimes be an essential component of psychiatric history taking.
2. An understanding of religion and spirituality and their relationship to the diagnosis, etiology, and treatment of psychiatric disorders should be considered as essential components of both psychiatric training and continuing professional development.
3. There is a need for more research on both religion and spirituality in psychiatry, especially on their clinical applications. These studies should cover a wide diversity of cultural and geographical backgrounds.
4. The approach to religion and spirituality should be person-centered. Psychiatrists should not use their professional position for proselytizing for spiritual or secular worldviews. Psychiatrists should be expected always to respect and be sensitive to the spiritual/religious beliefs and practices of their patients and of the families and carers of their patients.
5. Psychiatrists, whatever their personal beliefs, should be willing to work with leaders/members of faith communities, chaplains and pastoral workers, and others in the community, in support of the well-being of their patients, and should encourage their multidisciplinary colleagues to do likewise.
6. Psychiatrists should demonstrate awareness, respect, and sensitivity to the important part that spirituality and religion play for many staff and volunteers in forming a vocation to work in the field of mental health care.
7. Psychiatrists should be knowledgeable concerning the potential for both benefit and harm of religious, spiritual, and secular worldviews and practices and be willing to share this information in a critical but impartial way with the wider community in support of the promotion of health and well-being.

*Moreira-Almeida A, Sharma A, van Rensburg BJ, Verhagen PJ, Cook CC. WPA Position Statement on Spirituality and Religion in Psychiatry. World Psychiatry. 2016 Feb;15(1):87–8. https://doi.org/10.1002/wps.20304. PMID: 26833620; PMCID: PMC4780301 [9].

Very recently, the National Academies of Sciences, Engineering, and Medicine [10] issued a report that described "whole health" as physical, behavioral, spiritual, and socioeconomic well-being as defined by each individual and their family and community for themselves. The specification of spirituality as an element of health was notable. Whole health care was characterized as an interprofessional, team-based approach anchored in trusted relationships, aligning with a person's life mission, aspiration, and purpose. Furthermore, the report emphasized ensuring the well-being and whole health of care team members. Thus, the whole healthcare model seeks to shift the focus from a reactive disease-oriented medical care system to one that prioritizes disease prevention, health, and well-being.

Assessing Spirituality

In the current practice of health care focused on disorders, spirituality as well as other factors related to well-being are almost never evaluated. Interestingly, many patients would like to have conversations with their physicians about these topics, but, surprisingly, most of them have never been asked to discuss these areas. A systematic review of more than 20,000 medical reports found that R/S was addressed in healthcare consultations by one-third of physicians (median 32%), with a higher frequency reported by psychiatrists (48–78%, median: 50%). The most common obstacles reported included lack of time, insufficient knowledge or training, concerns about medical boundaries, cultural differences between patients and doctors, worries about colleague disapproval, and, for a minority of physicians, beliefs that R/S could have a negative effect on patient outcomes [11].

Evidence reinforces that even brief assessments provide useful information and benefits for mental health. In a study including 3141 general internal medicine hospitalized patients at the University of Chicago Medical Center, those who had discussions on their R/S concerns were much more likely to rate their care at the highest level of patient satisfaction [12].

A recent comprehensive systematic review assessed the evidence regarding spirituality and health and offered six implications regarding incorporation of spirituality in the care of patients with serious illnesses, confirming that we should (1) *incorporate spiritual care into care for patients with serious illnesses*; (2) *incorporate spiritual care education into training of interdisciplinary teams caring for persons with serious illnesses*; and (3) *include specialty practitioners of spiritual care in care of patients with serious illnesses* [13].

In research though, numerous instruments have been developed to assess spirituality and its association with health outcomes [14]. The Duke Religious Index and the Religious or Spiritual Coping Instruments are among the most widely used and specific measures of religious involvement available in scientific literature. The Brief Multidimensional Measure of Religiousness/ Spirituality is one of the most comprehensive and commonly employed instruments in this type of research [15]. These measures do have limitations including variable reliability and validity, but there is a need for testing and implementing routine assessment of spirituality with valid but pragmatic scales.

A systematic review analyzed 25 instruments developed for assessing R/S in clinical care [16]. The instrument that received the best evaluation

for clinical use was FICA, one that is easy to use and involves only four topics: F—faith, belief, and meaning; I—importance and influence of R/S for patient's life; C—community, if the patient is part of an R/S community; and A—address/action in care, and how to integrate R/S in the treatment and care plan.

Recently, Jeste et al. [17] developed and validated a 4-item measure of spirituality in a national-level sample of 1786 adults aged 20–82 years. These items, to be rated on a 1 (strongly disagree) to 5 (strongly agree) Likert scale, include the following:

1. My spiritual belief gives me inner strength.
2. There is no existence of the soul after death (reverse scored).
3. I feel that we are all connected on a higher level.
4. There is no overall purpose to life (reverse scored).

This spirituality measure correlated positively with well-being. More research is clearly needed to test the usability of this and other measures of spirituality in clinical practice, based on studies of populations diverse in age, sex, race, ethnicity, education, and socioeconomic status.

Wisdom and Spirituality

Wisdom has been known as a critical human quality since time immemorial. Practically, all the religions and all the major philosophies describe wisdom. For example, there are a number of books on wisdom in the Bible, including the Book of Job, Proverbs, Ecclesiastes, Psalms, Song of Songs, Wisdom (Wisdom of Solomon), and Sirach (Ben Sira or Ecclesiasticus). However, empirical research on wisdom began only in the 1970s at the Max Planck Institute in Berlin and the University of Southern California in Los Angeles, led by Baltes and Clayton, respectively. It has been growing rapidly. There were 2000 peer-reviewed papers on wisdom from 2010 to 2019 listed in the PubMed.

A critical question is how to define wisdom. Jeste et al. [17–21] have sought to do so using three different approaches.

A. *Conceptualization of Wisdom in the Indian Scripture*: Jeste and Vahia [21] conducted a qualitative–quantitative mixed-method study of wisdom in the Bhagavad Gita, an Indian scripture based on the Yogas, which were written several 1000 years BCE. It is considered a guide to wisdom in life. We performed independent reviews of English translations of the Gita by Swami Nirmalananda Giri and Zaehner/Goodall, followed by a back translation using Oxford English Dictionary, Roget's New Millennium Thesaurus, and Cologne Digital Sanskrit Lexicon. We employed Textalyser and NVivo software with an electronic version of the Giri translation and examined the contexts (verses) in which terms related to "wisdom" were used. The following components of wisdom were found to be most commonly listed in the Gita: knowledge of life, emotional regulation, compassion/sacrifice, insight/humility, decisiveness, love of the god (religiosity and spirituality), and lack of emphasis on materialistic pursuits. The Gita listed four levels of wisdom: nil or negative ("indulgence in devil or dark ways"), low ("passion or selfish and foolish ways"), moderate ("goodness"), and highest ("yogi"). According to the Gita, wisdom can be taught and learned, and one can improve ("upgrade") one's level of wisdom. An illustrative verse is # 32 in Chap. 9: *"For whosoever makes Me (God) his haven, base born though he may be; Yes, women too, and artisans, even serfs— Theirs it is to tread the highest way."*

B. *International Expert Consensus Using Delphi (Rand Panel) Method*: Jeste et al. [18] conducted a two-phase Delphi method survey of 30 international experts on wisdom, with 53 statements about behaviors. The experts were asked about similarities vs. differences among wisdom, intelligence, and spirituality on every one of these statements. We found a large consensus among the experts. They conceptualized wisdom as a complex, uniquely human trait, with advanced cognitive and emotional development, that is experience-driven, can be learned, and increases with age. Common components of wisdom in the expert consensus were rich knowledge of life, practical life skills, emotional regulation, social cognition, social cooperation and advising, insight, tolerance of ambiguity, value relativism, tolerance of diversity, openness to new experience, successful coping strategies, resilience, and sense of humor. Wisdom was thought to be different from intelligence (and, to a lesser extent, spirituality) on most relevant items. On only four characteristics (e.g., presence of skepticism, absence of religious participation) was wisdom was thought to be similar to intelligence and different from spirituality. In contrast, wisdom was viewed as being similar to spirituality but different from intelligence on 16 characteristics (e.g., humility, ego integrity, self-compassion, mindfulness, ethical conduct, reverence for nature).

C. *Systematic Review of Modern Western Scientific Literature*: Meeks and Jeste [22] conducted a systematic review of the empirical literature on wisdom which, as mentioned above, started in the mid-1970s. A subsequent review by Bangen et al. [23] found 24 articles on components of wisdom. Wisdom was generally thought to be a complex, multidimensional trait. The construct of wisdom was considered holistic, involving an integration of various components, i.e., the whole is greater than the sum of its parts. Behavior was felt to be the final determinant of wisdom. Wisdom was useful to society (prosocial behaviors) and to the self (greater happiness). Some studies suggested culture-based weight for different components of wisdom. The common components were pragmatic knowledge of life, social decision-making, emotional regulation, prosocial attitudes and behaviors, reflection and self-understanding, advising, dealing effectively with uncertainty and ambiguity, and value relativism and tolerance of diverse perspectives. Somewhat less common components included spirituality, openness to new experiences, and a sense of humor.

Comparing the result of the three different approaches to define wisdom, it is remarkable that a majority of the components were common to all three. These include knowledge of life, emotional regulation, prosocial behaviors, self-reflection, tolerance of ambiguity and diversity, decisiveness, and social advising. Somewhat less consistent were spirituality and openness to new experience. Notably, spirituality (and religiosity) were much more prominent in the Gita than in modern scientific literature. This finding is obviously not restricted to the Gita but would also apply to the scriptures from most other religions.

Loneliness Versus Wisdom and Spirituality

According to a British historian Fay Bound Alberti [24], the term "loneliness" did not exist in the English language until 1800. The closest word was "oneliness," which meant a state of being alone that was not undesirable, but rather a necessary space for reflection with god, and as god is always nearby, a person was never truly alone. The beginning of the nineteenth century was characterized by the start of the Industrial Revolution, which led to growth of the consumer economy, declining influence of religion, and popularity of evolutionary biology (Darwin's hypothesis of survival of the fittest). The result was that individualism and social anomie replaced traditional, paternalistic visions of a society in which everyone had a place.

Importantly, loneliness (perceived social isolation) has increased markedly during the last quarter century and has been called a Grand Challenge for the Society. It is also labeled a silent killer as it has increased the odds of mortality by 30% [25]. This is through increased risk of heart disease, diabetes, obesity, major depression with suicide, opioid and alcohol use, and Alzheimer's disease, and other dementias [26]. In the UK and Japan, new Ministries of Loneliness have been established during the last few years.

Several large cross-sectional studies have shown a consistently strong inverse correlation between loneliness and wisdom [17, 19, 27]. A prospective longitudinal study with a sample size of 1261 found that baseline wisdom/compassion scores predicted lower loneliness and better mental well-being 5–7 years later [28]. The negative relationship between loneliness and wisdom was seen not only in clinical studies but also in biological ones. EEG and gut microbiome studies showed significant opposite associations of biomarkers of loneliness and wisdom [27, 29].

In terms of the relationship of loneliness with various wisdom components, prosocial behaviors (empathy and compassion) had the largest (medium effect size) negative correlation with loneliness, whereas that for spirituality was small [17]. Conceptually, a spiritual person having connectedness with oneself, with nature, or with the transcendent would be less prone to feeling lonely when socially isolated. Increasing globalization and incredibly rapid advances in technology are upending long-held social mores and causing modern behavioral pandemics of loneliness, opioid abuse, and suicides. Wisdom (including compassion, self-reflection, emotional regulation, accepting diversity, spirituality) at individual and societal levels could be a behavioral antidote or vaccine to manage and prevent these pandemics.

R/S is commonly expressed and practiced in communities, and this community integration seems to be a significant factor in the impact of R/S on health. Recent editorials and commentaries by some epidemiology experts have discussed the importance of R/S social integration and regular attendance to R/S services for public health, including depression rates and general and suicide mortality [30, 31].

Empirical Science of Spirituality

A number of important scientific questions exist regarding spirituality. A basic question may relate to the rationale for a core spiritual belief, the survival after death. Moreira-Almeida et al. [32] have discussed in detail the empirical evidence regarding the survival of human consciousness after death, supported by studies on R/S experiences such as mediumship, near-death and out-of-body experiences, and reincarnation. They have also listed the limitations of the published studies and suggested future research of high quality.

Other aspects of spirituality that need more research include its neurobiology or neuroethology. Remarkably, the former Director of the National Institutes of Health, Francis Collins, believes that there may be a center in the brain related to a belief in a higher power. Palliative care, especially hospice care, has raised the importance of the role of faith-based health care. There is also growing interest in focusing on eudaimonic well-being as distinct from hedonic well-being. A vital component of eudaimonic well-being is a sense of meaning or purpose in life. Such a purpose may be related to prosocial behavior in general or could be tied to spirituality.

Spirituality and Mental Illnesses

A recent systematic review of research about the relationships between R/S and mental health identified a general protective effect of R/S [33]. The protective effects of religious or spiritual involvement were stronger for alcohol and substance abuse disorders, depression, and suicide risk. Another systematic review including only prospective research studies of depressive disorders reported that R/S was associated with less depression in 47% of studies versus greater depression in 11% of studies [34]. R/S importance may be capable of preventing incident depression in community individuals at risk in long-term follow-up [35] and of improving symptom remission and recovery in severely depressed individuals in tertiary care centers [36].

Spirituality encompasses connection—religious or otherwise—with a nonphysical entity or transcendent realm as perceived by the individual. It can have both positive and negative effects on people with mental illnesses. The unfavorable effects of negative R/S coping strategies or religious struggles for some individuals, for instance, are a well-recorded effect in individuals with

mood disorders [37], reinforcing the need of clinicians to be aware of and to deal with those questions in clinical practice.

Religious and/or spiritual commitment often provides a sense of meaning to life and helps people cope with consequences of a serious disease, thus enhancing personal wellness. A systematic review with meta-analysis found a moderate positive correlation between spirituality/religiosity and resilience in schizophrenia (r = 0.40; p < 0.01) [38]. Another study reported that intrinsic religiosity was associated with higher resilience scores, higher improvement of symptoms, greater quality of life, and lower suicide risk among severe depressed inpatients in Brazil [39].

Religion and spirituality might be a resource of recovery and social connection and support for individuals with chronic psychosis and serious mental illness. Mohr et al. [40] proposed different reasons why clinicians should be more aware of and integrate R/S issues in the treatment of serious mental illness patients [40]. For some patients, religion instills hope, purpose, and meaning in their lives, whereas for others, it induces spiritual despair. Patients may have religious delusions or hallucinations in acute episodes and crises, but in the long term, R/S generally provide meaning and support to many individuals. Religious practices influence social integration, suicidal risk, substance use, and treatment nonadherence. Higher level of religiosity and more frequent use of religious coping were associated with lower level of psychopathology and better self-reported quality of life in studies published from India [41].

Spirituality-Focused Interventions

A recent meta-analysis examined 57 randomized controlled trials (RCTs) to enhance components of wisdom, i.e., empathy/compassion/altruism, emotional regulation, or spirituality [28]. The study participants included people with mental illnesses, people with physical illnesses, and those from the general population. Nearly half (47%) of these studies reported significant enhancement of a wisdom component with moderate to large effect size. Meta-analysis of 15 RCTs on spirituality interventions showed a medium to large effect size increase in spirituality in people with terminal medical illnesses or psychiatric illnesses including opiate use disorders, depression, anxiety, and eating disorders. Several studies reported improvements in depression, anxiety, and well-being. A few reported improved suffering and distress, greater optimism and resilience, and fewer risk behaviors such as binging and HIV risk behaviors. Imagery, meditation, and group support improved meaning in life, self-awareness, connectedness with others, and a larger reality [42].

Recent literature has demonstrated the feasibility and potential benefits of R/S-integrated interventions for different mental health conditions. Spiritually integrated psychotherapies are understood as psychotherapy interventions that connect conventional theoretical techniques from different approaches with religious or spiritual backgrounds. It would be possible, for instance, to use CBT protocols for individuals with Christian, Jewish, Hindu, Buddhist, or Muslim traditions. Building on that, a meta-analysis of RCTs of CBT-adapted protocols for depression or anxiety demonstrated equivalent results compared to conventional techniques, with a potential additional benefit for spiritual well-being [43]. Another meta-analysis confirmed the benefits of spiritually integrated psychotherapies across different approaches, as a promising clinical tool and of special interest for more religious or spiritual individuals or for patients facing R/S struggles or spiritual suffering [44].

Recently, Keshavan et al. [45] discussed the psychotherapeutic aspects of Hinduism. They have drawn several parallels with modern approaches in psychotherapy such as focus on metacognitive awareness, balance, happiness, and intrinsic motivation. Huxter and Pizzuti [46] presented principles and practices of Buddhism relevant to mental health, especially the "four noble truths" that discuss the causes of suffering and ways to avoid and relieve it. The fourth truth focuses on freeing one from suffering and is composed of eight practices divided into three groups: wisdom, ethics, and meditation.

Positive Psychiatry

The present practice of medicine focuses entirely on asking our patients "What is wrong with you?" without ever asking "What do you like about yourself or what are your strengths?" Another question could be "What gives your life the most meaning?" Very often, the answers have to do with religion or spirituality. We inquire only about the risk factors and not about any protective or preventive factors. The treatment goal is strictly to reduce symptoms rather than to enhance the person's well-being. This is not useful either for the individual patients or for the overall healthcare system. Hundreds of studies have shown that positive factors such as strong social connections, resilience, optimism, and components of wisdom like compassion and spirituality have a significant positive impact on health, and therefore, they should be assessed and addressed as intervention targets. This is positive psychiatry, defined as the science and practice of psychiatry that focuses on the study and promotion of mental health and well-being through enhancement of positive psychosocial factors such as social relationships, wisdom, and resilience [20]. Even at the end of life, in palliative care settings, qualitative interviews show the presence of valued social connections, wisdom, and resilience [47]. Positive psychiatry practice is addition to (and not a substitute for) current practice. It should include assessment of well-being, personal strengths, resilience, wisdom, religiosity/spirituality, and social connections, by completing forms in the waiting room and online at home prior to visits [48, 49]. This should lead to identification of treatment targets and interventions.

Also important is social prescribing—one of the core pillars of the new UK model of personalized patient care. Social prescribing link workers focus on "what matters to me?" to co-produce a simple personalized care and support plan to connect people to activities, groups, and services in their community to meet the practical, social, and emotional needs that affect their health and well-being [50, 51].

Eastern Models of Spirituality and Religion

There are scores of formal religions and spiritual practices around the world. Two large divisions are the so-called Eastern and Western traditions [52], so-called because these are social constructs, not geographic, given that the earth is round and spinning. Eastern religions, beginning with Hinduism thousands of years ago, originated in the East, South, and Southeast of Asia. In contrast, the so-called Western ones, often called Abrahamic religions with a clear belief in a monotheistic god, originated in the Middle East and later spread to Europe, the Americas, and other places in the world. To confuse names a bit more, there is a Western denomination of Spiritism, differing from spirituality, which is an R/S movement including the teachings of Jesus and a focus on how spirits interact with the corporeal world. Moreover, there are also widespread native, indigenous, and aboriginal spiritual practices. Sometimes, there are syncretic combinations in a system. There can be many subgroups and denominations in large groups, and practices can change over time. Individuals can vary in the intensity and specificity of their beliefs. Migrations often result in populations in a diaspora as well as a parent country of origin. Most religions also have branches with varied degrees of fundamentalism or liberalism.

In all the valuable experiences and expressions of spirituality and religion discussed throughout this chapter, Eastern traditions have a particular history and focus, which seem distinct from Western ones. At the end of the last century, a well-known Eastern philosopher and statesman observed that Western traditions were inclined to dogma and the scientific exploration of the outer natural world, whereas Eastern religions emphasized openness to inner experiences and spiritual experimentation. He found the West generally more logical, and the East more mystical, though clearly with exceptions.

One particular belief separating East and West concerns the afterlife. Whereas Western religions such as Christianity, Islam, Shintoism, and Zoroastrianism often teach that one goes to Heaven or Hell forever, depending on what they did on earth, Eastern religions including Hinduism, Jainism, Buddhism, and Sikhism teach reincarnation, in which the physical body dies, but the soul comes back in another body, also depending on earthly deeds, with the goal of obtaining Nirvana. Sometimes, the mystical Kabbalah beliefs in Judaism are included in this group.

Psychiatric clinicians with appropriate curiosity and respect can be educated by their patients as to the importance of their religious and spiritual beliefs, and further studying the essence of the main religions and spiritual practices can help therapists in understanding the patient, establishing a therapeutic alliance, and including those beliefs in the treatment planning [53].

Interfaith experiences can also be enlightening. A well-known such interchange occurred in 1990 when a group of prominent American Jewish delegates went to Dharamshala in India to meet the XIV Dalai Lama of Tibet in exile [54]. The historical Buddha is a focus, but not a god, and Buddhism is often thought to be more of an Eastern spiritual practice than a religion. By comparison, Judaism is the first Abrahamic Western religion with a basis of ethical monotheism. Knowing the history of Jewish exile as well as the Buddhist focus on addressing suffering, the Dalai Lama wanted the help of the Jewish people as he said: "Tell me your secret, the secret of Jewish spiritual survival in exile."

From the other side, the Jewish delegation was especially interested in why so many Jews had turned to Buddhism starting in the 1960s as an adjunct to their Judaism or an alternative. Something spiritual seemed missing for these Jews that they found in Buddhism. What these delegates and so many others felt missing was the long practice of deep meditation in Tibetan Buddhism and other branches. For the chronicler of the trip, learning the Eastern meditative practices brought him back to the hidden history of meditation in Jewish mysticism [55]. Longer term, the connections made in the original trip continued over time as practitioners of each tradition learned from the other and found a model for interfaith cooperation. Meditation, of course, has come to be a common practice of stress reduction in America, as well as being useful for deeper personal introspection and inner transformation, a clear connection to mainstream psychiatry. After increasing his meditation practices, the chronicler became fascinated with the visualization practices found in Buddhism, but seemingly absent from Judaism. Exploring, he found the remnants, which led him to analyzing the visualization inevitably available in dreams, the oldest spiritual technology on the planet and a direct link to the Jewish psychiatrist Sigmund Freud, who analyzed his own dreams and made dream analysis a key in psychoanalytic psychotherapy [56]. The bestselling book of the meeting has been reprinted scores of times.

Summary

Spirituality has been appropriately gaining growing attention in healthcare and in empirical science. Psychiatry should be at the forefront of this movement, given the vital role of spirituality and religion in mental health as well as its variable effects on people with mental illnesses. Spirituality should be an excellent target for interventions focused on enhancing well-being as well as health of individuals and communities. Eastern models can contribute to Western understanding of spirituality and well-being. An expanded model of psychiatry to a bio-psycho-social-spiritual one will help to include the relevance of spirituality and religions.

References

1. Moreira-Almeida A, Bhugra D. Religion, spirituality and mental health: setting the scene. In: Moreira-Almeida A, Mosqueiro BP, Bhugra D, editors. Spirituality and mental health across cultures. Oxford: Oxford Cultural Psychiatry; 2021. p. 11–25.
2. Puchalski CM, Vitillo R, Hull SK, Reller N. Improving the spiritual dimension of whole person care: reaching national and international consensus. J Palliat Med. 2014;17(6):642–56. https://doi.org/10.1089/jpm.2014.9427. Epub 2014 May 19.
3. Badash I, Kleinman NP, Barr S, Jang J, Rahman S, Wu BW. Redefining health: the evolution of health ideas from antiquity to the era of value-based care. Cureus. 2017;9(2):e1018. https://doi.org/10.7759/cureus.1018.
4. Hankinson R. Magic, religion and science: divine and human in the Hippocratic corpus. Apeiron. 1998;31(1):1–34. https://doi.org/10.1515/APEIRON.1998.31.1.1.
5. de Brito Sena MA, Damiano RF, Lucchetti G, Peres MFP. Defining spirituality in healthcare: a systematic review and conceptual framework. Front Psychol. 2021;12:756080. https://doi.org/10.3389/fpsyg.2021.756080.
6. Dike C, Briz L, Fadus M, Martinez R, May C, Milone R, Nesbit-Bartsch A, Powell T, Witmer A, Brendel RW. Resource document on the interface of religion, spirituality, and psychiatric practice, vol. 210. APA Official Actions, American Psychiatric Association; 2022. p. 557.
7. Mosqueiro BP, de Abreu Costa M, Caribé A, Oliveira de Oliveira F, Pizutti L, Zimpel R, Baldaçara L, da Silva AG, Moreira-Almeida A. Brazilian psychiatric association guidelines on the integration of spirituality into mental health clinical practice: part 1. Spiritual history and differential diagnosis. Braz J Psychiatry. 2023;45(6):506–17.
8. Cook CCH. Recommendations for psychiatrists on spirituality and religion. Position statement PS03/2011. London: Royal College of Psychiatrists; 2011.
9. Moreira-Almeida A, Sharma A, van Rensburg BJ, Verhagen PJ, Cook CC. WPA position statement on spirituality and religion in psychiatry. World Psychiatry. 2016;15(1):87–8. https://doi.org/10.1002/wps.20304.
10. National Academies of Sciences, Engineering, and Medicine. achieving whole health: a new approach for veterans and the nation. Washington, DC: National Academies Press (US); 2023.
11. Best M, Butow P, Olver I. Doctors discussing religion and spirituality: a systematic literature review. Palliat Med. 2016;30(4):327–37. https://doi.org/10.1177/0269216315600912. Epub 2015 Aug 12.
12. Williams JA, Meltzer D, Arora V, Chung G, Curlin FA. Attention to inpatients' religious and spiritual concerns: predictors and association with patient satisfaction. J Gen Intern Med. 2011;26(11):1265–71. https://doi.org/10.1007/s11606-011-1781-y. Epub 2011 Jul 1.
13. Balboni TA, VanderWeele TJ, Doan-Soares SD, Long KNG, Ferrell BR, Fitchett G, Koenig HG, Bain PA, Puchalski C, Steinhauser KE, Sulmasy DP, Koh HK. Spirituality in serious illness and health. JAMA. 2022;328(2):184–97. https://doi.org/10.1001/jama.2022.11086. Erratum in: JAMA. 2022 Aug 23;328(8):780.
14. Monod S, Brennan M, Rochat E, Martin E, Rochat S, Büla CJ. Instruments measuring spirituality in clinical research: a systematic review. J Gen Intern Med. 2011;26(11):1345–57. https://doi.org/10.1007/s11606-011-1769-7.

15. Masters KS. Brief multidimensional measure of religiousness/spirituality (BMMRS). In: Gellman MD, Turner JR, editors. Encyclopedia of behavioral medicine. New York, NY: Springer; 2013. https://doi.org/10.1007/978-1-4419-1005-9_1577.

16. Lucchetti G, Bassi RM, Lucchetti AL. Taking spiritual history in clinical practice: a systematic review of instruments. Explore (NY). 2013;9(3):159–70. https://doi.org/10.1016/j.explore.2013.02.004.

17. Jeste DV, Thomas ML, Liu J, Daly RE, Tu XM, Treichler EBH, Palmer BW, Lee EE. Is spirituality a component of wisdom? Study of 1,786 adults using expanded San Diego wisdom scale (Jeste-Thomas wisdom index). J Psychiatr Res. 2021;132:174–81. https://doi.org/10.1016/j.jpsychires.2020.09.033.

18. Jeste DV, Ardelt M, Blazer D, Kraemer HC, Vaillant G, Meeks T. Expert consensus on the characteristics of wisdom: a Delphi method study. Gerontologist. 2010;50:668–80.

19. Jeste DV, Di Somma S, Lee EE, Nguyen TT, Scalcione M, Biaggi A, Daly R, Liu J, Tu X, Ziedonis D, Glorioso D, Antonini P, Brenner D. Study of loneliness and wisdom in 482 middle-aged and oldest-old adults: a comparison between people in Cilento, Italy and San Diego, USA. Aging Mental Health. 25:2149. https://doi.org/10.1080/13607863.2020.1821170.

20. Jeste DV, Palmer BW, Rettew DC, Boardman S. Positive psychiatry: its time has come. J Clin Psychiatry. 2015;76(6):675–83. https://doi.org/10.4088/JCP.14nr09599.

21. Jeste DV, Vahia I. Comparison of the conceptualization of wisdom in ancient Indian literature with modern views: focus on the Bhagavad Gita. Psychiatry. 2008;71:197–209.

22. Meeks TW, Jeste DV. Neurobiology of wisdom: an overview. Arch Gen Psychiatry. 2009;66:355–65.

23. Bangen KJ, Meeks TW, Jeste DV. Defining and assessing wisdom: a review of the literature. Am J Geriatr Psychiatry. 2013;21(12):1254–66. https://doi.org/10.1016/j.jagp.2012.11.020. Epub 2013 Apr 15. Erratum in: Am J Geriatr Psychiatry. 2014 Apr;22(4):e1.

24. Alberti FB. A biography of loneliness: the history of an emotion. Oxford University Press; 2019. p. 320.

25. Holt-Lunstad J, Smith TB, Baker M, Harris T, Stephenson D. Loneliness and social isolation as risk factors for mortality: a meta-analytic review. Perspect Psychol Sci. 2015;10(2):227–37. https://doi.org/10.1177/1745691614568352.

26. 2019 National Healthcare Quality and disparities report. Rockville, MD: Agency for Healthcare Research and Quality (US); 2020. https://www.ncbi.nlm.nih.gov/books/NBK579354/.

27. Nguyen TT, Zhang X, Wu T-C, Liu J, Le C, Tu X, Knight R, Jeste DV. Association of loneliness and wisdom with gut microbial diversity and composition: an exploratory study. Front Psychiatry. 12:648475. https://doi.org/10.3389/fpsyt.2021.648475.

28. Lee EE, Bangen KJ, Avanzino JA, Hou B, Ramsey M, Eglit G, Liu J, Tu XM, Paulus M, Jeste DV. Outcomes of randomized clinical trials to enhance social, emotional, and spiritual components of wisdom: a systematic review and meta-analysis. JAMA Psychiatry. 2020;77(9):925–35. https://doi.org/10.1001/jamapsychiatry.2020.0821.

29. Grennan G, Balasubramani PP, Alim F, Zafar-Khan M, Lee EE, Jeste DV, Mishra J. Cognitive and neural correlates of loneliness and wisdom during emotional bias. Cereb Cortex. 2021:1–12. https://doi.org/10.1093/cercor/bhab012.

30. Krause N. Invited commentary: explaining the relationship between attending worship services and mortality-a brief excursion into the contribution of social relationships in religious institutions. Am J Epidemiol. 2017;185(7):523–5. https://doi.org/10.1093/aje/kww180.

31. VanderWeele TJ, Balboni TA, Koh HK. Invited commentary: religious service attendance and implications for clinical care, community participation, and public health. Am J Epidemiol. 2022;191(1):31–5. https://doi.org/10.1093/aje/kwab134.

32. Moreira-Almeida A, de Abreu CM, Coelho HS. Science of life after death. Springer Publishing; 2022.

33. Koenig H, Al-Zaben F, VanderWeele T. Religion and psychiatry: recent developments in research. BJPsych Adv. 2020;26(5):262–72. https://doi.org/10.1192/bja.2019.81.

34. Braam AW, Koenig HG. Religion, spirituality and depression in prospective studies: a systematic review. J Affect Disord. 2019;257:428–38. https://doi.org/10.1016/j.jad.2019.06.063. Epub 2019 Jul 2.

35. Miller L, Wickramaratne P, Gameroff MJ, Sage M, Tenke CE, Weissman MM. Religiosity and major depression in adults at high risk: a ten-year prospective study. Am J Psychiatry. 2012;169(1):89–94. https://doi.org/10.1176/appi.ajp.2011.10121823. Epub 2011 Aug 24.

36. Mosqueiro BP, Caldieraro MA, Messinger M, da Costa FBP, Peteet JR, Fleck P, M. Religiosity, spirituality, suicide risk and remission of depressive symptoms: a 6-month prospective study of tertiary care Brazilian patients. J Affect Disord. 2021;279:434–42. https://doi.org/10.1016/j.jad.2020.10.028. Epub 2020 Oct 16.

37. Stroppa A, Colugnati FA, Koenig HG, Moreira-Almeida A. Religiosity, depression, and quality of life in bipolar disorder: a two-year prospective study. Braz J Psychiatry. 2018;40(3):238–43. https://doi.org/10.1590/1516-4446-2017-2365. Epub 2018 Feb 15.

38. Schwalm FD, Zandavalli RB, de Castro Filho ED, Lucchetti G. Is there a relationship between spirituality/religiosity and resilience? A systematic review and meta-analysis of observational studies. J Health Psychol. 2022;27(5):1218–32. https://doi.org/10.1177/1359105320984537.

39. Mosqueiro BP, da Rocha NS, Fleck MP. Intrinsic religiosity, resilience, quality of life, and suicide risk in depressed inpatients. J Affect Disord.

2015;179:128–33. https://doi.org/10.1016/j.jad.2015.03.022. Epub 2015 Mar 21.

40. Mohr S, Brandt PY, Borras L, Gilliéron C, Huguelet P. Toward an integration of spirituality and religiousness into the psychosocial dimension of schizophrenia. Am J Psychiatry. 2006;163(11):1952–9. https://doi.org/10.1176/ajp.2006.163.11.1952.

41. Triveni D, Grover S, Chakrabarti S. Religiosity among patients with schizophrenia: an exploratory study. Indian J Psychiatry. 2017;59(4):420–8. https://doi.org/10.4103/psychiatry.IndianJPsychiatry_17_17.

42. Hawks SR, et al. Review of spiritual health: definition, role, and intervention strategies in health promotion. Am J Health Promot. 1995;9(5):371–8. https://religionandpsychiatry.org/main/wpa-position-statement-on-spirituality-and-religion-in-psychiatry/.

43. de Abreu Costa M, Moreira-Almeida A. Religion-adapted cognitive behavioral therapy: a review and description of techniques. J Relig Health. 2022;61(1):443–66. https://doi.org/10.1007/s10943-021-01345-z.

44. Captari LE, Hook JN, Hoyt W, Davis DE, McElroy-Heltzel SE, Worthington EL Jr. Integrating clients' religion and spirituality within psychotherapy: a comprehensive meta-analysis. J Clin Psychol. 2018;74(11):1938–51. https://doi.org/10.1002/jclp.22681. Epub 2018 Sep 16.

45. Keshavan MS, Gangadhar BN, Pandurangi AK. Hinduism. In: Moreira-Almeida A, Mosqueiro BP, Bhugra D, editors. Spirituality and mental health across cultures. Oxford: Oxford Cultural Psychiatry; 2021. p. 201–18. https://doi.org/10.1093/med/9780198846833.003.0013.

46. Huxter M, Pizzuti L. Principles and practices of Buddhism in relationship to mental health. In: Moreira-Almeida A, Mosqueiro BP, Bhugra D, editors. Spirituality and mental health across cultures. Oxford: Oxford Cultural Psychiatry; 2021. p. 219–35. https://doi.org/10.1093/med/9780198846833.003.0014.

47. Montross LP, Joseph J, Edmonds EC, Palinkas LA, Jeste DV. Reflections on wisdom at the end of life: qualitative study of hospice patients aged 58-97 years. Int Psychogeriatr. 2018;30(12):1759–66. https://doi.org/10.1017/S1041610217003039.

48. Thomas ML, Bangen K, Palmer BW, Martin AS, Avanzino JA, Glorioso DK, Daly RE, Jeste DV. A new scale for assessing wisdom based on common domains and a neurobiological model: the San Diego wisdom scale (SD-WISE). J Psychiatr Res. 2019;108:40–7. https://doi.org/10.1016/j.jpsychires.2017.09.005.

49. Thomas ML, Palmer BW, Lee EE, Liu J, Daly R, Tu XM, Jeste DV. Abbreviated San Diego wisdom scale (SD-WISE-7) and Jeste-Thomas wisdom index (JTWI). Int Psychogeriatr. 2022;34(7):617–26. https://doi.org/10.1017/S1041610221002684.

50. Morlett Paredes A, Lee EE, Chik L, Gupta S, Palmer BW, Palinkas L, Kim HC, Jeste DV. Qualitative study of loneliness in a senior housing community: the importance of wisdom and other coping strategies. Aging Ment Health. 2020 Jan;10:1–8. https://doi.org/10.1080/13607863.2019.1699022.

51. Vahia IV, Depp CA, Palmer BW, Fellows I, Golshan S, Thompson W, Allison M, Jeste DV. Correlates of spirituality in older women. Aging Ment Health. 2011;15:97–102.

52. Radhakrishnan S. Eastern religions and Western thought. Oxford University Press; 1990.

53. Moore T. Soul therapy: the art and craft of caring conversations. HarperOne; 2021.

54. Kamenetz R. The Jew in the lotus: a Poet's rediscovery of Jewish identity in Buddhist India. HarperOne; 1994.

55. Kamenetz R. Afterward, in the Jew in the lotus. HarperOne; 2007.

56. Kamenetz R. The history of last Night's dream. HarperOne; 2008.

Part II

Specific Eastern Religious and Spiritual Traditions

Basic Aspects and Clinical Implications of Hinduism

8

Neil Krishan Aggarwal

Introduction: Affirming the Diversity of Hinduism

Hinduism is one of the world's largest religions. According to the Pew Research Center's projections from 2021, there are more than 1.1 billion Hindus around the world [1], with 94% in India, 2% in Nepal, and 1% in Bangladesh [2], constituting nearly 1.05 billion [3], 21.6 million [4], and 14.3 million people [5], respectively. The world's largest Islamic republics, Indonesia and Pakistan, also have the world's fifth and sixth largest Hindu populations with nearly 4.6 million [6] and 4.4 million people [7], respectively. Finally, Hindus in the diaspora number nearly 3.3 million in the United States [8], 1.03 million in the United Kingdom [9], 828,000 in Canada [10], and 684,000 in Australia [11]. These figures demonstrate the global distribution of a religion that historically emerged in South Asia.

The acculturation and socialization experiences of Hindus vary widely. A survey on religion that enrolled 30,000 households in India across 17 languages in 2019 and 2020 offers the most recent indications about sociodemographic characteristics [1]. In the United States, Hindus have attained higher levels of education (15.7 years of schooling) compared to all other religious groups, but Hindus are among the least educated groups (~10 or more years of schooling) in India [1]. Nearly 98% of Hindus believe in god, with approximately 61% believing that there is a single god who has multiple manifestations and 7% believing that there are many gods [1]. Although reincarnation is often taught as an essential doctrine, only 41% of all Hindus believe in it, and this figure falls to 31% among the college-educated [1]. These statistics should prompt us to ask how a single chapter could encompass this human diversity.

In fact, social scientists have critiqued diversity, equity, and inclusion (DEI) initiatives in health care for assuming that group-based characteristics are relevant to individual patients. Anthropologists have challenged "the beliefs and behaviors" method of cultural competence for minoritized racial, ethnic, religious, and gender groups that present lists of "dos and don'ts" for providers, which ignores variations in life experiences within these groups and overestimates differences across groups [12]. The "the beliefs and behaviors" method also risks pathologizing unfamiliar patient behaviors through group-based stereotypes that providers may interpret as "noncompliant" or "non-adherent" with treat-

N. K. Aggarwal (✉)
New York State Psychiatric Institute, New York, NY, USA

Columbia University Medical Center, New York, NY, USA

Committee on Global Thought, Columbia University, New York, NY, USA
e-mail: Neil.Aggarwal@nyspi.columbia.edu

ments [13]. Even worse, a focus on individual beliefs and behaviors can ignore political, economic, and social determinants of mental health such as the stigma of mental illnesses; access to stable food, housing, and transportation; immigration policies; and neighborhood infrastructure or financial resources that can be more relevant to how patients think, feel, and behave than the demographic groups to which they belong [14]. Finally, given that cross-cultural psychiatry and psychology began during European colonialism in the 1800s to comprehend, hierarchize, and subjugate peoples in the Global South [15], any list of recommendations for people should interrogate the politics of who produces knowledge and why to avoid perpetuating inaccuracies [16]. These arguments raise epistemological questions about how we represent religious traditions, especially Hinduism.

Debating Who Speaks for Hinduism in the Secular Academy

Questions of accurate representation are important to people from all faith traditions. For Hinduism, it is especially relevant because non-Hindus produced the first forms of knowledge in secular universities. An article in the *Journal of the American Academy of Religion* on introductory textbooks on Hinduism posed thought-provoking questions about how to read, i.e., interpret, Hindu beliefs and practices:

> Is authentic Hinduism only in India, or in New Jersey? Or maybe even Singapore? What counts as legitimate "Hindu" knowledge? Does it have to be written down or transmitted orally? Does it have to come from someone who practices? Can it be televised? Does the internet count? Does it have to be free of colonial impurities? Can it be modern? Does it have to be "proper," fitting an ethical or normative notion of what a religion ought to be? Is it socially constructed or a perennial essence? ([17], p. 717)

Christian missionaries who targeted Hindus for conversion, not Hindus themselves, introduced theories and methods that have disseminated in university-based studies of Hinduism.

As the scholar above writes, "A scriptural typography has deep roots in the study of Hinduism harking back to the days of Christian missionaries. It concentrates on Sanskrit texts and tends to picture Hinduism as having a creative Vedic period, followed by a philosophical period, a descent into a decadent period of polytheism, and a final period of devotional reconciliation" ([17], p. 734). The Euro-American *academe* has represented Hinduism in four ways: (1) as a textual tradition with a historical trajectory that reifies scripture, philosophy, and theology; (2) as a civilization centered on Sanskrit religious literature with a distinct socio-cosmic order and theological movements; (3) as a collection of local practices—some of which have nothing to do with Sanskrit or scriptures—to interpret rituals, identities, and communities around the world; and (4) a unified society within which groups debate power, resources, and institutions [17].

Starting with the 1990s, Hindu scholars of Hinduism challenged these ideas. Three social trends prompted questions about who should authoritatively speak for Hindus: the rise of (1) scholars claiming that no single entity called Hinduism ever existed, (2) diasporic South Asian students studying Hinduism in North America, and (3) a social conservative movement known as Hindutva ("Hinduness") in India that has sought to exclude Christians and Muslims from political power [18, 19]. Practicing Hindus researching Hinduism in universities have not recognized themselves in scholarship that non-Hindus produce because the reliance on historical events and sacred texts omits practices that are more central to everyday lives such as giving gifts; compositions in regional languages outside the ambit of Sanskritic, Brahminical, male-centered learning; hymns of women and lower-caste Hindus; and the performing arts [20]. Some Hindu scholars have objected to any non-Hindus researching Hinduism, with one writing:

> The modern academy claims theory as thoroughly Western and thus constructs the rules by which the Hindu world has been theorized. A Western or modern education prevents many Hindu scholars from writing or speaking from a "real" and authentic Hindu or Indic position and perspective. Those

who do dare to speak from a traditional Hindu perspective are criticized for not making sense. Alternatively, their arguments are "suitably translated" or reduced to some "nativist" discourse by Western (and many Westernized Hindu) academics. More often, their ideas are dismissed as naive, contradictory, and illogical. This positions today's Hindus in North America in a difficult space both in relation to the general Indic populations and within the Western academy ([21], p. 273).

Hindu scholars have different solutions about who should speak authoritatively for Hinduism. One practitioner of Mādhava Vedanta who is a professional philosopher of religion notes that across sects with learned traditions, spiritual teachers who have obtained religious, intellectual, and hierarchical status by attending monasteries and following strict rules to interpret texts acquire *adhikāra* ("eligibility") and *āptatvā* ("reliability") in expertise [22]. While many such experts exist, they too often tend to be high-caste Brahmin men atop a social hierarchy that has excluded others and whose views are not widespread [22]. Another practitioner of Advaita Vedanta, also a philosopher of religion, has subverted the insider-outsider dichotomy by arguing that insiders can study their traditions with critical distance while outsiders can acquire "perceptual interiority" through identification with Hindu traditions [23]. Within Hinduism, Advaita Vedanta instructs that dualities lead to false assumptions about the nature of worldly existence [23]. Applying this concept in studying Hinduism may appeal to some, but it does not address centuries of grievance from the violent colonization of South Asia.

Non-Hindu scholars of Hinduism have recognized their privileged status as white academics of European ancestry who receive salaries to teach Hindu students in North America wishing to learn more about Hinduism. Some have written about the ethics of staying silent when interpreting beliefs and practices that they find unfamiliar (polytheism), odious (widow burning), or contentious among Hindu sects (caste) [24, 25], presenting the multiplicity of opinions within Hinduism while reserving personal judgments for private settings outside classrooms. Others suggest that

scholars not born as Hindus can compensate for a lack of knowledge through fieldwork in South Asia, including Hindu voices in their scholarship, being aware of how one's scholarship impacts Hindus and non-Hindus alike, and listening to Hindu debate traditions [26].

Recently, a team of Hindu and non-Hindu scholars of Hinduism has proposed a method known as "interdialogue" (*samvāda*). Disputing the essentialization in terms such as "Hindu" and "non-Hindu" or "insider" and "outsider," they acknowledge that all of us possess complex, diverse identities—a stance with roots in the Sanskrit philosophical tradition of Hinduism [27]. As they write, "In all of its complexity in the Sanskrit tradition, *samvāda* conveys the idea of a transformation through conversation. In the *samvāda*s of early and classical India, there might be two or more speakers, but the participants were many—witnesses, audiences, praisers, and detractors. And all acknowledged the social transformation that takes place" ([27], p. 289). In *samvāda*, each person advances arguments only after representing other positions accurately:

> Ancient Indian philosophers, despite their use of polemic against opponents (*purvapaksha*), are also patient and detailed in laying out their views. Even the destructive dialectic of the Advaitin Sri Harsha, which seeks openly to refute a variety of positions, nevertheless is faithful in the construction of the opponent's argument. Seldom is it possible to criticize Sri Harsha on the grounds that he misrepresents his opponent; the best comeback is to find flaws in his arguments or to develop better theories that escape his objections ([27], p. 292).

Operationalizing this method requires presenting concepts about Hinduism that reflect internal and external perspectives. Here, cultural psychiatrists have drawn from anthropology in differentiating between *etic* outsider and *emic* insider understandings [28]. An etic understanding can detect concepts that are otherwise taken for granted within a community in searching for cross-cultural universalistic frameworks, whereas an emic understanding can highlight concerns within a community to which outsiders may not have access [28]. Accordingly, this chapter presents etic-emic perspectives on Hinduism from non-Hindu and Hindu scholars of religion, interrogates extant scholarship on clinical recommendations for Hindu patients, and offers a technique for providers to explore the identities of Hindu patients.

One core tenet in cross-cultural psychiatry is clinical reflexivity, the process of accounting for the provider in developing knowledge about patients [29]. This introspection can make transference and countertransference dynamics apparent, whether providers are working with patients from similar or different demographic backgrounds [30]. Therefore, I acknowledge life experiences that affect the production of this chapter. After completing medical school, I obtained a graduate degree in South Asian studies from Harvard University, where my coursework focused on studying the textual interactions among Hindus, Muslims, and Sikhs in South Asian languages. During my psychiatric residency training, I served as the Hindu Fellow through the Yale University Chaplain's Office. After residency, I completed a postdoctoral fellowship in clinical applied medical anthropology, and I continue to research cultural psychiatry through applied anthropological methods at Columbia University among minoritized South Asian populations in New York City. I am all too aware of the irony that I have acquired *adhikāra* and *āptatvā* to speak for Hinduism in elite American universities whose credentials would not be recognized as sufficient among Hindu institutions in South Asia. Nonetheless, as a cultural psychiatrist and social scientist, I work in the secular academy. My experiences have sensitized me to tensions in etic vs. emic perspectives and textual vs. anthropological methods in studying religion. Rather than minimizing these tensions or pretending that they do not exist, I suggest that a more constructive way is for providers to commit to ongoing inquiry in educating themselves about Hinduism while remaining open-minded to the unique lives of individual patients. Providers reading this chapter should engage in clinical reflexivity to explore their reactions to Hinduism as they work with Hindu patients.

The Challenges in Representing Hindu Beliefs and Practices

Hinduism differs from other faith traditions. In the nineteenth century, the academic creation of "world religions" posited that each religion should have a single god, founder, an organized community of priests, a canon of sacred texts, and defining beliefs, which Hinduism does not have [31]. Unlike Judaism, Christianity, Islam, Buddhism, Jainism, and Sikhism, Hindus do not believe that their religion has a founder. There is no canon of texts which all Hindus affirm. There is no consensus of prophets, saints, or spiritual teachers for all Hindus. Hindu sects vary in whether they believe in a single god, several gods, many gods, or no god at all. The variation in beliefs and practices among Hindus captures the shortcomings of cultural competence and DEI initiatives that claim to accurately depict minoritized groups.

Through *samvāda*, etic and emic representations of Hinduism can be scrutinized. A comprehensive literature review of such representations is outside the scope of this chapter, but the following examples come from popular textbooks in university settings that have been peer reviewed and from a Hindu organization representing Hindu interests in the United States. They have acquired *adhikāra* and *āptatvā* to speak for Hinduism, but to different audiences and for different goals. These representations typify what some consider to be the basic tenets of Hinduism, though they still fall short in capturing the lived experiences of over a billion people.

Some non-Hindu scholars who take the civilizational approach have treated Hinduism as the product of European colonialism. The following passage illustrates a view of Hinduism in relation to non-Hindu Europeans:

The English word "Hinduism" is of fairly recent coinage, not much more than a couple of centuries old. It is not a translation of some early Indian term purporting to give a self-description of Indian religion or culture. It is a Western invention, created for a specific purpose. But it was not entirely plucked out of thin air. Part of this name—the "Hindu" element—is derived from the name of the great river, the Indus, which runs along the northwest of the subcontinent with its tributaries. The word "Indus" itself seems to have been derived from the description which ancient inhabitants of this region, the so-called Āryans, gave to this riverine system, recorded at least as long ago as the second millennium BCE. This area is historically important for our purposes because along its banks (or former banks) there are sites where civilization in the Indian subcontinent had an early flowering, in the technical sense of "civilization," with urban centers and their civic, sociopolitical, and communicational infrastructure, together with various forms of architectural, commercial, artistic, and ritual expression ([32], pp. 9–10).

This scholar posits that Āryans descended from Europeans despite admittedly "fragmentary" linguistic and archaeological evidence: "These people(s) seem to have incorporated aspects of early European ancestry and ways of life and in the course of time mingled to greater or lesser degree through intermarriage and otherwise with the inhabitants of the Indus civilization. In time—over centuries—their developing language and culture spread hegemonically, though unevenly, over the entire subcontinent" ([32], p. 12).

Critics have challenged this civilizational approach for projecting analytical biases onto the study of Hinduism. One skeptic, a Hindu professor who researches the European construction of Hinduism, writes that "an inability to view Hinduism on its own terms has shaped the study of comparative religion" and led British colonial "scholars to seek out comparable features, such as monotheism, a salvational scheme, and notions of the afterlife, in other religions" ([33], p. 25). British colonial administrators who studied Hinduism established terms that still endure. In 1845, the Lex Loci Act codified separate laws for Hindus and Muslims, the former derived from Sanskrit texts that British Orientalist scholars translated, resulting in a scriptural unity that foreigners imposed across diverse Hindu sects [34]. In 1901, Herbert Hope Risley (1851–1911) applied the categories of caste and separate Aryan and Dravidian races to all Hindus in British India as the Commissioner of the 1901 census [35]. Prior to the British colonization of India from 1757 to 1947, Hindus did not live under a unitary political administration, so the effort to define Hinduism as a single entity through a canon of scriptures emerged from the practical need to subjugate diverse social groups [33]. No such exigency exists today, raising questions about why anyone should force such unity across diverse human experiences.

Other non-Hindu scholars dispute the idea of Hinduism as "a Western invention." The characterization below exemplifies the "local practices" approach to representing Hindus:

> On the one hand, there is the Sanskritic tradition of brahmanical [brahman = the traditional, priestly highest caste] orthodoxy, flowing from the ancient revelation of the Veda, concerned with correct ritual procedures, the maintenance of caste boundaries, and the interpretation of scripture. This is a decisive constraint on the traditions that comprise Hinduism. On the other hand, there is a great proliferation of decentered traditions, often founded by a charismatic teacher or guru, and communities expressed in vernacular languages that cannot be defined by a central, brahmanical tradition and which are often set against that tradition ([36], p. 4).

This characterization belongs to the "great tradition" formulation of the anthropologist Robert Redfield from the 1950s. Redfield contended that "There are two kinds of people, peasants and a more urban (or at least manorial) elite" and that "The lower kind of people recognize, in certain respects, the political authority of the other and also their 'guidance in the moral sphere'" ([37], p. 60). Consequently, he suggested that "In a civilization there is a great tradition of the reflective few, and there is a little tradition of the largely unreflective many. The great tradition is cultivated in schools or temples; the little tradition works itself out and keeps itself going in the lives of the unlettered in their village communities ([37], p. 70). Redfield's binary is retained above in a "Sanskritic tradition" concerned with scriptural interpretation and "decentered traditions" in communities, with scholars calling the Hinduism of non-Brahmins "a mixture of folk elements with elements from the greater and Sanskritic tradition" ([38], p. 46). By the late 1980s, Indian historians created the Subaltern Studies movement to critique this form of scholarship across the social sciences for privileging the views of political and economic elites, challenging "higher" and "lower" levels of culture or degrees of "backwardness" [39]. On an experiential level, this makes sense—why should anyone's Hinduism be adjudged "centered" or "decentered," and for what reason?

The Hindu American Foundation (HAF), an educational and advocacy group in the United States founded in 2003, articulates an emic view of Hinduism through informational sheets. Like many Hindu and non-Hindu scholars, HAF interprets Hinduism as a textual tradition within a historical trajectory, noting, "Hinduism has always encompassed a wide range of beliefs and traditions, but all are unified by a respect for the Vedas, Upanishads, and Epic texts, and shared metaphysical concepts such as samsara, karma, dharma, and moksha" [40]. This formula has two main components: scriptures and beliefs. With respect to scriptures, HAF notes, "Some Hindus see the Vedas as texts expounding on rituals and Gods, whereas others see them as teaching metaphysical and spiritual truths about God and the soul," dating to at least 3000 years ago [41]. The Upanishads were composed between 800 and 200 BCE and contain contradictory viewpoints as "different texts forwarding monist, dualist, and non-theist perspectives on God" [40]. The epics, the Ramayana and Mahabharata, date from 200 BCE to 800 CE and have "focused largely on dharma, or righteous conduct, often in morally uncertain circumstances" [40]. Hindus do not share a single view about the nature of god, as HAF writes:

> Hindu understandings of God range from non-dualistic (the universe and the Absolute are not two) to qualified non-dualism (that the universe is different from but dependent on God and inseparable from God) to dualistic (that the universe is both dependent and different from God). These understandings also range from philosophies of pantheism (all of existence is the Absolute) to panentheism (all of existence is within the Absolute), to theism (the Absolute is external to all of existence) …. God in Hinduism is understood as beyond gender although capable of taking on both masculine and feminine qualities and forms. Some examples of different manifestations include Brahma, the Creator; Vishnu, the Preserver; and Shiva, the Destroyer. Female forms include Goddesses such as Lakshmi, the Goddess of Wealth; Saraswati, the Goddess of Knowledge; and Parvati, the Goddess of Strength [42].

HAF defines all four metaphysical concepts above. *Samsāra* is the cycle of reincarnation as an individual soul passes through multiple lives [43]. *Karma* is one's entirety of thoughts, words, and actions that produce reactions, experienced either in this life or in future lives [43]. *Moksha* is the state of liberation achieved through rituals, selfless service toward all, remembering a chosen divinity through love, and/or working through all karma to reach a state of peace and compassion toward all [43, 44]. *Dharma*, often translated as "duty," is the ethical foundation for life that consists of right actions toward spiritual advancement, transmitted through scriptures [45]. Hindus debate which practices are considered right and which scriptures are canonical, but all agree that *dharma* is essential to daily living [45].

HAF's representation provides an insider perspective, but still cannot represent all Hindus. For instance, worshippers of Lord Shiva may revere texts known as the *Āgamas* more than the Ramayana and Mahabharata which illustrate aspects of *dharma* through narratives of Lord Rama and Lord Krishna, respectively [46]. Worshippers of Hindu goddesses prioritize the *Devi Bhagavata Purana* and *Kalika Purana* as much as, if not more than, the Vedas and Upanishads [47]. And while sects founded after charismatic leaders such as the Dadupanthis, Kabirpanthis, Ravidasis, Swaminarayans, and Udasis from the 1500–1800s CE acknowledge certain shared scriptures, they prioritize the writings of their founders over others [48].

Finally, some etic and emic scholars view Hindus as a unified community despite the differences in groups that identify as Hindus. This quote exemplifies such argumentation:

> On a Hindu view, anyone's understanding of truth—even that of a guru regarded as possessing superior authority—is fundamentally conditioned by the specifics of time, age, gender, state of consciousness, social and geographic location, and stage of attainment. People see things differently, which enhances the nature of religious truth rather than diminishing it. It also suggests that people have much to learn from one another, or at least that they should respect their differences; hence there is a strong tendency for contemporary Hindus to affirm that tolerance is the foremost religious virtue. On the other hand, even cosmopolitan

Hindus living in a global environment recognize the fact that their religion has developed in the specific geographical, social, historical, and ritual climates of the Indian Subcontinent ([49], p. 11).

These scholars contend that "at least five elements give shape to Hindu religion: doctrine, practice, society, story, and devotion" ([49], p. 12). Doctrine is "enunciated and debated in a vast textual tradition anchored to the Veda (meaning 'knowledge'), the oldest core of Hindu religious utterance, and organized through the centuries primarily by members of the scholarly Brahmin caste" ([49], p. 12). Practice, often known as *puja*, finds its roots outside Vedic texts and consists of rituals to worship God through icons or images in homes or temples with food offered symbolically to offer thanks for one's current circumstances [49]. With respect to society, these scholars reference the caste system to write, "Few would dispute the perception that Indian society has been notably plural and hierarchical both in concept and in fact" ([49], pp. 13–14). Story is the means by which diverse Hindu groups articulate and debate *dharma* through common narratives: "For at least two millennia, people in almost all corners of India—and now well beyond—have responded to certain prominent stories of divine play and divine/human interaction. These concern major figures in the Hindu pantheon: Krishna and his beloved Radha, Rama and his wife Sita and brother Lakshmana, Shiva and his consort Parvati, and the great goddess Durga or Devi as a slayer of the buffalo demon Mahisa" ([49], p. 14). Finally, devotion or *bhakti* is the way that many Hindus adore the divine by remembering the words of saints writing in vernacular languages outside of Sanskrit [49].

Even this representation, despite affirming a healthy respect for internal differences, does not contain the totality of Hindu experiences. Sects like the Ramnamis which have traditionally emerged from low-caste groups with no access to formal education do not read the Veda and prioritize *bhakti* instead [50]. Reformist movements such as the Arya Samaj railed against the *puja* of icons and images as superstitious and favored a return to Vedic rituals [51]. Hindu reformist

groups such as the Brahmo Samaj [52] and leaders like Mohandas "Mahatma" Gandhi [53] have militated against the caste system. Therefore, not all five elements—doctrine, practice, society, story, and devotion—shape Hinduism, at least not in the same ways for all Hindus.

This brief review of how Hindu and non-Hindu scholars represent Hinduism reveals an abiding interest in the search for common features, a vestige of the "world religions" project that European scholars initiated during the colonial era. But as we have seen, there is no way to characterize all people who identify as Hindus without misinterpreting real-world data. The next section analyzes how this search for common features affects ways that scholars write about Hinduism in clinical settings.

The Clinical Implications of Representing Hinduism as a Homogenous Entity

The tendency to interpret Hinduism as a single tradition affects the clinical scholarship on recommendations for "dos and don'ts" in mental health settings. On May 7, 2023, I searched the medical database PubMed for recommendations pertaining to Hindus without any restriction on the date of publication. I paired the term "Hindu*" [for "Hindu" and "Hinduism"] with "mental" OR "psychiatr*" [for "psychiatry" and "psychiatric"] OR "psycholog*" [for "psychology" and "psychological"] to elicit as many results as possible, which produced 1128 listings. I read the titles and abstracts of each result, analyzing any article that offered clinical recommendations for providers who work with Hindus. I excluded studies that only enrolled Hindu participants without providing recommendations, provided clinical recommendations in nonmental health fields such as internal medicine or bioethics, and addressed a specific Hindu sect. Only four studies met the inclusion criterion. Table 8.1 lists all studies by reference number, source of knowledge about Hinduism, representation of Hinduism, and clinical recommendations for Hindu patients.

Table 8.1 Clinical recommendations for Hindu patients in mental health settings

Reference	Source of representation	Example of the representation	Recommendation
[54]	Textual sources in English	"In Hinduism, there is the belief that all humans pass through four life stages: student, householder, retirement, and finally, sannyas, a stage unattached to the world and without expectations. The student acquires knowledge but also character. The householder marries and focuses on family, work, and duty to the community. A retired person focuses more inwardly. A person becomes the sannyasin 'who neither loves nor hates anything' (*juthani*) with internal reflection and greater knowledge" (p. 202)	"The focus on child and adolescent development as a separation–individuation process that moves the child into an independent life with individual goals may run contrary to family cultural values and to the Hindu and Buddhist views of interconnectedness. For the Hindu family, however, when therapy can be seen as being compatible with an evolution toward the higher self and is consistent with the shared sense of family belonging, the goals can be complementary" (p. 216)
[55]	Textual sources in English	"The Hindu philosophical beliefs of transmigration of the soul, re-birth and fatalism, the different nature and quantum of guilt feeling in the Indian culture, and the differences in the need for confidentiality and inactivity exercised by the therapist, especially with regard to decision-making for the patient, and environmental manipulation render Indian psychotherapy vastly different from the western model" (p. S143)	"The Indian patients expect the therapist to play an active and authoritarian role, making difficult the maintenance of 'therapeutic neutrality,' an important part of western practice of psychotherapy. The western models of psychotherapy encouraging independence are redundant in the Indian population as dependency is a social norm among Indians" (p. S143)
[56]	Textual sources in English	"Dowry is a custom in Hindu marriage since times immemorial. According to Dharmashastra, the meritorious act of '*kanyadan*' is not complete until the bridegroom is given a '*Varadakshina*'" (p. S244)	"Over the years dowry has turned into a widespread social evil. Surprisingly, it has spread to other communities, which were traditionally non-dowry receiving communities. Demand for dowry has resulted in cruelty, domestic violence, and death by homicide or suicide" (p. S244)
[57]	Textual sources in English	"Misinterpretation of this metaphorical description in the Rigveda of the anthropomorphized origins of the four *varnas* led to creation of a system of hierarchy [sic] and was (erroneously) championed as a Divine Design [ca. 900 B.C.–600 B.C.]. In this hierarchy *Brahmanas* were on top, *Kshatriyas* below, *Vaishyas* next, and *Shudras* at the bottom" (p. 363)	"Caste hierarchy could manifest in and out of analytic situations and could lead to withdrawal from authority figures including the analyst. Subtle manifestations of repulsion are often revealed by what is not brought into analysis (hinted at by habits of vegetarianism or of taking the shoes off before entering the office or before lying down on the couch). One manifestation of the derivative of feeling condemned by heredity is the fear that 'I am unclean for life', which represents the belief that 'I am untouchable for life'. While all could be dealt with in analysis—even without reference to caste related transference-resistance manifestations—awareness and attention to these could help the dyad to get to the core faster" (p. 377)

These studies exhibit similar trends. First, each relies on texts produced hundreds of years ago as an authoritative source of knowledge about Hinduism. Hence, they all approach Hinduism as a static textual tradition. No article engages with commentaries produced in Sanskrit, regional languages, or English to see how Hindus have dynamically interpreted these texts throughout history or as a vibrant contemporary tradition [58]. Second, each article presents Hinduism as a monolithic entity. There is no attempt to point out the vast diversity in beliefs, practices, scriptural traditions, and institutions. Third, each article risks inadvertently blaming Hindus for difficulties that health providers could encounter, a shortcoming of many cultural competence programs that are developed for unfamiliar patient populations [59]. Texts are cited to anticipate problems with adolescent identity development [54], suicide [56], and transference-countertransference [55, 57]. Finally, Hindus are assumed to model behaviors off scriptures. This assumption reflects the enduring "world religions" approach to Hinduism [31] whereby texts—rather than practices and/or social position—are considered central to devotional life. Mental health providers would benefit from alternate approach that is experience-near to patients.

Samvāda as a Person-Centered Approach to Working with Hindus

Samvāda is a method that providers can adopt with Hindu patients. The Sanskrit word is composed of the prefix *sam* ("together") and the root stem *vāda* ("speaking"), implying that people are speaking together. Hinduism does not have a single set of doctrines and practices that binds all sects, but for centuries, the scriptural tradition has valued a Hindu's ability to understand multiple perspectives on an issue through *samvāda* [49]. Speaking together with Hindu patients about what matters in care is consistent with current cultural competence and DEI initiatives.

In particular, *samvāda* aligns with the cultural formulation approach in mental health settings. Based on concerns that busy clinicians would not complete cultural assessments with patients without usable questions, the DSM-5 Cross-Cultural Issues Subgroup created a series of interviews and a 16-item core Cultural Formulation Interview (CFI) that was field tested with 321 patients and 75 clinicians in six countries [60]. Rather than expecting providers to memorize "dos and don'ts" for myriad social groups, the CFI treats the patient as an informant in his/her/their life to ask about cultural views of health and illness with the expectation that all of us con-

struct hybrid identities based on belonging to multiple groups [61].

The American Psychiatric Association has made these interviews [62, 63] available to providers free of cost to promote clinical implementation and dissemination. The core CFI contains these questions for providers to ask patients about identities:

> Sometimes, aspects of people's background or identity can make their problem better or worse. By background or identity, I mean, for example, the communities you belong to, the languages you speak, where you or your family are from, your race or ethnic background, your gender or sexual orientation, or your faith or religion.
>
> 8. For you, what are the most important aspects of your background or identity?
>
> 9. Are there any aspects of your background or identity that make a difference to your problem?
>
> 10. Are there any aspects of your background or identity that are causing other concerns or difficulties for you? [62]

A CFI interview known as the "Supplementary Module for Spirituality, Religion, and Moral Traditions" also consists of 16 questions, which asks patients how faith plays a role in everyday life. This supplementary module asks patients a variety of questions about how they and family members personally identify with a faith tradition and the role of religious practices in daily life. For instance, the questions below take a person-centered approach to religion:

> *Role of spirituality, religion, and moral traditions*
>
> 5. What role does [NAME(S) OF SPIRITUAL, RELIGIOUS OR MORAL TRADITION(S)] play in your everyday life?
>
> 6. What role does [NAME(S) OF SPIRITUAL, RELIGIOUS OR MORAL TRADITION(S)] play in your family, for example, family celebrations or choices in marriage or schooling?
>
> 7. What activities related to [NAME(S) OF SPIRITUAL, RELIGIOUS OR MORAL TRADITION(S)] do you carry out in the home, for example, prayers, meditation, or special dietary laws? How often do you carry out these activities? How important are these activities in your life?
>
> 8. What activities do you engage in outside the home related to [NAME(S) OF SPIRITUAL, RELIGIOUS OR MORAL TRADITION(S)], for example, attending ceremonies or participating in a [CHURCH, TEMPLE OR MOSQUE]? How often do you attend? How important are these activities in your life? [63]

In clinical settings, the core CFI and this supplementary module have helped providers understand how patients view the relationship of their religious outlook to mental illnesses [64] and social supports/stressors [65]. The interviews align with *samvāda*, to speak together, so that social transformation occurs in the clinical encounter. This method implements a person-centered approach to providers learning about Hinduism in the daily lives of patients rather than making erroneous assumptions or inadvertently propagating group-based stereotypes.

Finally, Hindu providers have written extensively on similarities between the *guru-shishya* ("teacher-disciple") relationship and psychotherapy. Some have found inspiration in Sanskrit texts such as the Bhagavad Gita [66–68] and the Ramayana [69]. Others have observed that Hindu models of the self and relationships have influenced schools of psychotherapy such as mindfulness and transpersonal psychology that are commonly in use with non-Hindus in secular mental health contexts shorn of their religious roots [70]. The scholarship is divided in terms of how to use concepts of Hinduism for psychotherapy with Hindus. Acknowledging that there are few case studies of psychotherapy with Hindus, some believe that psychotherapists can draw upon concepts like *karma* from Hinduism to encourage Hindus with a fatalistic approach to life to take personal responsibility for their actions [71]. Others suggest that providers obtain explicit informed consent by asking patients about their religious beliefs and practices, broaching particular topics of interest, and requesting permission to include such topics within therapy [69]. This informed consent process may avoid one form of countertransference known as the "clinical anthropological syndrome" where the provider is overly curious and eager to demonstrate awareness of a patient's cultural background at the expense of directly addressing the presenting clinical problem [30].

Conclusion

This chapter has reviewed representations of Hinduism in religious studies and mental health scholarship. Non-Hindus initiated the academic study of Hinduism as part of the British colonial project to missionize and subjugate non-Christian populations in South Asia during the eighteenth through twentieth centuries. Influenced by postcolonial theories, Hindus and non-Hindus have questioned who speaks authoritatively for Hinduism as this imperial legacy has attempted to negate the vast diversity of Hindu experiences. By taking a person-centered approach through *samvāda*, mental health providers can help Hindu patients speak for themselves in articulating views on identity, illness, and health.

References

1. Evans J. 7 facts about Hindus around the world. Pew Research Center. 2022. https://www.pewresearch.org/short-reads/2022/10/26/7-facts-about-hindus-around-the-world/.
2. The global religious landscape. Hindus. Pew Research Center. 2012. https://www.pewresearch.org/religion/2012/12/18/global-religious-landscape-hindu/.
3. Office of the Registrar General & Census Commissioner, India. C-15: Religious community by age group and sex: India. Ministry of Home Affairs, Government of India. 2011 Census of India. https://censusindia.gov.in/census.website/data/census-tables.
4. Nepal profile. Ministry of Foreign Affairs, Government of Nepal. n.d.. https://mofa.gov.np/about-nepal/nepal-profile/.
5. Bangladesh Bureau of Statistics. In: Population & Housing Census—2011. Statistics and informatics division, Ministry of Planning. Dhaka: Government of People's Republic of Bangladesh; 2014.
6. Data umat berdasar jumlah pemeluk agama menurut agama. 2018. Biro Hubungan Masyarakat Data, dan Informasi. https://web.archive.org/web/20200903221250/https://data.kemenag.go.id/agamadashboard/statistik/umat.
7. Hasnain K. Pakistan's population is 207.68m, shows 2017 census result. Dawn; 2021.
8. Public Religion Research Institute. The 2020 census of American religion. Washington, DC: PRRI; 2020.

9. Office for National Statistics. CT0341—Religion by ethnic group by main language. National Archives, Government of the United Kingdom. 2011 Census. https://webarchive.nationalarchives.gov.uk/ukgwa/20160105160709/http://www.ons.gov.uk/ons/about-ons/business-transparency/freedom-of-information/what-can-i-request/published-ad-hoc-data/census/ethnicity/ct0341-2011-census.xls.

10. Statistics Canada. The Canadian census: a rich portrait of the country's religious and ethnocultural diversity. Government of Canada; 2022. https://www150.statcan.gc.ca/n1/daily-quotidien/221026/dq221026b-eng.htm.

11. Australian Bureau of Statistics. Census of population and housing: general community profile. Government of Australia. 2021. https://www.abs.gov.au/statistics.

12. Kleinman A, Benson P. Anthropology in the clinic: the problem of cultural competency and how to fix it. PLoS Med. 2006;3(10):e294.

13. Santiago-Irizarry V. Culture as cure. Cult Anthropol. 1996;11(1):3–24.

14. Metzl JM, Hansen H. Structural competency: theorizing a new medical engagement with stigma and inequality. Soc Sci Med. 2014;103(1):126–33.

15. Littlewood R. Psychiatry's culture. Int J Soc Psychiatry. 1996;42(4):245–68.

16. Aggarwal NK. Mental health in the war on terror: culture, science, and statecraft. New York: Columbia University Press; 2015.

17. Grieve GP. Staking out the field: a henotheistic review of supplemental readers for the study of Hinduism. J Am Acad Relig. 2008;76(3):716–47.

18. Caldwell S, Smith BK. Introduction: who speaks for Hinduism? J Am Acad Relig. 2000;68(4):705–10.

19. Smith BK. Who does, can, and should speak for Hinduism? J Am Acad Relig. 2000;68(4):741–9.

20. Narayanan V. Diglossic Hinduism: liberation and lentils. J Am Acad Relig. 2000;68(4):761–79.

21. Tilak S. Taking back Hindu studies. In: Hawley JS, Narayanan V, editors. The life of Hinduism. Berkeley: University of California Press; 2006. p. 271–87.

22. Sarma D. Let the Āpta (Trustworthy) Hindu speak! J Am Acad Relig. 2000;68(4):781–90.

23. Sharma A. Who speaks for Hinduism? A perspective from Advaita VedĀnta. J Am Acad Relig. 2000;68(4):751–9.

24. Hawley JS. Who speaks for Hinduism: and who against? J Am Acad Relig. 2000;68(4):711–20.

25. Harman W. Speaking about Hinduism and speaking against it. J Am Acad Relig. 2000;68(4):733–40.

26. McDermott RF. New age Hinduism, new age orientalism, and the second-generation south Asian. J Am Acad Relig. 2008;76(3):721–31.

27. Patton LL, Ram-Prasad C, Acharya K. Hinduism with others: inter-logue. In: Hawley JS, Narayanan V, editors. The life of Hinduism. Berkeley: University of California Press; 2006. p. 288–99.

28. Tseng W-S. Handbook of cultural psychiatry. San Diego: Academic Press; 2001.

29. Good BJ, Herrera H, Good MJ, Cooper J. Reflexivity and countertransference in a psychiatric cultural consultation clinic. Cult Med Psychiatry. 1982;6(3):281–303.

30. Comas-Diaz L, Jacobsen FM. Ethnocultural transference and countertransference in the therapeutic dyad. Am J Orthopsychiatry. 1991;61(3):392–402.

31. Lopez DS. Pandit's revenge. J Am Acad Relig. 2000;68(4):831–5.

32. Lipner J. On Hinduism and Hinduisms: the way of the banyan. In: Mittal S, Thursby GR, editors. The Hindu world. New York: Routledge; 2004. p. 9–34.

33. Viswanathan G. Colonialism and the construction of Hinduism. In: Flood G, editor. The Blackwell companion to Hinduism. Oxford: Blackwell; 2003. p. 25–44.

34. Viswanathan G. Outside the fold: conversion, modernity, and belief. Princeton: Princeton University Press; 1998.

35. Smith D. Orientalist and Hinduism. In: Flood G, editor. The Blackwell companion to Hinduism. Oxford: Blackwell; 2003. p. 45–63.

36. Flood G. Introduction: establishing the boundaries. In: Flood G, editor. The Blackwell companion to Hinduism. Oxford: Blackwell; 2003. p. 1–19.

37. Redfield R. Peasant society and culture: an anthropological approach to civilization. Chicago: The University of Chicago Press; 1956.

38. Singer MB. When a great tradition modernizes; an anthropological approach to Indian civilization. London: Pall Mall; 1972.

39. Guha R, editor. A Subaltern Studies Reader, 1986–1995. Minneapolis: University of Minnesota Press; 1997.

40. Hindu American Foundation. The history of Hinduism. https://www.hinduamerican.org/wp-content/uploads/2019/12/The_History_of_Hinduism.pdf.

41. Hindu American Foundation. Hindu scriptures. https://www.hinduamerican.org/wp-content/uploads/2019/12/Scriptures2.0_0.pdf.

42. Hindu American Foundation. Hindu concepts about God. https://www.hinduamerican.org/wp-content/uploads/2019/12/HinduConceptsAboutGod2.0_2.pdf.

43. Hindu American Foundation. What is karma? https://www.hinduamerican.org/wp-content/uploads/2019/12/KarmaMokshaandSamsara2.0_0.pdf.

44. Hindu American Foundation. How do Hindus worship? https://www.hinduamerican.org/wp-content/uploads/2019/12/HowHindusWorship2.0.pdf.

45. Hindu American Foundation. What is dharma? https://www.hinduamerican.org/wp-content/uploads/2019/12/Dharma2.0_1.pdf.

46. Sivaraman K. Śaivism in philosophical perspective. Delhi: Motilal Banarsidass Publishers; 1973.

47. Foulston L, Abbott S. Hindu goddesses: beliefs and practices. Liverpool: Liverpool University Press; 2009.

48. Lorenzen DN, editor. Religious movements in South Asia 600–1800. Oxford: Oxford University Press; 2006.
49. Hawley JS, Narayanan V. Introduction. In: Hawley JS, Narayanan V, editors. Life of Hinduism. Berkeley: University of California Press; 2006. p. 1–29.
50. Lamb R. Rapt in the name: the Ramnamis, Ramnam, and untouchable religion in Central India. Albany: State University of New York Press; 2002.
51. Hardiman D. Purifying the nation: the Arya Samaj in Gujarat 1895–1930. Indian Econ Soc History Rev. 2007;44(1):41–65.
52. Kopf D. The Brahmo Samaj and the shaping of the modern Indian mind. Princeton: Princeton University Press; 1979.
53. Gandhi M. A vindication of caste. https://ccnmtl.columbia.edu/projects/mmt/ambedkar/web/appendix_1.html.
54. Black N. Hindu and Buddhist children, adolescents, and families. Child Adolesc Psychiatr Clin N Am. 2004;13(1):201–20.
55. Avasthi A, Kate N, Grover S. Indianization of psychiatry utilizing Indian mental concepts. Indian J Psychiatry. 2013;55(Suppl 2):S136–44.
56. Sharma I, Pandit B, Pathan A, Sharma R. Hinduism, marriage and mental illness. Indian J Psychiatry. 2013;55(Suppl 2):S243–50.
57. Vallabhaneni MR. Indian caste system: historical and psychoanalytic views. Am J Psychoanal. 2015;75(4):361–81.
58. Patel D. Source, exegesis, and translation: Sanskrit commentary and regional language translation in South Asia. J Am Orient Soc. 2011;131(2):245–66.
59. Carpenter-Song EA, Schwallie MN, Longhofer J. Cultural competence reexamined: critique and directions for the future. Psychiatr Serv. 2007;58(10):1362–5.
60. Lewis-Fernández R, Aggarwal NK, Hinton L, Hinton DE, Kirmayer LJ. DSM-5 handbook on the cultural formulation interview. Washington, DC: American Psychiatric Publishing; 2016.
61. Aggarwal NK. Hybridity and intersubjectivity in the clinical encounter: impact on the cultural formulation. Transcult Psychiatry. 2012;49(1):121–39.
62. American Psychiatric Association. Cultural formulation interview. https://www.psychiatry.org/File%20Library/Psychiatrists/Practice/DSM/APA_DSM5_Cultural-Formulation-Interview.pdf.
63. American Psychiatric Association. Supplementary modules to the core cultural formulation interview (CFI): 5. Spirituality, religion, and moral traditions. https://www.psychiatry.org/getmedia/aca8f5a2-9b1b-456c-a3b7-f7f852edcf7c/APA-DSM5TR-CulturalFormulationInterviewSupplementaryModules.pdf.
64. Pearton T, van Staden W. The core cultural formulation interview in yielding religious content among patients suffering from a current major depressive episode. J Relig Health. 2021;60(4):2465–83.
65. Goyal S, Gupta B, Sharma E, Dalal PK, Pradeep Y. Psychiatric morbidity, cultural factors, and health-seeking behaviour in perinatal women: a cross-sectional study from a tertiary care Centre of North India. Indian J Psychol Med. 2020;42(1):52–60.
66. Reddy MS. Psychotherapy—insights from Bhagavad Gita. Indian J Psychol Med. 2012;34(1):100–4.
67. Bhatia SC, Madabushi J, Kolli V, Bhatia SK, Madaan V. The Bhagavad Gita and contemporary psychotherapies. Indian J Psychiatry. 2013;55(Suppl 2):S315–21.
68. Pandurangi AK, Shenoy S, Keshavan MS. Psychotherapy in the Bhagavad Gita, the Hindu scriptural text. Am J Psychiatry. 2014;171(8):827–8.
69. Jacob KS, Krishna GS. The Ramayana and psychotherapy. Indian J Psychiatry. 2003;45(4):200–4.
70. Miovic M. An introduction to spiritual psychology: overview of the literature, east and west. Harv Rev Psychiatry. 2004;12(2):105–15.
71. Sharma AR, Tummala-Narra P. Psychotherapy with Hindus. In: Richards PS, Bergin AE, editors. Handbook of psychotherapy and religious diversity. Washington, DC: American Psychological Association; 2014. p. 321–45.

Utilizing Ancient Hindu Scriptures to Conceptualize and Manage Anxiety Disorders

Shuchi Khosla

Introduction

Om dyauh shantir-antariksham shantih—Yajurveda 36.17 [1]
Meaning: May Peace prevail in the entire universe.

My life's journey began in the middle Himalayas, being born as the great-granddaughter of Acharya Ramdev (1881–1939), a renowned religious scholar, historian, and the founder of "*Kanya Gurukul Mahavidyalaya* (1932)" one of the first institutions of formal education for women in erstwhile British India. This history of scholarship of my family in the "*Satya Sanatana Vedic Dharma*" likely prompted my parents to encourage my memorization of the stories of *the Ramayana and the Mahabharata* in Hindi and "*Havan Mantra Sangraha*" in Sanskrit, all before the age of 5. The expectation of proficiency in Sanskrit and prioritization of an enduring pursuit of literacy in *Vedic* (ancient Hindu scripture) teachings were communicated early.

The protracted course to becoming a Harvard-trained psychiatrist mandated a change of address every few years, taking me to many regions in India and the United States for opportunities for higher education. In return, I was rewarded with an immersive experience in the two countries' diverse languages, cultures, and history.

The melodies of *Garhwali* and *Kumaoni* poets of the Himalayan mountains celebrating the union of their diverse populations in a spirit of activism for statehood of *Uttarakhand*, the vibrance of the fields of Punjab reminiscing the valor of the *Sikh gurus*, the tales of bravery of the *Gurjars* (backward class) to rival those of the *Rajputs* (forward caste) by the natives of the *Thar* Desert, the funeral of a gender-nonconforming young adolescent who completed suicide in small-town *Uttar Pradesh* and the social ostracizing of their family in the aftermath, the *susegad* (serene) *Goan* spirit of the spectacular *Konkan* coast that cloaks within its silence, imprints left by four and a half centuries of Portuguese colonial rule, the Midwestern spirit of Detroit as it responded to an economic recession and then to a pandemic, and the celebration of diverse leadership as an asset by a room full of Boston *Brahmins*—solemnizing many experiences like these have been formative in shaping my diasporic identity, that of an Indian embracing America within her and of an American proud of her Indian heritage.

Continuing research for references to mental illness in *Hindu* scriptures at various stages of my education has left me pleasantly surprised at the wealth of such data. The cultural education provided by lived experience, interactions with patients from the Indian and Indian American

S. Khosla (✉)
Harvard Medical School, Boston, MA, USA
e-mail: skhosla2@mgb.org

© The Author(s), under exclusive license to Springer Nature Switzerland AG 2024
H. S. Moffic et al. (eds.), *Eastern Religions, Spirituality, and Psychiatry*,
https://doi.org/10.1007/978-3-031-56744-5_9

communities, questions put forth by astute listeners during presentations on *"Mental Illnesses in the Vedas"* in the community, and data obtained from research into the *Hindu* scriptures inform the writing of this chapter.

Translating from ancient *Sanskrit* puts scriptural text at high risk for interpretive bias. I have endeavored to engage religious scholars to confirm these interpretations wherever possible. It is recommended that the reader view the content of this chapter as not immune to the implicit biases driven by my identity as an immigrant, *Hindu/Arya-Samaji*, female, and Indian/American psychiatrist.

Journey of Hinduism: From *Dharma* to Religion

yada yada hi dharmasya glanir bhavati bharata abhyutthanam adharmasya tadatmanam srijamyaham—Shrimad Bhagavad Gita 4.7 [2]

Meaning: O descendant of Bharat, whenever there is a decline in dharma and increase in adharma, in those times I will manifest.

In his book "Blunders in International Business (1974)" [3], David A. Ricks shared a story of Parker, later refined by Roger E. Axtell, a former company employee. The company, when launching its quick-drying, leakage-free ink in Latin America in the 1950s, had to promptly redact its posters with its tagline "To avoid embarrassment—Use SuperQuink" in Spanish as *"Para evitar embarazo compra SuperQuink"* which translates to "To avoid pregnancy buy SuperQuink" [4]. This exemplifies *"lost in translation,"* as does the use of the nineteenth-century term *Hinduism* (coined by Raja Ram Mohan Roy in 1816) to describe a "righteous way of life" written in texts from fifteenth century BCE or the theorizing of an *Indo-Aryan* invasion based on the linguistic interpretation of these texts, by the Western-European scholars of the 1800s with limited scholarship in its cultural and traditional context [5].

The term *Hindu* has its roots in Old Persian, an eponym given by the *Persian Achaemenids* implying a geographic identifier for those who inhab-

ited the lands around the *Sindhu* (Indus) river, first found in the inscriptions of *Darius the Great* (*Darius I*), who crossed the Himalayas to invade India in the sixth century BCE. The inhabitants of the Indus Valley, starting in the late Bronze Age, began compiling *Mantras* (hymns) about *Dharma* (the righteous way of life) that had been passed in an oral tradition for over a thousand years. The *Sanskrit* language does not have a word for "religion" in its vocabulary, and the *Vedas* do not have the term *Hindu*. It took 22 centuries for the followers of *"Satya Sanatana Vedic Dharma"* to start to identify as *Hindu* during the *Mughal* rule in the 1500s, and three centuries later, under the British *Raj*, *Hinduism* officially became a religion with over 100 sects and 1000 scriptures.

Hinduism and the Hindu Scriptures: Chronology and Classification

Tsmaadyjyatsrvehuth richah samani jjyire, Chhndaan si jjyire tsmaady justsmaadjaayt.— Yajurveda 31.7

Meaning: Oh mankind, you must learn about the all-knowing supreme soul that created the Rig, Sam, Yajur and Atharva-Vedas through reading them.

Darwin's finches of the Galapagos are an iconic example of rapid diversification in response to an unstable challenging environment with a competition for resources. An analogous diversification is observable in the *Hindu* scriptures in the *post-Vedic* period starting in the sixth century BCE as it negotiated the prolonged geopolitical crisis of more than 200 foreign invasions. The region in 2400 years, from the invasion by the Persians in 538 BCE to its independence from the *British Raj* in 1947, documents 700 years of indigenous and 1700 years of foreign rule. The foreign empires that ruled the region include the *Persians Achaemenids* (530 BCE–330 BCE), the *Macedonians/Indo-Greeks* (200 BCE–300 CE), the *Turko-Afghans* (975 CE–1520 CE), the *Mughals* (1526 CE–1707 CE), the East India Company (1756 CE–1856 CE), and the British *Raj* (1857 CE–1947 CE).

The periods of foreign rule influenced changes that appear to be incorporated within the scriptures during the interspersed periods of rule by the Indian dynasties, including the *Maurya* empire (320 BCE–181 BCE); the *Gupta*, *Chalukya*, and *Gurjar-Pratihara* empires (300 CE–975 CE); and smaller regional dynasties (1707 CE–1756 CE).

Various priests, scholars, and religious philosophers have classified the *Hindu* scriptures differently. From a content-driven perspective of this chapter, a five-category classification of *Hindu* scriptures based on the period in which they were written is functional:

1. Scriptures written before the *Achaemenid* empire—These include *Vedas* (1500–900 BCE), *Manusmriti* (1400–800 BCE), and *Vedangas* (900–700 BCE).
2. Scriptures written during the *Mauryan* empire—These include *Up-Vedas* (500 BCE–200 BCE) and *Darshans* (500 BCE–200 BCE).
3. Scriptures written during the *Macedonians* and *Indo-Greek* rule—*Itihas* (300 BCE–200 BCE) *including Ramayana and Mahabharata*, and *Puranas* (100 CE–250 CE).
4. Scriptures written during and shortly after the *Gupta* period—*Smriti-Dharma Sutras* (300 CE–800 CE) and *Agamas* (800 CE–1100 CE).
5. Interpretive religious texts written in the modern era—eighteenth century onwards.

In the modern era, during the rule of the East India Company (1756–1856), and the British *Raj* (1857–1947), while much of Europe negotiated the relationship between church and state [6], *Hinduism* experienced multiple social-religious reform movements closely tied to those associated with India's struggle for independence (Fig. 9.1).

These reformist movements brought forth varied philosophical reinterpretations of the ancient *Hindu* scriptures, as applicable to the times. These included among others *Brahmo Samaj* founded by Raja Ram Mohan Roy in 1828, *Arya Samaj* founded by Swami Dayanand Saraswati in

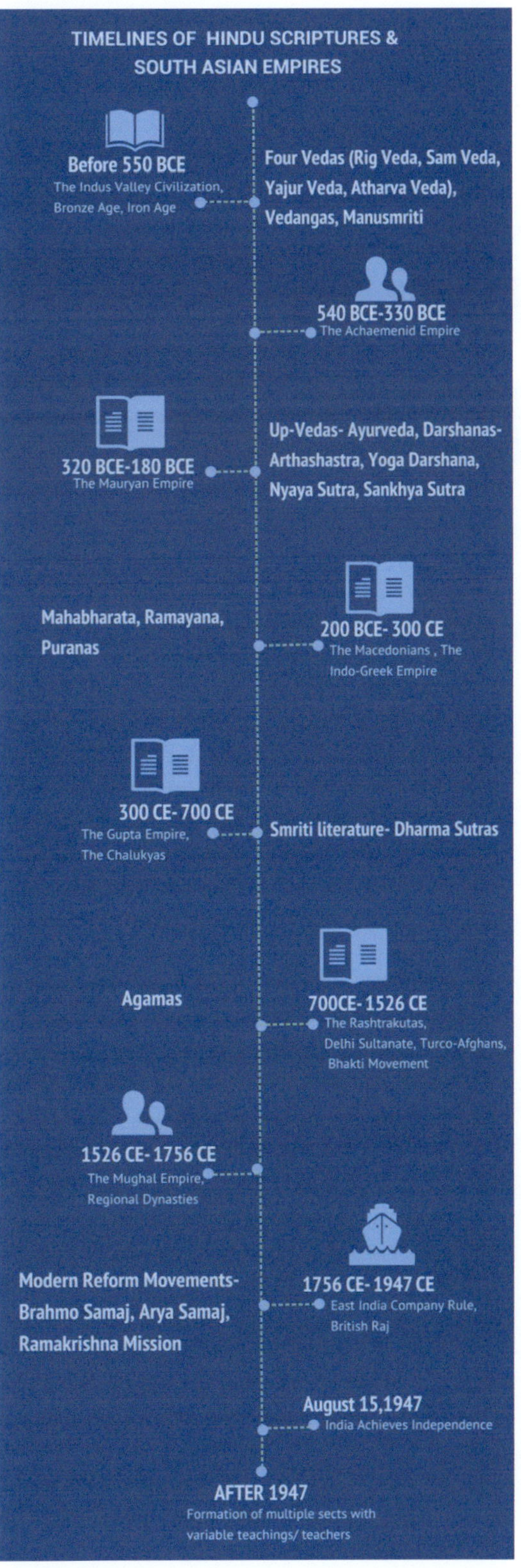

Fig. 9.1 Timeline of Hindu scriptures and South Asian empires [7–17]

1875, and *Ramakrishna Mission* founded by Swami Vivekananda in 1897.

Since the mid-twentieth century, a young independent India has seen the emergence of many religious leaders, saints, and spiritual guides who have established additional sects within Hinduism, each with philosophical differences in their interpretation of the ancient *Hindu* scriptures and an additional collection of new religious texts. Most prominent among these are *Sai Baba of Shirdi, Sathya Sai Baba, Sri Aurobindo, Paramhansa Yogananda, Maharishi Mahesh Yogi, Swami Gyanvatsal, Shree Rajneesh—Osho, Sadhguru Jaggi Vasudev, Mata Amritanandamayi, Brahmakumari Shivani, Baba Ramdev, Shri Shri Ravi Shankar*, among others.

The most powerful invention of the twentieth century, the Internet, and the social media revolution it brought, has allowed the spiritual messages and writings of many modern-day saints to be popularized worldwide. This has led to an expansion in the number of Hindu sects and scriptures at an unprecedented pace. It is plausible that the time lapse between the writing of this chapter and the publishing of the book may witness the addition of more than one Hindu religious sect and/or scriptural text.

Conceptualizing the Anatomy of Belief System of a Hindu Patient: Five-Category Classification

The first step to understanding the belief system of a *Hindu* patient is to appreciate that the sheer number of variables involved makes it akin to finding the solution to the 1974 invention of Hungarian sculptor and professor of architecture Erno Rubik. There is the perfect permutation for everyone, albeit the process of finding it may be labor intensive. For conceptualization, it is useful to break down the complex modern *Hindu* identity into five categories and understand that a patient may identify with one or more of them in varying proportions. The categories include the spiritual *Hindu*, the scriptural *Hindu*, the cultural *Hindu*, the ritualistic *Hindu*, and the amalgamated *Hindu*.

The Spiritual Hindu

The spiritual Hindu may be atheistic, monotheistic, or polytheistic. The focus for this type of *Hindu* is the teachings of *Hinduism*. They will often have a spiritual guide, a *sadhu* or a *rishi*, whose messaging on anxiety will be relevant to this patient's understanding of anxiety (Table 9.1) [18–20].

Many of those are focused on *yoga*, and yoga-based meditation for managing anxiety symptoms, a magnificent culturally congruent form of mindfulness that can be incorporated into CBT-based psychotherapeutic treatment as described further in the chapter.

The Scriptural Hindu

The scriptural *Hindu's* beliefs are directly determined by the scripture(s) they have read and follow. These include the followers of *Vedas, Vedanta, Puranas, Ramayana, Mahabharata,* and *Shrimad Bhagavad Gita*. The *Vedas* and *Vedantic* literature describe multiple anxiety disorders. The *Puranas, Ramayana, Mahabharata,* and *Shrimad Bhagavad Gita* all describe characters with various anxiety disorders [21]. These are detailed further in the chapter under their respective subheadings. Engaging with the scriptural *Hindu* around anxiety disorders can focus on sharing references from the texts and incorporating passages from the texts into therapy as demonstrated by Dr. Keshavan in his case study in which he incorporated verses from *Shrimad Bhagavad Gita* as a part of the psychotherapeutic intervention [22].

The Cultural Hindu

The cultural *Hindu* often belongs to the community of over a million diasporic individuals born in the United States or moved here early, with

Table 9.1 Massaging on anxiety from some modern spiritual guides

Guru	Messaging on anxiety
Shri Shri Ravi Shankar	Top four lesser known ways to beat anxiety: 1. Give yourself much deserved rest from anxiety with meditation 2. Chase your worries away with the spirit of enthusiasm 3. Freedom from pills with side effects 4. Make your worries bigger
Sai Baba of Shirdi	"Do not be anxious about what you have, what you have been, or what awaits you in the future. Be content with what you have."
Sathya Sai Baba	"Anxiety is removed by faith in the Lord; the faith that tells you that whatever happens is for the best and that the Lord's will be done. Quiet acceptance is the best armor against anxiety, not the acceptance of the heroic."
Sri Aurobindo	Integral yoga as an approach to anxiety management
Paramhansa Yogananda	"When the consciousness is kept on god, you will have no fears; every obstacle will then be overcome by courage and faith."
Maharishi Mahesh Yogi	Transcendental meditation for anxiety
Swami Gyanvatsal	YouTube series on "zero stress, zero tension, peaceful life"
Shree Rajneesh—Osho	"The desire is nothing but an escape from the state of anxiety. Desires don't create anxiety, as ordinarily is believed. Anxiety creates desire. Man is anxiety."
Sadhguru Jaggi Vasudev	Yoga for management of anxiety disorders
Mata Amritanandamayi	"Immobilization, caused by ceaseless waves of thoughts: That is what we call anxiety. When this happens, it is like we pay interest on a loan even before taking it!"
Brahmakumari Shivani	Regular practice of Rajyog meditation
Baba Ramdev	Yoga and Ayurvedic herbs are treatments

immigrant *Hindu* parents. They relate to Indian food, culture, festivals, and holidays but not as much to the religion or scriptures. Data suggests that this population is at a higher risk of inter-generational caste and immigration-based trauma often transmitted through the beliefs of their parental generation. They are at a higher risk for invalidation and stigmatizing attitudes from family figures regarding their anxiety disorder [23]. Depending on age, enmeshment, and approachability, this type of patient would benefit from family education. If the family includes scriptural or spiritual *Hindus*, they may benefit from the strategies mentioned earlier.

ciated with certain special days and seasons. Some literature suggests that religious scrupulosity in these patients may put them at a higher risk of obsessive-compulsive spectrum disorders [21, 24]. From a management standpoint, these patients may not be aware of the content of the *Vedic* scriptures but will often engage around the *Puranic* stories of their chosen deity, and examples of their deity exhibiting anxiety symptoms can be reassuring. Additionally, *Pranayama* (breath practice) from structured forms of yoga, like the *Patanjali Yoga* described later in the chapter, can prove to be an easily acceptable, culturally congruent grounding technique incorporated in exposure-response prevention.

The Ritualistic Hindu

The ritualistic *Hindu* is often steeped in tradition, endeavoring to precisely perform the prescribed practices. Many of these come from the *Agamas* as described later in the chapter. Classically, the ritualistic Hindu will identify with one of the four denominations—*Shaivism*, *Shaktism*, *Vaishnavism*, or *Smartism*. This patient will describe elaborate fasts and temple prayers asso-

The Amalgamated Hindu

The amalgamated *Hindu* is often the most complex. He or she may follow a blending of religious traditions, values, and understanding. The most common amalgamations are seen with *Buddhism*, *Jainism*, and *Sikhism*. For such a patient, culturally congruent mindfulness meditation—*Vipassana* for *Buddhism*, *Dhyana* for

Jainism, and *Surat Shabd Yoga* for *Sikhism*—may be explored [25].

It is expected that there will be patients who fit into more than one or none of these categories [26]. The purpose of these is not rigidification or stereotyping, but rather a pragmatic approach to the patient with religious and cultural humility to engage with their complex *Hindu* identity in formulation and treatment.

Vedas and Anxiety

yuñjate mana uta yuñjate dhiyo viprā viprasya bṛhato vipaścitaḥ, vi hotrā dadhe vayunāvid eka in mahī devasya savituḥ pariṣṭutiḥ.—*Rig Veda 5.81.1*

Meaning: Those desirous of a calm mind must join their mind to the universal soul, as that will make the mind tranquil, and the person will become blissful and enlightened and filled with knowledge.

Shruti, meaning "that which was heard," is the name given to the most ancient scriptures of *Hinduism* called *Vedas*. The *Vedas* are the collection of ancient knowledge, passed down in oral tradition as hymns among the Indus Valley's ancient inhabitants. They were compiled and written down in the *Kuru* kingdom starting in the mid-second millennium BCE.

The *Mantra Samhita* (a compendium of 20,416 hymns) was systematized into four books based on subject matter between 1500 and 900 BCE: *Rig Veda* (10,589 mantras on *Gyan/Knowledge*), *Sam Veda* (1975 mantras on *Karma/Duties*), *Yajur Veda* (1875 mantras on *Upasna/Meditation*), and *Atharva Veda* (5977 mantras on physical/medicinal science).

In addition to the *Mantra Samhita*, the *Vedas* contain three interpretive sections. *Brahmans* (a commentary on the *Mantra Samhita*), *Aranyaks* (the esoteric interpretation of the mantra *Samhita* by the forest dwellers), and *Upanishads* (an uncomplicated summary of the deepest knowledge of the *Vedas*) complete the four sections of a *Veda*.

The *Mantras* (hymns) were composed in *Vedic* (preclassical) *Sanskrit*, following variable grammatical rules. The *Rishis* (scholars) of the time agreed over the content (semantics and pragmatics) but had divergent opinions on the form (syntax, morphology, and phonology) of the language. This led to the development of different *Vedic* schools called *Shakhas* (branches) and the writing of different recensions of *Vedas* presenting with variation in form yet a remarkable consistency in content.

There are variable versions of how many of these ancient *Vedic* schools existed. The total documented in *"Mahabhashya" of "Maharishi Patanjali"* is widely accepted and details 21 *Shakhas* of *Rig Veda*, 101 of *Yajur Veda*, 1000 of *Sam Veda*, and 9 *Shakhas* of *Atharva Veda*. Each recension of the *Veda* includes a *Mantra Samhita*, a *Brahman*, an *Aranyak*, and one or more *Upanishads* developed by the *Rishis* of the *Shakha*.

The *Vedas* describe the existence of one God, "the supreme soul." They describe three eternal elements—mind, matter, and soul. They describe the purpose of human life as fourfold—*Dharma* (righteousness), *Artha* (industry and prosperity of the society), *Kama* (comforting oneself with physical and emotional pleasure), and *Moksha* (eventual liberation of the soul from the cycle of life) [1]. The *Vedic* literature describes the "mind" as distinct from the "brain." More than 60 synonyms are used in the *Vedas* for anxiety, ranging in severity from "anxious excitement" to "paralyzing panic" and fear.

In the *Rig Veda*, the 81st *Mantra* of the fifth *Adhyaya* (chapter) prescribes the path to mental tranquility as the union of the mind with the universal soul, which is the same as the definition of *Yoga* in *Patanjali Yoga Darshan* [27].

In the *Yajur Veda*, the first six *Mantras* of the *Shiv-Sankalpa Sukta* (the 34th chapter) are dedicated to the "mind," describing the pursuit of "a tranquil mind" as *Dharma*.

In the *Chandogya Upanishad* of the *Sam Veda*, a section of the third *Adhyaya* (chapter) is entirely dedicated to the mind. It describes the mind, its power, and the importance of meditation to calm anxiety and decrease distractibility.

The sixth *Adhaya* (chapter) of the *Atharva Veda* is focused on "nonnormative behavior" and mentions multiple mental illnesses, including anxiety disorders. It classifies the "abnormal behavior" as "less severe" or "more severe." The "less severe" category includes *Krodh* (anger), *Moh* (attachment), *Shok* (deep sadness/depression), and *Dushswapna* (anxious dreams/nightmares). The "more severe" category includes *Unmad* (psychosis), *Apasmar* (seizure), *Bhay* (phobias), and *Grahi* (hysterical conversion). True to its prescriptive nature, recommendations for *Bheshaj* (medication) and *Mantra Jap* (meditation) are also given [28, 29].

The themes of anxiety and the need for its management to facilitate a tranquil mind are seen across all four *Vedas* and reflect the prioritization of mental health in that era. As the *Vedas* were written before the *Achaemenid* invasion, they are considered free of foreign influence, superior to all other texts, and the primary source, and the supreme authority on *Dharma* by most sects of *Hinduism*. Even though reading the *Vedas* is no longer a common practice among *Hindus*, the reverence toward them is widespread. When shared with the modern *Hindu*, acknowledging mental illness in *Vedic* texts may help combat some stigma surrounding mental health treatment.

Vedangas (the Explanatory Limbs of *Vedas*) and Anxiety

The *Rishis* of the various *Shakhas*, along with completing the compilation of the *Vedas*, compiled a vast amount of derivative work in the period. Among these are the six *Vedangas* (explanatory limbs) that supplement the *Vedas*. These include *Siksha* (phonetics), *Vyakaran* (grammar), *Chhandas* (prosody), *Nirukta* (etymology), *Jyotish* (astronomy), and *Kalpa* (rules/practices) [30]. Among these, the *Dharmasutras* (descriptions of *Dharma*) of *Rishi Vasishtha* and *Srauta Sutras* (interpretations of Shruti) of *Rishi Bharadwaj* describe ways to prevent and manage anxiety [31].

Up-Vedas (the Subsidiary *Vedas*) and Anxiety

Sattvamatma Shareeram Cha Trayametatridandavat—Ayurveda Charak Samhita 1.46

Meaning: Mind, Self, and Body. These three make a tripod on which the living world stands.

Four *Up-Vedas* form a subsidiary of the *Vedas*: *Ayurveda* (the treatise on health science, sixth century BCE–fourth century CE), *Dhanurveda* (the treatise on warfare—900 BCE), *Arthashastra* (the treatise on statecraft, political science, and economic policy—297 BCE), and *Gandharva Veda* (the treatise on melody/music—200 BCE). The *Ayurveda* consists of two books *Charak Samhita* (a treatise on ancient medicine) and *Sushrut Samhita* (a treatise on ancient surgery).

Diseases of the *Manas* (the mind) [32] have been described in both *Sushrut Samhita* and *Charak Samhita*. *Sushrut Samhita* prescribes guidelines on *Unmad Pratished* (preventing psychosis) in postsurgical delirium [33].

Charak Samhita lists a variety of mental illnesses and a full spectrum of anxiety disorders: *Chittodvega* (generalized anxiety) [34], *Bhay* (phobia), *Vishad* (panic), *Apatanaka* (conversion disorder), and *Atatwabhinivesa* (obsessions and compulsions). The symptomatology of each of these is described, and the prescribed treatment includes *Daivavyapasraya-Chikitsa* (spiritual treatment), *Yuktivyapasrya-Chikitsa* (medicinal treatment), and *Sattvavajaya-Chikitsa* (psychotherapy) [33, 35].

Ayurveda, a subsidiary of *Atharva Veda*, established many important *Vedic* philosophies directing the ideology of *Dharma*. Consideration of "spiritual health" and "mental health" as separate domains put one in the purview of the priests and the other in the purview of the physician. Contrary to the *Agamas* (later interpretive texts written in seventh–eleventh centuries), it described mental illness as a treatable *"Manovikar"* (a disorder of the mind) rather than a "character flaw." It acknowledged the mind-body connection by stating, *"The body follows the mind and mind follows the body."* It described psychiatric disorders in the same classification as physical disorders and considered multiple factors (biological, nutritional, psychological, trauma, social, and spiritual) as *Avashyak* (necessary) to a psychiatric formulation [36].

This ensured that in ancient times, physicians directed psychiatric diagnosis and treatment (for medicinal care and psychotherapy), and priests were added as a part of the treatment team (for spiritual therapy) [37]. This body of literature, now widely drawing fascination from the Western world, has existed within the *Hindu* scriptures for 3000 years before Freud and can provide an important relational point to the *Hindu* patient.

Manusmriti (the Ancient Dharma-Law), *Smriti-Dharmasutra* (the Remembered Texts), and Anxiety

One of the older texts of the second millennium BCE, "*Manusmriti*," is a name that may generate strong emotions and may prove anxiolytic or anxiogenic depending on the context in which it is used. It has been closely (but not accurately) linked to India's caste system. *Manu* wrote his laws based on observing the social order of his time. The *Vedic* society was a *Varna* (class)-based society. The *Varna* of an individual was based on their conduct, character, wisdom, motivation to pursue knowledge, and industry. The expectations of conduct, behavior, and productivity of each of these classes are detailed in his book. *Varna* was not attached to hereditary lineage. *Manu* wrote at length about keeping the classes "authentic" and "reclassifying" individuals as many times as necessary to determine their place in the social order based on their attributes. He was a proponent of class-switching rather than the intermingling of classes. The stated purpose was to allow individuals to marry within their class, such that they are "understood" by their partner, sharing the same lived experience, leading to a harmonious marriage.

As the son of a Shudra may attain the rank of a Brahman if he were to possess his qualifications, character, and accomplishments, and as the son of a Brahman may become a Shudra, if he degrades in his character, inclinations, and manners, even so, must it be with him who springs from a Kshatriya; even so with him who is born of a Vaishya. In other words, a person should be ranked with the Class whose qualifications, accomplishments, and character he possesses—Manusmriti 10:65 [27].

The opinions of *Manu* were also shared by *Apastamba*, a philosopher of the *Vedic* time, who writes in his *Sutra*, "*A lower classman may, by leading a virtuous life, rise to the level of a higher classman and he should be ranked as such. In like manner, a higher classman can, by leading an immoral life, degrade to the lower class and should be considered as such.*"

Despite this clear messaging, the *Manusmriti* continues to be linked to the caste system, which is widely propagated as having its origins in the *Vedas* with no evidence of the same. Rather, we know that this profession-based social classification, designed to facilitate marriage with the flexibility of change, continued well into the *Mauryan* Empire (320–185 BCE). This is described by the Greek historian *Megasthenes* in his book *Indica* (compiled by *Arrian of Nicomedia*), who wrote the account upon visiting *Pataliputra*, the capital of *Chandragupta Maurya*. "*The society was classified into seven classes—philosophers, farmers, soldiers, herdsmen, artisans, magistrates, and councilors.*"

It was not until the *Gupta* period (300–800 CE), often called the Golden Age of *Hinduism* based on the large number of interpretative/derivative scriptures generated during this time, that the caste system became incorporated in scriptures, prompting the start of caste-based endogamy. The most convincing evidence of this emerged from the recent work of a team of three Indian geneticists (*Partha Majumder, Analabha Basu,* and *Neeta Sarkar Roy*) published in the Proceedings of the National Academy of Sciences (PNAS) in 2015 [38]. The team used genomic reconstruction models to determine the beginning of endogamy in the Indian population. Their models predicted that there was "free gene flow" among the ancestral populations until about 1575 years ago, which abruptly ended between 319 CE and 550 CE, during the middle of the *Gupta* Empire. This is congruent with the previously known time in which "untouchability" began, based on the writings of the Chinese traveler, *Faxian*, who traveled to India between 399 CE and 412 CE in search of *Buddhist Scrolls*. *Faxian* noted in his book, "A Record of Buddhist Kingdoms," the plight of *"Chandalas"* (the lower caste people) in the *Gupta* Empire.

This *Gupta* period corresponds to the writings of *Smriti-Dharmasutras*, which describe the rules of the caste system. These scriptures, written over the 500 years of the *Gupta* dynasty rule, vary widely in their interpretations of class and caste and the description of the *dharma-law*. There are 18 *Brahman* (upper caste) *Rishis* credited with writing these (*Yajnavalkya, Atri, Vishnu, Harit, Aushanasi, Angirasa, Yama, Samvartta, Katyayana, Brihaspati, Parashar, Vyasa, Shankha, Likhit, Daksh, Gautam, Satatap, Vashishth*), who appear to describe the law, as they observed it, under the rule of different emperors of the *Gupta* dynasty. Based on their linguistic patterns and content, scholars have dated Smriti-Dharmasutras at least 1500 years after Manusmriti. Linguistically, they are written in classical *Sanskrit*, typical of the *Gupta* period. From a content standpoint, all of them mention *"Puranas"* as an authority on *"Dharma."* The *"Puranas"* (described later in the chapter) are dated to the post-*Vedic* era, written during and after the *Macedonian/Indo-Greek* empire (320 BCE–240 CE). *Smriti* texts are considered secondary in authority to *Shruti* texts [39].

This reinterpretation of scriptural history is an important part of understanding the cultural tradition of *Hinduism*. The caste system, inaccurately publicized as from the *Vedas*, has led to over a thousand years of systemic mistreatment of *Hindus* by fellow *Hindus*, predisposing 70 generations of *Hindus* to intergenerational trauma. This context may be helpful for the psychiatric practitioner in understanding a *Hindu* patient who self-identifies as "lower caste" or "upper caste" as this may inform the etiology of their anxiety, guilt, and/or challenges in building a trusting therapeutic alliance.

Darshans (Philosophy), *Itihas* (Tales of Ancient Kingdoms), *Puranas* (the Pantheon), and Anxiety

True wisdom comes to each of us when we realize how little we understand about life, ourselves, and the world around us.—Socrates

In 327 BCE, when Alexander began his "India Campaign," he brought Greek influences of food, culture, and literature to the land. Many a food blogger has talked about the Indian *Raita* (a yogurt sauce) being a cousin of Greek *Tzatziki* (a yogurt dip), and many an essay draws parallels between the cultures of ancient Greece and ancient India. Written as a derivative literature of the *Upanishads, Darshans* (written during the *Mauryan* Empire), *Itihas*, and *Puranas* (written during the *Macedonian* and *Indo-Greek* empires) perhaps embody the most remarkable similarities to the ancient Greek writings of philosophy and mythology. Philosophy and mythology seek to answer similar questions about the universe, God, and being. The philosophical texts, *Darshans*, seek to answer the questions with observation, reason, and argument, while the mythological texts, *Itihas* (tales of ancient kingdoms) and *Puranas* (stories of deities of the Pantheon), seek to answer the questions using inspiration and revelations. Anxiety and anxiety disorders appear in both philosophical and mythological literature. *Darshans* details the etiology of anxiety disorders and recommendations for prevention and management. In *Itihasic* and *Puranic* literature, characters exhibit the symptoms of various anxiety disorders and sometimes suffer the lasting consequences of untreated anxiety. Additionally, multiple heroes in the stories perform psychotherapy interventions leading to positive outcomes.

Darshans (Philosophical Texts)

There are six orthodox schools of *Hindu* philosophy: *Samkhya*, *Yoga*, *Nyaya*, *Vaisheshika*, *Mimasa*, and *Vedanta*. In addition, some scholars mention three heterodox schools of *Hindu* philosophy: *Buddhism*, *Jainism*, and *Charvaka*. There is some debate about whether heterodox schools are a part of *Hindu* religious schools of philosophy versus independent philosophies of ancient India coexisting with and separate from *Hinduism*. However, considering that *Buddhism*, *Jainism*, and *Charvaka* (atheism) have independent religious identities in modern times, this chapter focuses on the six orthodox schools of *Hinduism* that accept the *Vedas* as canonical texts.

These are further grouped into three classes based on content: *Nyaya-Vaisheshika* (laws of physics and material creation with rationale), *Samkhya-Yoga* (need for mental well-being and prescribed processes to attain it), and *Mimamsa-Vedanta* (knowledge of spiritual integration with the divine and actions to help attain it).

The writings in *Samkhya Darshan* attributed to *Kapila Muni* and *Yoga Darshan* attributed to *Maharishi Patanjali* are the most valuable from a mental health standpoint. *Swami Vivekananda* described *Maharishi Kapila* as the "greatest psychologist the world has ever known" based on the reading of *Samkhya Darshan*. *Samkhya* describes mental suffering as due to the engagement of *Purush* (consciousness—the unemotional, thinking, observing entity) with the *Prakriti* (material, environmental world). As environmental influences (information from sensory perception, negative emotion) start to overpower our consciousness (the thinking/observing entity), mental suffering worsens. *Moksha* (liberation) is defined as the separation of *Purush* from *Prakriti*. This may remind the reader of cognitive behavioral therapy and dialectical behavioral therapy concepts of the separation of emotions from thought or the negotiation between the emotional and rational mind. *Patanjali's Yoga Darshan* provides the pathway to achieving *Moksha*, the separation of *Purush* and *Prakriti*, through *Ashtanga Patanjali Yoga* (eight-limb yoga). The eight limbs

of *yoga* (*yama*, *niyama*, *asana*, *pratyahara*, *pranayama*, *dharana*, *dhyana*, and *samadhi*) are steps to achieve sustained detachment of consciousness from the environment such that the inner self can observe all feelings and sensations without judgment. This is congruent with the modern definition of mindfulness. According to *Patanjali*, when an individual with the continual practice of *yoga* can achieve complete detachment of consciousness from the environment, they will achieve *Moksha*. *Patanjali Yoga Darshan* is the oldest known document on *yoga*, which has since diversified into many other forms.

In managing anxiety disorders of *Hindu* patients, engaging the patient in the writings of *Samkhya Darshan* that describe the principles of and utilize *pranayama* (breath practice) and other elements of yoga as mindfulness techniques can prove to be safe, effective, and culturally congruent interventions.

Itihas (*Ramayana* and *Mahabharata*) and *Puranas* (Pantheon)

The mythological literature in the Hindu scriptures consists of 2 epics, *Ramayana* (from the kingdom of *Kosala*) and *Mahabharata* (of the *Kuru* kingdom), and 18 *Puranas* (6 *Puranas* glorifying Lord *Brahma*, 6 *Puranas* glorifying Lord *Vishnu*, and 6 *Puranas* glorifying Lord *Shiva*). All these mythological texts were passed down in oral tradition for a few hundred years before being written down in *Sanskrit* for the first time in late *Maurya*, the early *Macedonian* empire. They were rewritten in the *Gupta* period first in *Sanskrit* and then in *Hindi*. They also became the source for a vast amount of derivative literature called *Agamas*, starting in the seventh century CE. *Ramayana*, attributed to *Maharishi Valmiki*, is the story of Prince *Ram* [40] from *Ayodhya*, in the *Kosala* kingdom, with the message of victory of good over evil as *Ram* fights the demon *Ravana* to rescue his wife, *Sita*. In the story, *Ram* shoots *Ravana's* brother *Marrich* with an arrow through his heart. Marrich exhibits symptoms congruent with post-traumatic stress disorder in the aftermath [37].

Mahabharata, attributed to *Maharishi Ved Vyas*, is the story of a war between *Kauravas* and *Pandavas* to establish *Dharma* (the righteous path) over *Adharma* (the unrighteous path). The story has many complex characters and situations that reflect anxiety disorders. The most memorable, however, is an incident central to the plot. Before the war, the great warrior *Arjuna* realizes that he will need to fight his own family and teachers in the war and develops the symptoms of a panic attack. At that moment, *Shri Krishna* uses the *Shrimad Bhagavad Gita* as a psychotherapeutic tool to treat *Arjuna's* anxiety and helps him work through his cognitive distortions of emotional reasoning, overgeneralization, catastrophizing, personalization, and blame among others [41]. *Shrimad Bhagavad Gita*, although a part of the *Mahabharata*, is read by many *Hindus* as a free-standing text, and readings from this can be utilized as a part of culturally congruent cognitive behavioral therapy [2]. Similarly, within the *Puranic* texts, there are examples of *Brahma*, *Vishnu*, and *Shiva* all evidencing the symptoms of anxiety disorders in many stories resolved with yoga meditation and psychotherapy engagement. The videos of dramatization of anxiety symptoms by the characters of *Itihas* and *Puranas*, many of which have been converted into movies and television series, are an effective tool in helping patients identify anxiety symptoms. Additionally, since many revered characters in these stories exhibit anxiety symptoms, their use helps to normalize the occurrence of anxiety disorders and prevents them from being viewed as a "character flaw."

Agamas (*Tantric* Texts) and Anxiety

The *Gupta* empire, often referred to in history as the "Golden Age of *Hinduism*," ended around 550 CE with a series of invasions by the "White Huns," the nomadic tribes of central Asia. The *Guptas* were succeeded by several smaller dynastic empires that lived in political unrest and frequent wars. In 712 CE, the Arabs, in the *Umayyad* campaign, after the successful conquest of *Sindh*, moved to conquer kingdoms to the east of the Indus River. The next 300 years saw repeated invasions from the Arabs, the Turks, the *Turko-Afghans*, and the Mongols. The most significant were those of *Mahmud* of *Ghazni*, who is reported to have invaded India no less than 17 times between 1000 CE and 1025 CE, and *Muhammad* of *Ghor* who invaded India 7 times between 1175 CE and 1205 CE. During these invasions, many cities were ravaged, temples destroyed and looted, women kidnapped and raped, and men taken and sold as slaves [42]. During this period of religious angst, the *Agamas* were written, starting after the White *Huns* invasions in the mid-first millennium CE and continuing through the invasions of *Muhammad* of *Ghor* in 1175 CE [43]. The word *Agama* means "tradition." The voluminous *Agama* literature includes 28 *Shaiva Agamas*, 64 *Shakta Agamas*, 108 *Vaishnav Agamas*, and many *Up-Agamas*. These texts vary in their religious philosophies and contain detailed manuals of rules and rituals on the building of temples, idols, traditions, and *Puja* (religious prayer). There is often a focus on performing the ritual "correctly" to please the deity and the anxiety of the "incorrect" ritual causing displeasure to the deity with resultant misfortune being brought upon the individual, encouraging religious scrupulosity. The *Agamas* are different from the texts of *Puranas* even as they share deities. In *Agamas*, the deities are presented as a symbol of strength, and anxiety is viewed as a personal failing. There are variations of yoga in the *Agamas* like "*kundalini* yoga"; however, their purpose is to "ready one's mind" to engage in the rituals of worship, as opposed to being attached to a goal of self-actualization. *Agama* literature and its influence should be considered in conceptualizing obsessive-compulsive spectrum disorders in a *Hindu* patient who describes "rituals" and "traditions" as central to their religious beliefs. Patients may find meditation rituals an adaptive coping skill when dealing with nonreligious environmental stressors.

Using This Chapter to Build a Religiously Informed Culturally Congruent Psychiatric Formulation and Treatment Plan

The cursory reading of the chapter can help a reader understand how the conceptualization of anxiety and anxiety disorders evolved through the transitions in religious scriptures. The reader may potentially use this information in various educational and clinical settings. The following four-step approach may be helpful from a diagnosis and management standpoint.

Step 1: Understanding the Patient's Hindu Identity

It is imperative to approach the patient without preconceived assumptions or judgment. Open-ended questions followed by complex reflections are effective in helping the patient educate the psychiatrist about their *Hindu* identity. Phrases from the cultural formulation interview like "For you, what are the most important aspects of your background or identity?" can be used. If the patient mentions being a Hindu as important to their identity, it is helpful to follow up with "What does being a *Hindu* mean to you?". Allow the patient to share the aspects of Hinduism that influence their identity, and seek clarifications to see if/where they fit in the five-category classification of the *Hindu* belief system.

Step 2: Identifying a Spiritual Guide, a Deity, or a Scripture

Most patients should identify one or more spiritual guides, deities, or scriptures. Sometimes, they may just share the deity or the spiritual guide, so it is reasonable to ask if they are aware of the scripture associated with the deity. The chapter offers a fair amount of data in this regard. Considering there were no deities in the Vedas, all the deities mentioned can be found in the Puranas. Similarly, if unable to find a spiritual

guru in Table 9.1 (earlier in the chapter), it may be reasonable to research the spiritual guides and their messaging using other sources like the Internet.

Step 3: Sharing the Relevant Content with the Patient

This can be achieved in a multitude of ways. One can share the written message or a recorded lecture of the spiritual guide with their message on anxiety. Most Puranas have been turned into TV series and movies. Sharing clips of these stories and allowing the patient to recognize anxiety symptoms in their revered deity are a highly effective way to engage the patient in recognizing and identifying those symptoms. In my clinical practice, I have used the videos of *"Arjun Vishad"* in BR Chopra's *Mahabharata* to demonstrate panic symptoms, which have been well-received by many patients. Another way to share the relevant content is to integrate scripture readings into therapy sessions as described by Dr. Keshavan, where he used passages from Bhagavad Gita incorporated effectively into psychotherapy.

Step 4: Incorporating Culturally Congruent Therapeutic Techniques into Treatment

Almost all patients who describe religion as important to their identity can share one or more meditative aspects or practices that help them feel calm or grounded. Mindfulness, a core technique in anxiety management, can be effectively and creatively replaced by almost any meditative practice. In my clinical work, I have used "OM breathing" as a substitute for square breathing, in which the patient says the word *"OM"* during the last part of the exhale, to good effect. Similarly, breath practice or "pranayama" of Patanjali yoga, "Mantra Jap" or recitation of mantras, or passages of the Puranas that many patients have memorized can all be effective mindfulness techniques.

Conclusion

In summary, the Hindu identity is diverse and complex and may have varying contributions to a patient's anxiety disorders making it a consideration in the psychiatric formulation.

The knowledge of the timeline of different Hindu scriptures, and the messaging on anxiety disorders within this chapter, can help a psychiatrist develop confidence in navigating the nuances that the interplay of the culture-religion-caste-language quartet might bring. This chapter is intended to be a starting and a jumping-off point in approaching the topic of religion with a Hindu patient, following the patient's lead in the exploration of their beliefs, and engaging them in culturally congruent treatment planning.

References

1. Garg VS. Know the Vedas. New Delhi: Arya Pratinidhi Sabha. 2018.
2. Gurudutt. *Guru-Dutt-Bhagwat-Geeta.*
3. Ricks DA. Blunders in international business. 1st ed. Grid, Inc.; 1974.
4. Marketing_Management_in_Practice (1).
5. Truschke A. Hindu: a history. Comp Stud Soc Hist. 2023;65(2):246–71. https://doi.org/10.1017/S0010417522000524.
6. Haupt H-G. Religion and nation in Europe in the 19th century: some comparative notes 1. 2008.
7. Cousins LS. The dating of the historical Buddha: a review article. J R Asiat Soc. 1996;6(1):57–63. https://www.jstor.org/stable/25183119 (not open access).
8. Basham AL. The wonder that was India: a survey of the culture of the Indian sub-continent before the coming of the Muslims. London: Sidgwick and Jackson; 1954. Reprint, London: Picador; 2004
9. Thapar R. The later Mauryas. In: Aśoka and the decline of the Mauryas. Oxford University Press; 2012. p. 229–47.
10. Bhandare S. Numismatics and history: the Maurya-Gupta interlude in the Gangetic Plain. In: Olivelle P, editor. Between the empires: society in India 300 BCE to 400 CE. New York: Oxford University Press; 2006. p. 67–112. Oxford Scholarship Online, 2011. https://doi.org/10.1093/acprof:oso/9780195305326.003.0004.
11. Quintanilla SR. History of early stone sculpture at Mathura, ca. 150 BCE–100 CE. In: Studies in Asian art and archaeology, vol. 25. Leiden: Brill; 2007. https://brill.com/view/title/13083.
12. Thapar R. Early India: from the origins to AD 1300. Berkeley, CA: University of California Press; 2002.
13. Wink A. Al-Hind, the making of the indo-Islamic world. Leiden, New York: Brill; 1990.
14. Sastri KA, Nilakanta. A history of South India: from prehistoric times to the fall of Vijayanagar. 3rd ed. London: Oxford University Press; 1966.
15. Davidson RM. Indian esoteric Buddhism: a social history of the tantric movement. New York: Columbia University Press; 2002.
16. Grousset R. The empire of the steppes: a history of Central Asia. New Brunswick, NJ: Rutgers University Press; 1970.
17. Bhandare S. Money and the monuments: coins of the Sada dynasty of the coastal Andhra region. In: Shimada A, Willis M, editors. Amaravati: the art of an early Buddhist monument in context. London: British Museum; 2016. p. 37–45.
18. https://www.artofliving.org/us-en/meditation/meditation-for-you/cope-up-with-anxiety-with-meditation.
19. Sri Sathya Sai Speaks, vol 1, 1953–1960.
20. https://teachingsofmasters.wordpress.com/2013/02/18/osho-on-anxiety-and-desire/.
21. Weiss MG, Sharma SD, Gauk RK, Sharma JS, Desai A, Doongaji DR. Traditional concepts of mental disorder among Indian psychiatric patients: preliminary report of work in progress. Soc Sci Med. 1986;23:379.
22. Pandurangi AK, Shenoy S, Keshavan MS. Psychotherapy in the Bhagavad Gita, the Hindu scriptural text. Am J Psychiatry. 2014;171(8):827–8. https://doi.org/10.1176/appi.ajp.2013.13081092.
23. Badrinathan S, Kapur D, Kay J, Vaishnav M. Social realities of Indian Americans: results from the 2020. Indian American Attitudes Survey; 2021.
24. https://iocdf.org/faith-ocd/living-with-ocd-religious-traditions/religious-scrupulosity-in-hinduism/.
25. Bioethics of Sikh and Hindu traditions.
26. Hunt J, et al. Race and beliefs about mental health treatment among anxious primary care patients. J Nerv Ment Dis. 2013;201(3):188–95. https://doi.org/10.1097/NMD.0b013e3182845ad8.
27. Saraswati D. Rig Vedadi Bhashya Bhumika. New Delhi: Vijaykumar Govindram Hasanand; 2018.
28. Pandey SK, Pandey SK. The abnormal behaviour and psychotherapies in Atharva Veda. https://doi.org/10.13140/RG.2.2.34722.99523/1.
29. Kumar D, Chandra P. Atharvaveda Samhita. Delhi Sanskrit Academy; 1972 reprint.
30. Bhimansak Y. Sanskrit Vyakaran Shastra Ka Itihas Bhag 3. Haryana; 1973.
31. Sheth HC, Gandhi Z, Vankar GK. Anxiety disorders in ancient Indian literature. Indian J Psychiatry. 2010;52(3):289–91. https://doi.org/10.4103/0019-5545.71009.
32. Madlur A, Joshi JR. Vata—the Niyanta and Praneta of Manas. J Ayurveda Integr Med Sci. 2023;8(4):74–7. https://doi.org/10.21760/jaims.8.4.11.
33. Kulkarni A. Review of Mana and Manas Roga from classical ayurvedic texts. World J Pharm Res. 2022; https://doi.org/10.20959/wjpr20223-23290.

34. Agrawal S, Bhakuni H, Kishor Joshi R. A systemic review on Chittodvega and its management. IRJAY. 2020;3:1–11.
35. Devkarni V, editor. Ayurveda. 3rd ed. Ajmer: Paropkarni Sabha. 2003.
36. Behere PB, Das A, Yadav R, Behere AP. Ayurvedic concepts related to psychotherapy. Indian J Psychiatry. 2013;55(Spec Suppl):310. https://doi.org/10.4103/0019-5545.105556.
37. Mental health in ancient India and its relevance to modern psychiatry.
38. Basu A, Sarkar-Roy N, Majumder PP. Genomic reconstruction of the history of extant populations of India reveals five distinct ancestral components and a complex structure. Proc Natl Acad Sci USA. 2016;113(6):1594–9. https://doi.org/10.1073/pnas.1513197113.
39. Saraswati D. KashiShastrartha. Ajmer: Paropkarni Sabha; 1869.
40. Vidyalankar M. Maryada Purushottam Shriram ka Prerak Swaroop. New Delhi: Vaidik Prakashan; 2017. Available: www.thearyasamaj.org.
41. Bhawanilal. ShriKrishnaCharit. New Delhi: Govindram Hasanand; 1981.
42. Raza SJ. Hindus under the Ghaznavids. Proc Indian History Congress. 2010;71:213–25. http://www.jstor.org/stable/44147488.
43. Sethi RR, Saran P, Bhandari DR. The March of Indian history. Ranjit Printers & Publishers; 1951. p. 269.

Basic Principles and Clinical Aspects of Buddhism in Psychotherapy

Kenneth Po-Lun Fung, Soyeon Kim, and Josephine Pui-Hing Wong

Introduction

Buddhism is one of the oldest major religions in the world, with its roots tracing back to the fifth century BCE and practiced by approximately 7% of the world's population [1]. In psychology and mental health, it has become more relevant than ever with the rise in awareness and popularity of mindfulness-based psychological interventions in the West. This chapter highlights the fundamental principles and tenets of Buddhism, examines its evolution in modern societies, and considers its application to psychotherapy.

K. P.-L. Fung (✉)
Department of Psychiatry, University of Toronto, Toronto, ON, Canada

Asian Initiative in Mental Health Program, Toronto Western Hospital, Toronto, ON, Canada
e-mail: ken.fung@uhn.ca

S. Kim
Psychiatry and Behavioral Neuroscience, McMaster University, Hamilton, ON, Canada

Waypoint Research Institute, Waypoint Centre for Mental Health Care, Penetanguishene, ON, Canada
e-mail: Kims102@mcmaster.ca

J. P.-H. Wong
Daphne Cockwell School of Nursing, Faculty of Community Services, Toronto Metropolitan University, Toronto, ON, Canada
e-mail: jph.wong@torontomu.ca

Fundamental Principles and Tenets of Buddhism

Buddha Gautama reached enlightenment and delivered his first teaching on the *Turning of the Dharma Wheel* in Deer Park more than 2500 years ago [2]. Since then, the Buddha's teachings and suttas have spread and taken roots in Asia and around the world. Buddhism, as an organized religion and a philosophical system, has evolved into diverse traditions. However, the basic principles and tenets of Buddhism remain to be the Middle Way, the Four Noble Truths, and the Eightfold Path. Zen master and spiritual teacher Thich Nhat Hanh wrote in *The Heart of Buddha's Teaching* that "Buddha was not a god. He was a human being like you and me" [3] (p. 3). This awareness that all persons can reach enlightenment through the sustained disciplined practice of *connecting to* and *manifesting the Buddha nature within* lays an important foundation for understanding Buddhist philosophy and spiritual teaching.

The Four Noble Truths

The Four Noble Truths and the Noble Eightfold Path are complex principles that work together as a unifying framework of *dhamma-vinaya* (dhamma teaching and disciplined practice) to facilitate understanding ways to reach enlightenment [4].

The Four Noble Truths are as follows:

1. The First Noble Truth is that there is *dukkha*, which has loosely been translated into *suffering* in English. Dukkha refers not merely to bodily pain and psychological suffering. It also refers to everything that can produce suffering due to "the universal law of impermanence," which means that even "high and sublime states of happiness are subject to change and destruction" [4] (p. 29). In other words, when we become attached to the delusion of permanence, all states of existence can eventually become unsatisfactory and are seeds of dukkha.

2. The Second Noble Truth is *samudaya*, which refers to the origin, roots, and nature of dukkha, and lies in our human tendency towards craving and attachments. Ignorance of the true nature of things gives rise to wrong perceptions and afflictions and brings much of our suffering [3, 5]. The three poisons, or the roots of suffering, are greed, hatred, and ignorance.

3. The Third Noble Truth is *nirodha* (Pali/Sanskrit) or the cessation of suffering. Nirodha is possible when we let go of our cravings and attachments and refrain from doing things that bring suffering to ourselves and other sentient beings. The universal true nature of things, as described in the Three Dharma Seals, includes *impermanence* (nothing is static or stays the same), *non-self* (there is no separate independent self or entity), and *nirvana* (true liberation from suffering through the extinguishment of ignorance). Nhat Hanh [3] dispels the simplistic and reductionistic discourses around *life is suffering*, which may lead to misinterpretation of Buddhism as nihilistic pessimism. He points out that the impermanence of all phenomena, including suffering, makes all things possible.

4. The Fourth Noble Truth reveals the path of liberation from dukkha. The Buddha called this the *Noble Eightfold Path* of right practices: right view, right intention, right speech, right action, right livelihood, right effort, right mindfulness, and right concentration [5]. The word "right" refers to ways of practices that are beneficial to reaching nirvana [3]. The eightfold path is sometimes divided into three basic units: moral virtue (right speech, action, and livelihood), meditation (right effort, mindfulness, and concentration), and wisdom (right view and intention).

The Middle Way and the Noble Eightfold Path

The Middle Way is one of the key principles in Buddhist practice. In everyday living, the Middle Way refers to avoiding engaging in excessive sensual indulgence or painful ascetic practices, which become barriers to enlightenment when there is no integration of the two extremes [4]. The solution is the *Noble Eightfold Path* as revealed in the fourth noble truth, which offers a balanced spiritual path towards awakening. Bodhi [4] highlights the internal unity of the dhamma-vinaya (doctrine-discipline) of the Noble Eightfold Path, which includes:

1. Right view (samyag-dṛṣṭi) based on a deep understanding of the Four Noble Truths and the Three Dharma Seals, as well as the ability to distinguish wholesome roots or seeds (kushala mula) from unwholesome roots in the depth of our stored consciousness.

2. Right intention/right thinking (samyak-saṃkalpa) is aligned with right view and directs our active engagement and action in the world.

3. Right speech (samyag-vāc) is to engage in deep listening, speaking truth with compassion, and communicating in ways that bring joy and eliminate suffering.

4. Right action (samyak-karmānta) is the practice of nonviolence and includes the Buddhist principles of reverence for life, generosity, commitment to social justice, ethical sexual responsibilities, and mindful consumption.

5. Right livelihood (samyag-ājīva) is to earn our living without having to transgress our ideals of love and compassion or cause suffering in

self and others. Since we are all interconnected, right livelihood is not only a personal matter but also a part of our collective karma.

6. Right effort (samyag-vyāyāma) requires the wisdom of recognizing and differentiating *unwholesome* (unconducive to liberation) and *wholesome* (conducive to liberation) actions. There are four right efforts: (a) prevent any unwholesome action to arise; (b) once it has arisen, find a way to put an end to it; (c) cause wholesome action to arise when it has not already arisen; and (d) find ways to strengthen and sustain right action once it has arisen.

7. Right mindfulness (smriti) is returning to the present moment, staying in the here and now, paying bare attention without any judgment or interpretation, and looking deeply into the true nature of things. It enables us to experience true liberation directly in the form of understanding, compassion, and healing.

8. Right concentration (samyak-samādhi) is the cultivation of a one-pointed mind of evenness. There are two kinds of concentration: (a) in active concentration, we are fully present in the here and now and welcome whatever comes along, and (b) in selective concentration, we choose one object and focus on it without distraction. Concentration keeps our mind still and enables us to look deeply. However, to be liberated from dukkha, we must integrate right view and right intention in our practice [3, 5–7].

The Middle Way and Dependent Origination

From the perspective of metaphysics and knowledge about the truth, the Middle Way refers to avoiding the extremes of *eternalism and absolutism*, i.e., believing in the absolute and real permanence of individuals or things, or *annihilationism and nihilism*, believing that nobody and nothing really survives or exists. The solution is dependent origination (因緣生起, dependent arising/conditioned genesis/interdependent arising), *paṭiccasamuppād (pratītya-samutpāda)*, a key Buddhist doctrine that all beings and things are interdependent. Nhat Hanh [8] coined the term *interbeing* to help illuminate this principle that things come into existence or go out of existence when the conditions are right. He explains the notions of self and non-self in the contexts of time and space:

> The insight of interbeing is that nothing can exist by itself alone, that each thing exists only in relation to everything else.... Interbeing means emptiness of a separate self, however, impermanence also means emptiness of a separate self. Looking from the perspective of space, we call emptiness 'interbeing'; looking from the perspective of time, we call it 'impermanence'" (p. 45).

To illustrate the concept of interdependent arising, Thich Nhat Hanh invites us to look deeply into ordinary things in our everyday lives. For example, the existence of the flower is dependent on the non-flower elements (e.g., water, clouds, rain, sunshine), and therefore, the flower is empty of a separate self-being [9]. Emptiness is not to be misinterpreted as nonexistence; rather, it means "to be full of everything but empty of a separate existence" [10] (p. 11), that nothing exists independent of other things. The non-dualistic concept of interbeing gives clarity to the principle of the Middle Way to avoid the extreme views of nihilism and eternalism, which give rise to wrong perceptions and afflictions and perpetuate our stuckness in dukkha [10].

Socially Engaged Buddhism

Drawing from Buddha's teachings, Nhat Hanh [3] emphasizes that true liberation from dukkha comes from our full engagement with the world and direct practices of the Noble Eightfold Path, which can be supported by taking refuge in the *Three Jewels*—the Buddha (the teacher), the Dharma (teachings), and the Sangha (the community). Taking refuge is not an idea, a belief, or a proclamation. It is a practice to "cultivate mindfulness, concentration, and insight" that enables us to deal with challenging situations, maintain our mindful stability, and gain clarity on the true nature of our struggles [11] (p. 16). The Three Jewels, together with the right view of interdependent arising and interbeing, are key principles that inform socially engaged Buddhism, drawing on Buddhist principles as critique and corrective to the social, political, economic, and environmental problems of the modern world [12]. For example, Harris [13] coined the term "eco-Buddhism," which describes a movement that views Buddhism as intrinsically environmentalist. Dalai Lama furthered this view linking the congruence between Buddhist and environmental ethics [14].

Buddhism can be seen to potentially have a powerful positive impact on society. With this macro interdependent lens, we will provide an overview and a sampling of the impact of social, historical, cultural, and political context on the development of Buddhism from a modern global perspective.

Buddhism in Modern Contexts

Originating from the Ganges valley, India, in the sixth century BCE, Buddhism has spread throughout Asia, resulting in three main branches (Fig. 10.1): Theravada (Southeast Asia including Sri Lanka, Burma, Thailand, Laos, and Cambodia), Mahayana (East Asia including China, Korea, and Japan), and Vajrayana, a subsect of Mahayana (Northern Asia including Tibet, Nepal, Bhutan, and Mongolia). All three branches are based on the Four Noble Truths, but differ in focus and emphasis. Throughout the centuries, Buddhism has been infused into other social and cultural facets in Asia, transforming bidirectionally [15]. For example, Buddhism has vastly influenced Chinese society and philosophy, including Daoism and Confucianism's philosophical systems embedded in Chinese culture, and vice versa [15]. In the past two centuries, Buddhism has expanded beyond Asia, spreading to Europe and North America, hybridizing with the traditions of Western modernity, including Christianity, Judaism, and Western psychology, and has become a global religion [16]. With remarkable adaptability, Buddhism has taken on new forms and blended with other religions and cultures in modern societies.

Mahayana Buddhism

Mahayana, "Great Vehicle," accepts scriptures and teachings of early Buddhism as well as those not included by Theravada Buddhism, such as the sutras. Mahayana Buddhism is practiced mostly in China, Korea, Vietnam, and Japan. Its goal is the liberation of all sentient beings. Mahayana proclaims the possibility of universal salvation, including the path of the bodhisattva to become enlightened, and in this process, those on the path nearing enlightenment voluntarily and compassionately stay in Samsara to help all living beings until there is no more suffering. Its teachings include the theory of emptiness, the Yogacara tradition of Buddhist philosophy and psychology, and *Buddha nature*, the inherent potential for any sentient being to become the Buddha.

Buddhism in Modern China

It is estimated that about 1 in 5 people in China, or about 240 million people, is Buddhist, making Buddhism the largest institutionalized religion in China, the country with the largest number of Buddhists worldwide. It is not uncommon for many Chinese people to practice a mix of multiple religions, including Buddhism, Daoism, and folk religion, which have cross-fertilized each other in their development over the years. Even for those not formally engaging in Buddhist religious practice, Buddhism has been infused in Chinese cultural patterns of thoughts, language, and actions [17]. For example, it is not uncommon for Buddhist terms such as *Kuhai* ("the bitter sea"), meaning life's difficulties, to be used in the common vocabulary. Buddhism has been restricted, controlled, and persecuted by the communist government and was nearly eradicated during the Cultural Revolution (1966–1976) [18, 19]. While there continues to be regulatory control, there has been a revival of the religion since, at times, enjoying active support from the government, as Buddhist charitable organizations and temples provide services to vulnerable populations, and Buddhism continues to have major cultural and spiritual influence and significance.

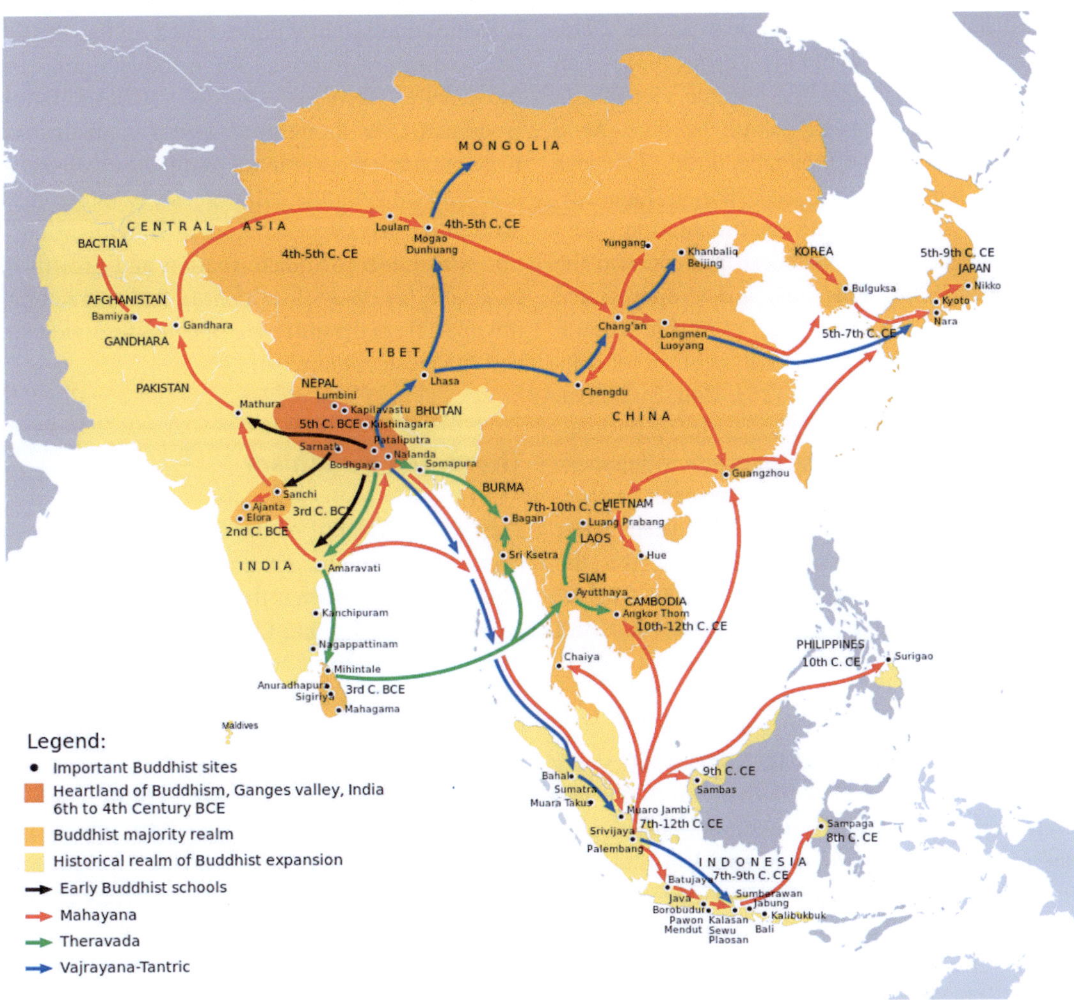

Fig. 10.1 [CC BY-SA 3.0, via Wikimedia Commons] The expansion of Buddhism, originated from India in the sixth century BCE to the rest of Asia until the present

Buddhism in Modern Japan

Buddhism represents Japan's largest religion [20]. Buddhism is a vibrant part of Japanese people's daily life nowadays as it is considered a cultural heritage shown not only in its faith and doctrine but also in Japanese art (e.g., temple architecture and the Buddhist images of the Asuka, Hakuho, and Tempyo eras) [20, 21]. From its introduction in 552 AD through the Nara, Heian, and Tokugawa periods, as a state religion, Buddhism flourished under the Shogunate regime, and various Buddhist sects were formed in Japan, with newer schools emerging during the Kamakura period (1185–1333). As Japan began modernization and industrialization in the Meiji period (1968–1912), adopting Western capitalistic civilization, Buddhism was severely persecuted with the policy of *"haibutsu kishaku"* (abolishing and demolishing Buddhism) [21]. To increase fit with the modern nation-state, legal reform, new lay movements, and ritual adaptations were undertaken [22]. Currently, *Jōdo Buddhism* (浄土教) is the largest sect, a branch of *Pure Land Buddhism*, with about 22 million followers [23]. Other large sects include *Nichiren*, *Shingon*, and *Zen*, with 11, 5.5, and 5.3 million followers, respectively. For the West, Zen is particularly well-known. It originated in China during the Tang dynasty, known as the *Chán School* (Chánzong 禪宗) [24]. From China, Chán spread south to Vietnam and became Vietnamese *Thiền*, northeast to Korea to become *Seon Buddhism*, and east to Japan, becoming Japanese *Zen*, as Chán is pronounced Zen in Japanese, meaning "contemplation" or "meditation." Zen Buddhism has had a profound influence on the Japanese. Military class and artists appreciated its doctrine, and it was a focal point for samurai culture and art from the twelfth century until its abolition in the Meiji era [25]. Zen Buddhism precipitated the integration of Chinese philosophy, especially Neo-Confucianism, into Japanese culture and commercial endeavors, such as shipping lines that controlled trade between Japan and China. Zen Buddhism was introduced to the Western world in the 1800s by a Zen Master, Suzuki, and has gained much popularity in North America and Europe [24].

Buddhism in Modern Korea

Buddhism was introduced to Korea 1700 years ago during the Three Kingdoms period and has been infused into Korean culture, art, philosophy, and mindset as a central philosophical tradition. From the Three Kingdoms period until the Chosun Dynasty, Buddhism was the dominant political and ruling ideology. Throughout the colonial era, Buddhist teaching and values were infused as a pillar doctrine for the unified nation, considered a protective force from foreign enemies and natural disasters (i.e., *Hoguk Bulgyo*, Buddhism for national protection; patriotic Buddhism). For example, Buddhist monks participated in and led Korean liberation initiatives from Japanese colonialism [26, 27]. Korean Buddhism suffered from the pressure to cooperate with Western modernity and Japanese colonization (religious invasion) [28]. Despite these challenges, Korean Buddhism has remained resilient and a spiritual resource [29]. For example, in protest against the Japanese regime's control and to overcome challenges with modern ideology, *Minjung Bulgyo* (People's Buddhism) emerged. *Minjung Bulgyo* continues to influence modern Korean society as a form of socially engaged Buddhism by championing climate

activities and social welfare based on the altruistic teachings of Buddha [30]. Another significant movement, *Hoetong Bulgyo* (Consolidation Buddhism), is thought to infuse a distinctive Korean characteristic in its preference to harmonize and consolidate different sects rather than promoting divisiveness. Korean Buddhism continues to undergo transformation and growth in its search for distinctive identity and characteristics apart from the influence of Chinese Buddhism and Japanese colonialism [30].

Theravada Buddhism

Theravada, "School of the Elders," is the oldest tradition of the three main Buddhist branches. Theravada Buddhism is the official religion of Sri Lanka, Myanmar, and Cambodia and the dominant religion in Laos and Thailand. Like Mahayana, the central Theravada Buddhist doctrine includes the Four Noble Truths and Eightfold Path and concepts such as karma and rebirth, which teaches that those not fully awakened will be reborn and karma will determine the life experience of the present life in Samsara. Theravada tends to focus on the monastic pursuit of Nirvana compared to Mahayana's focus on the Bodhisattva ideal.

Buddhism in Modern Thailand

Since the third century BCE, Buddhism has deeply influenced Thai culture and society. Nearly 95% of the population is Theravada Buddhist. They often visit a temple or attend Buddhist ceremonies and worship the Triple Gems: the Buddha, the Dharma, and Sanha [31]. Thailand has the second largest Buddhist population in the world after China and has two official monastic orders: Dhammayuttika Nikiya and Maha Nikaya. Thai Buddhism has faced significant challenges and has revolutionized the Theravada Buddhism tradition in the context of political changes in the modern era [32, 33]. Modernization of Thai Buddhism began in the early twentieth century when King Mongkut, a monk himself, founded a new order called Dhammayuttika Nikaya [34]. With the reforms, more strict disciplines, such as not using money or storing food, were applied; superstitious and folk elements were removed; and the Thai sangha became more centralized and controlled by the state. However, some of these reformations have also been criticized for linkages with politics and nationalist ideology, diminishing their revolutionary vision [33]. Dhammayuttika Nikaya accounts for less than 10% of the country's monks but holds the most political power. In the late twentieth century, with various movements and reforms, including by the Bhikkhu Buddhadasa, Buddhist meditation gained popularity among laypeople beyond the monastics [35].

Vajrayana Buddhism

Vajrayana, "diamond or thunderbolt" (*vajra* in Sanskrit), emphasizes its efficient and expedient path to enlightenment. Vajrayana originated in northern India around the fifth century CE and spread across the Himalayan region, including Tibet, Nepal, and Mongolia. Vajrayana, derived from Mahayana Buddhism, shares some common views with Mahayana. While it upholds the Mahayana bodhisattva ideal, tantric practices and esoteric rituals, like mantric formulas and incantations, are central to achieving physical, mental, and spiritual breakthroughs.

Buddhism in Tibet

Tibetan and Nepalese Buddhism are based on the Mahayana (Vajrayana) conceptual foundation that emphasizes universal altruism [36]. They are also characterized as tantric (e.g., deity yoga, Six Dharmas of Naropa) and highly ritualistic. For example, they focus on ritual practices involving visualizations of deities, repetition of mantras, and hand movements (mudra) to bring deities' power [37]. Tibet became independent under the 13th Dalai Lama government in 1912 until it was annexed by China in 1950. The most significant challenge for Tibetan Buddhism was the Chinese rule, which resulted in the exile of the Dalai Lama and 100,000 people, including a large proportion of Tibetan high clergy, in 1954 [38]. The

Chinese Cultural Revolution (1966–1976) further oppressed Tibetan Buddhist tradition and destroyed monasteries and temples until, in the 1980s, religious liberalization was initiated. Despite oppression, Tibetan Buddhists persisted in attempting to revive the tradition [36, 37]. In the 1960s, during his exile, Dalai Lama proposed reforming Tibetan Buddhism, focusing on universalism, ecumenism, and the rational character of Buddhism. In the twenty-first century, through public teachings of the Tibetan lamas, Tibetan Buddhism has spread worldwide in countries such as Mongolia, Nepal, Siberia, Russia, North America, and Europe and continues to stand [38].

Buddhism in Modern Western Societies

Unlike the Asian view of Buddhism as a religion, ritual, cultural tradition, philosophy, and way of life, Buddhism in the West is perhaps perceived as "Eastern wisdom" [39] and as a way to achieve mental and spiritual fulfillment [40]. In North America, Buddhism was first introduced by Buddhist teachers and missionaries such as Soyen Shaku, a Rinzai Zen master from Japan, in 1893 at the World's Parliament of Religions. A few years later, D.T. Suzuki, his disciple, came to promote Rinzai Zen Buddhism, which gained popularity in North America [24, 41]. Amidst Western modernization characterized by state capitalism, Buddhism was regarded as a philosophy for "sober, compassionate, disciplined, mercantile, and literate polities" [40].

Western psychological adoption of Buddhism tends to focus mostly on secular aspects that address perceived psychological needs, such as reducing stress, regulating emotions, and achieving mental well-being. For example, Ekman and Friesen [42] indicate that people can gain more control over their emotions by becoming aware of their automatic appraisals through Buddhist meditation (p. 74). Kabat-Zinn [43] further defined secular mindfulness as a practice that involves focusing on the present moment while acknowledging and accepting one's feelings, thoughts, and bodily sensations without judgment. Over the past two decades, Buddhism's perspective on emotions and meditation's benefits in regulating emotions have gained popularity in America [42]. Mounting scientific research has demonstrated its benefits, from fortifying the immune system to reducing stress and anxiety to improving overall well-being, as mindfulness-based programs have been employed to mitigate emotional challenges [44–46].

Another active function of Buddhism in Western society, as described earlier, is socially engaged Buddhism, coined by Thich Nhat Hanh and Gary Snyder in the 1960s [47]. It incorporates the practice of embodying the living bodhisattva ideals, including dana (charity) and seva (social service) [41]. Socially engaged Buddhism "extends Buddhism's focus from individual suffering to the suffering of unjust structures and systems and aims to achieve both individual and collective liberation" [48]. Gleig [48] further points out the changes in the demographics of Buddhists and the increased focus on inter-racial/cultural connections to address colonialism, racism, and intersectionality in modern Buddhism worldwide. In the modern world, technologies such as Internet-based platforms (e.g., social media) facilitate connections across countries and organizations, allowing the development of new modalities/formats of Buddhist practices. For example, an engaged Buddhist organization, the Buddhist Peace Fellowship (BPF), was founded in the United States in 1978. BPF actively addresses issues such as structural racism and anti-blackness in the United States based on Buddhist doctrine [49]. Further, connections between engaged Buddhists and Native American Indigenous communities have been fostered and strengthened in the modern era [48].

Is there a distinct Western Buddhism? This question was raised at a conference in Stockholm in 1993 [50], and the conclusion, consistent with general Buddhist philosophy, was that there is no distinctive "European Buddhism." Modern Buddhism can be approached from a global perspective, reflecting the transcultural flow and contextual conditions (national, geographical, social, historical, political, etc.). Similarly, the Dalai Lama indicated that "Buddhism naturally takes new forms in each culture," while Zen master Thich Nhat Hanh said, "The forms of Buddhism must change so that the essence of Buddhism remains unchanged. This essence consists of living principles that cannot bear any specific formulation" [51]. Gleig [48] highlights the unique contextual influence on modern Buddhism's evolution and transformation in our society. Modern societies have evolved based on their unique political, economic, and sociocultural contexts, and Buddhism adapts to society's unique needs based on its doctrine. Western modernity, characterized by a capitalistic, Eurocentric, stressed-out, and multitasking culture, has adapted Buddhism to provide an individual, science-based, secular meditation rather than traditional, spiritual, and religious experience. An American Tibetan Buddhist, Lama Surya Das, envisioned that the future American Buddhism would encompass (1) dharma without dogma; (2) a lay-oriented sangha; (3) a meditation-based and experiential tradition; (4) gender equality; (5) a nonsectarian tradition; (6) an essentialized and simplified tradition; (7) an egalitarian, democratic, and nonhierarchical tradition; (8) a psychologically astute and rational tradition; (9) an experimental, innovative, inquiry-based tradition; and (10) a socially informed and engaged tradition [52].

Buddhism and Psychotherapy

As there are diverse schools of Buddhism to draw from, aspects of Buddhism, as a religion, philosophy, psychology, or a set of meditative practices, may all be potentially usefully integrated into psychotherapy. This may vary depending on the training, cultural and religious background, and philosophical orientation of the therapist; the client's background; the problem being addressed; and the psychotherapy model being used.

The potential of Buddhism to have implications in psychotherapy dates back to classical psychoanalysis since the work of Carl Jung [53]. For example, while there are significant differences, his proposal of the controversial collective unconscious, i.e., an unconscious shared by all humans, has correspondence to the store consciousness in Yogacara Buddhism, in that there is a common vision of expanding beyond an individual autonomous focus towards a shared collective perspective. A number of psychotherapists have also attempted to integrate Buddhism into psychotherapy, such as psychodynamic therapy by Mark Epstein. Mindfulness-based stress reduction (MBSR) marks a pivotal moment in which mindfulness was utilized as a secular practice for chronic pain and in Western psychology [43]. The third-wave psychotherapies, such as mindfulness-based cognitive therapy (MBCT), dialectical behavioral therapy (DBT), and acceptance and commitment therapy (ACT), are all evidence-based approaches invoking acceptance and mindfulness principles and practices [54]. In particular, ACT, one of the most versatile transdiagnostic and non-pathologizing psychological interventions that have shown benefits to clinical and nonclinical populations, has close correspondence with Buddhism [55–57]. Further, ACT has inspired other related therapies consistent with Buddhism, such as mode deactivation therapy (MDT), which draws from ACT and schema therapy [58]. The relationship between ACT and Buddhism will be examined in more detail.

Buddhism and Acceptance and Commitment Therapy (ACT)

Acceptance and commitment therapy (ACT) is based on relational frame theory (RFT), a behavioral theory about how we come to acquire and develop language (and hence cognition) and its resulting impact on how we function daily in the world [59]. From a Buddhist perspective, it is a theory about how we come to form attachments in our minds as thoughts and networks of meaning; how they can acquire functional properties (e.g., evoke desire, fear, aversion) and become powerfully salient for us; and then, based on our learning history, how they can functionally impact on our everyday behaviors, which include not only overt actions but also feelings and thoughts.

RFT, through deictic relational framing, accounts for the process of forming an illusory autonomous "self," learned developmentally through our capacity for perspective-taking, i.e., learning to differentiate and discriminate between "I" vs. "you," "mine" vs. "yours," "here" vs. "there," and "now" vs. then, through multiple

exemplar training [59]. Like other relational framings, this process is reinforced over the years with further attachment to "self-knowledge" through basic underlying behavioral processes, namely mutual entailment, combinatorial entailment, and transformation of stimulus functions. In Yogacara and Zen Buddhism, this process of creating a self is similar to the emergence of the *manas-vijnana*, or mind consciousness, which arises from the perception of mental objects, seeds in the store consciousness:

> The nature of manas is delusion. It is born from the blocks of ignorance that are present as seeds in our store consciousness. It is always there, grasping the idea of self and the idea of nonself. It is always discriminating: this is me, this is mine, this is self; that is not me, that is not mine, that is not self. With or without our conscious awareness, that is the work of manas, and it works continuously [6] (pp. 98–99).

In both RFT and Buddhism, the illusion of a distinct self arises as a natural process without necessarily presupposing a true separate autonomous self.

RFT is embedded in functional contextualism (FC), or radical behaviorism, a philosophy of science, and its goal is to help predict and influence behaviors using an empirical approach [59]. Its root metaphor is an "act in the context", meaning that any life event and actions cannot be understood separately from its context, including current and past events, situations, and environment. The truth criterion is workability rather than striving for some objective truth. FC is based on American pragmatism, which is highly informed and influenced by Buddhism. In addition to mindfulness, the importance of realizing that we have a limited view of the larger context, including our history (i.e., past learning or habits and resulting karma), and the priority given to present experience over thoughts and dogmatic beliefs are distinct characteristics of Buddhism and FC, and hence ACT. Thus, ACT therapists do not necessarily emphasize the need to seek more objective truths as in many other therapies (which may often paradoxically deepen stuckness in our biased delusions) but seek to encourage the patient to mindfully reflect on their present experience and contingencies and make contextual changes towards "workability" as a criterion of success.

Like Buddhism in normalizing and embracing our natural state of pain and suffering, ACT aims to increase psychological flexibility through the training of six core psychological processes or skills [59]. Through **defusion**, we seek to increase our capacity to treat our thoughts as mere thoughts rather than objective reality. This includes our internalized rules, judgments, and reasons, regardless of how logically sound they are, i.e., there is no distinction between rational and distorted thoughts in this context. **Acceptance** is the willingness to make room for our internal experiences, including our thoughts and feelings, regardless of whether they are labeled positive or negative. **Contact with the present moment** helps us not to get stuck in our minds, ruminating about the past or overwhelmed by a feared future. **Self-as-context** offers an alternative to self-as-content, in which we become identified and locked into labels and concepts about ourselves, as they are merely thoughts, ideas, concepts, and self-narratives. **Values** are freely chosen qualities that we believe in and serve as a guide for the life we want to lead and become the yardstick for "workability." **Committed action** refers to persistent behavior patterns in the service of values, even in the face of internal obstacles.

While there are common techniques, metaphors, worksheets, and therapeutic strategies, ACT can be flexibly applied in a variety of different ways as long as the ACT processes are being advanced. It can be applied as a short-term or long-term intervention and as individual therapy or group intervention. To further our discussion, composite disguised cases will illustrate how some of the ACT principles consistent and informed by Buddhist teachings may be integrated into psychotherapy.

Case Vignettes

Mr. Chan was a Chinese-Canadian man presenting with depression. He felt distressed being caught in an ongoing conflict between his wife and their adult daughter, Anna, who was born in Canada. His wife had long-standing severe clinical depression, which had improved somewhat with treatment but remained symptomatic. For years, he played the role of the "good cop" to mediate the relationship between his wife and daughter. He had been telling Anna not to take her mom's critical comments and temper personally. He has also asked his wife to reflect on what it would be like if Anna were to cut off their relationship. In a recent family outing, however, Mr. Chan blew up after years of restraint, and Anna was angry at both of them. He began to have passive suicidal thoughts and lost interest in everything.

Initially, Mr. Chan felt demoralized and that all his efforts over the years seemed meaningless and futile, and he was left with uncertainty about what to do, utterly directionless. He talked about feeling "numb" towards Anna. One night, Anna went out to a family dinner as a sign of reconciliation and agreed to stay overnight at their home, avoiding a late-night commute back. However, she refused to sleep in her old room but chose to sleep on the couch. Although he glossed over this incident in passing, we explored his supposed feeling of "numbness." He had a wealth of feelings about his love for his daughter and wished she could feel at home at their house again. He recalled tearfully how he was holding on to his daughter's hand when she was in her teens, both of them mouthwatering and eyeing hotdogs at a street stand but unable to afford to buy them. He then vowed to do his best to provide for his family. He and his wife worked day and night as immigrants and had not been able to spend much time with their daughter, and at times, lost their temper with her. We talked about how he might communicate that with his daughter, acknowledging language and cultural differences between traditional high-context Chinese and low-context Western communication, where emotions are expressed explicitly. Exploration and loosening of these internalized cultural rules and scripts help elucidate their problems communicating and the courage it would take to break through their habitual way of communicating.

Regarding Mr. Chan's feelings of powerlessness and giving up, we examined how, with his strong value on family, he focused intently on changing his wife and daughter's behaviors over the years and defined his success based on the state of their problematic relationship. It was as if he was coming across a huge tree obstructing his path, and he had relentlessly been attacking it to no avail, especially as the tree had strong roots developing over many years. As he considered this, he began to see the alternative of going around the tree rather than insisting on going through it. If the tree was no longer treated as an obstacle, he could be watering it with compassion, which might bear different kinds of fruit. We discussed the value of his actions towards his family members as being embedded in the process of his actions rather than the outcomes and how the value of compassion towards his wife, daughter, and himself can sustain his continuing efforts to reach out rather than withdraw.

In further exploration of his self-image of impotence, it emerged that Mr. Chan's father died when he was only an infant, and his younger sister drowned at the age of 6, both tragedies he could not stop. His mother blamed his older sister Lin for his sister's death, which caused a rift between Lin and Mr. Chan. As we enlarged the focus beyond his daughter and wife, we explored how he might be able to take the initiative to reach out to Lin with compassion, another area of his life in which he felt utterly powerless. The work on compassion and interdependence was gradually expanded to include his relationships with his friends and the local Chinese immigrant community.

Anna was a 38-year-old woman, born in Canada, an IT specialist, living with her same-sex partner, and presenting with anxiety, chronic low-grade depression, and occasional cutting. Growing up, she found her mother's depression and volatile emotions frightening, as her mother often beat her with a bamboo stick. Otherwise, she hardly saw her parents. Her last therapist had told her that her parents were abusive, toxic, racist, and homophobic, and she was encouraged to establish clear boundaries with them. She was strongly encouraged to get in touch with her anger at her parents, but she was ambivalent about this and quit therapy.

We initially began with the idea that deliberately getting in touch with her anger or other emotions may or may not be necessary or helpful. With validation, she talked about her traumatic childhood experiences at home. At school, she described being envious of other "beautiful blonde hair and blue-eyed" students who seemed to have loving parents. She was ashamed of her poor, non-English-speaking parents and her Chinese cultural identity, fearing that authorities might take them away from her. She felt alone and isolated until she made some Asian friends at school. We observed her full spectrum of emotions without judgment, noticing the coming and going of intense emotions, from sadness to fear, and finally, her ambivalence about anger. She felt that she "should" feel angry, as per her previous therapist, and yet, she felt that her anger would be destructive, like "lava," and that anger at her parents would be against her personal and cultural values.

With mindfulness practice, we began to explore the idea of being able to have "transformed" emotions, including justified anger. This suddenly clicked. She previously visualized herself as a small, helpless child hugging herself in the dark. Now, this image of her was enveloped by "transformed anger" as a circle of fire, not to burn others but to bring illumination, strength, and safety. Further, recognizing that in this present moment, she was actually older than her mother many years ago, the aversive function of the memories of her mother as a figure of terror also changed, becoming less intimidating. Anna visualized welcoming her mother into the ring with her, having compassion for her mother, who was suffering from depression. Anna began to see hope for reconciling with her parents.

Beyond family issues, Anna began to defuse from internalized inferiority about her Asian culture and sexuality and felt empowered to have justified and transformed anger about systemic and internalized racism and homophobia, especially as she considered how this similarly had affected other children. Instead of fearing that this anger would lead to violent protests, she began to consider other ways of championing social change towards compassion and tolerance, embracing her hybrid cultural values from the East and West and having a sense of self-as-context that is neither bounded by narrow self-identities and narratives nor by the confusion in trying to find the elusive absolute "true" self.

Case Reflection

At this point, it is perhaps helpful for the reader to reflect on the two cases presented and any emerging perceptions.

1. What resonates most with you … as a therapist? … a child? … a parent? … an Asian/non-Asian? … a member identified with a majority or minority group in society? … an ACT/non-ACT therapist? … a Buddhist/non-Buddhist?
2. Consider next the kind of questions that may naturally arise with the two cases. Missing details that would seem to matter to you. Why would they matter?
3. Are there any evaluations and judgments that may arise, such as whether the cases are interesting or not, well written or not, helpful or not, etc.?
4. Finally, how may the cases be useful in your own personal or professional life? Are the cases about ACT, Buddhism, or anything else, such as alternative ways of interpreting and perceiving the stories?

Case Discussion

As alluded to throughout this chapter and more specifically by the preceding reflective section, the most relevant aspects of ACT and Buddhism to any therapist are, first and foremost, how they are perceived, understood, embodied, and utilized by the therapist and the patient. Here, we present one of an infinite number of ways to formulate the cases.

The most challenging aspect of both cases was the initial engagement. Mr. Chan had always resisted psychological treatment, seeing himself as the rational anchor of the family, while his wife was the identified mental health patient. Anna, more Westernized, embraced psychotherapy and yet found embedded Western values in therapy evoked ambivalence, inner conflict, and, eventually, disillusionment. They both opened up to the therapist and reported sharing experiences in ways they did not think possible, breaking out of their habitual ways of behaving, just as it may be possible for streams and rivers to find new channels to flow through if we explore and dig together, extending the Buddhist metaphor for habits and our conditioned actions in life.

The empirical literature has emphasized the importance of common factors in psychotherapy, particularly the importance of building a therapeutic alliance, which includes alignment of the therapeutic goals and tasks, as well as forming a bond. One key question is then how ACT and Buddhist principles may enhance this. There may not be one answer, but it includes having a compassionate, nonjudgmental stance and a nonpathologizing approach towards viewing suffering; being present in the relationship; connecting with the shared humanity; and maintaining hope by not becoming overly attached to the apparent manifested dilemma and problem. These qualities are not exclusive to mindfulness, ACT, or Buddhism but are strengthened immeasurably by them. From this perspective, the invitation to become mindful is not only a technique to teach the patient, nor a discipline residing solely in the therapist, but also arises in a compassionate therapeutic relationship in each **present moment**.

At the heart of **defusion** and **acceptance** in ACT is to be able to let go of the attachments to our rules, judgments, reasons, and stories, which is reflected in our mired attempts to categorize, label, judge, evaluate, make sense of, and solve, even when they are not helpful. This may include Mr. Chan, Anna, or even Anna's previous therapist's labeling and evaluation of each family member, their actions, thoughts, and emotions. Even as each new detail emerged that "explained" the narrative (e.g., Mr. Chan's and Anna's trauma, cultural and generational differences), they need to be held on to lightly and appreciated for their function, rather than literally, as they were but a part of a web of interconnected karma or causes and effects.

Related to defusion and acceptance and consistent with RFT, the Buddhist concept of non-dualism can facilitate these ACT processes. We tend to see things dualistically: good or bad, success or failure, sick or healthy, exists or not exists, etc. Buddhism transcends dualism and opens up all possibilities, such that one may appreciate something as good, bad, both, neither, and all (i.e., encompassing other seemingly unrelated phenomena). Rather than seeking to be consistent in absolute terms, a non-dualistic perspective allows the therapist and patient to explore all these possibilities in different contexts openly. Consider the binary concepts that the two cases seemed to present, e.g., Mr. Chan's efforts to change someone else (wife and daughter's relationship) are important/futile; expression of emotions in the family is good/bad/necessary/unnecessary; Mr. Chan is a success/failure; Mr. Chan's relationship with his sister is relevant/irrelevant to his relationship with his daughter and wife; Anna's anger is good/bad; Anna's relationship with her mother is related/unrelated to structural racism; and Anna's therapist's Western values or her parents' traditional Asian values are helpful/harmful.

Integral to a non-dualistic perspective is interdependence, i.e., there is no pure absolute, any one thing that exists independent of all other things; things are also impermanent. This readily applies in our therapeutic work with emotions, relationships, and problems.

For Mr. Chan, the moment of joy from the birth of Anna gave rise to his wish to hang on to joyful relationships in the family, which gave rise simultaneously to suffering, from the fear of losing this relationship to his frustration with how their relationships have evolved, to his hopelessness in inevitable conflicts. Depending on the context, his family values motivated him towards self-sacrifice while also bringing him pain and suffering and, at one point, the wish to give up everything. The possibility of transformation from joy to suffering and vice versa is powerful. In Buddhism, **mindfulness** enables us to intentionally grow wholesome seeds (e.g., compassion and love) and transform unwholesome seeds (e.g., anger, hate). Anna's anger came from a place of hurt. Anger can be seen as "bad" and to be avoided as one of the three poisons in Buddhism, or "good" as justified moral outrage or "secondary" emotions and to be in touch within certain schemas in Western psychology or, in Anna's case, to be transformed as a source of courage and compassion for herself, her mother, and all other children who might experience the same.

Interdependence also gives insight into the appreciation of no-self or emptiness. In ACT, the **self-as-context** process helped free Mr. Chan's and Anna's self-narratives as impotent victims. But as described, it also enlarged the scope of concern from the self to relationship with others in the immediate family and beyond. The two stories seem to relate to one another, expanding the context and scope of cause and effect. Yet, it is uncommon, except with family therapists, for traditional individual psychotherapists to work with both father and daughter as described due to various reasonable rationales (aside—Were they really related? Does this matter in disguised cases?). Even beyond this, both cases are related to social and cultural issues, from the plight of immigrants to structural racism that impacts identity, values, and worldview (aside—Is this the therapist's concern? If there is socially engaged Buddhism, should therapists be socially engaged?)

This brings us finally to the **values** and **committed action**. While we continuously work to detach and undermine everything, at the same time, the Middle Way guides us against moral relativism and grounds us in our values and actions. From a Buddhist perspective, living and operating in the conventional truth (vs. the ultimate truth) allow us to reorient Mr. Chan and Anna towards their values (of love and compassion) in a deeper way, with an expanded scope and taking pragmatic actions in more effective workable ways (or skillful means in Buddhism) in their lives, interwoven with their families, communities, and the society at large.

Concluding Reflections

The practice of psychotherapy is a modern Western secular endeavor aimed at alleviating psychological suffering and promoting psychological growth and (self)-actualization. Buddhism is an ancient Eastern religion aimed at alleviating human suffering and promoting spiritual growth and (self)less enlightenment. They both continue to evolve across time, space, and contexts. In many ways and at many levels, they cannot be more similar and/or more different. As in all things, they "inter-are."

The mental health practitioner, regardless of discipline and background, may find benefits in exploring the integration of Buddhist wisdom into their personal lives and professional practice. There is an important caveat in recognizing a Western individualistic and low-context cultural worldview bias, including the construct of the psychological self, that contrasts with a more collectivistic and interdependent vision of Buddhism. A piecemeal decontextualized understanding and use of Buddhism and its practices may potentially lead to more harm and suffering. Skillful use, on the other hand, may lead to psychological and/or spiritual growth for the individual, family, community, and humanity.

This chapter provides the reader with a particular instance of a glimpse into the potential relationship between psychotherapy and Buddhism. It is but a knock on the door. We hope that it will lead to doors being opened, connections being made, and possibilities being realized.

References

1. Hackett C, et al. The global religious landscape. Washington, DC: Pew Research Center; 2012. p. 80.
2. Gadjin N, Blum ML. The Buddha's life as parable for later Buddhist thought. Eastern Buddhist. 1991;24(2):1–32.
3. Nhat Hanh T. The heart of Buddha's teaching. Parallax Press; 1998.
4. Bodhi B, Truths N. Noble path: the heart essence of the Buddha's original teachings. Simon and Schuster; 2023.
5. Bodhi B. The noble eightfold path: way to the end of suffering. Pariyatti Publishing; 2006.
6. Nhat Hanh T. Understanding our mind. Parallax Press; 2006.
7. Nhat Hanh T. Awakening of the heart: essential Buddhist sutras and commentaries. Parallax Press; 2011.
8. Nhat Hanh T. The other shore: a new translation of the heart sutra with commentaries. Parallax Press; 2017.
9. Holst MA. "To be is to inter-be": Thich Nhat Hanh on interdependent arising. J World Philos. 2021;6(2):17–30.
10. Nhat Hanh T. The art of living: peace and freedom in the here and now. HarperCollins; 2017.
11. Nhat Hanh T. Interbeing: the 14 mindfulness trainings of engaged Buddhism. Parallax Press; 2020.
12. Makransky J. Applied Buddhism: past and present. Can J Buddhist Stud. 2022;17:8–32.
13. Harris I. How environmentalist is Buddhism? Religion. 1991;21(2):101–14.
14. Lama HD. A Tibetan Buddhist perspective on spirit in nature. In: Spirit and nature. Princeton University Press; 1992. p. 109–23.
15. Garfield JL. Buddhism and modernity. In: The Buddhist world. Routledge; 2015. p. 294.
16. McMahan DL. Buddhism in the modern world. Routledge; 2012.
17. Fisher G. Buddhism in China and Taiwan. In: Buddhism in the modern world. Routledge; 2012. p. 69–88.
18. Berkwitz SC. Buddhism in world cultures: comparative perspectives. ABC-CLIO; 2006.
19. Welch H. The Buddhist revival in China. Harvard University Press; 1996.
20. Covell SG. Buddhism in Japan. In: Buddhism in world cultures: comparative perspectives. ABC-CLIO; 2006. p. 219.
21. Ienaga S. Japan's modernization and Buddhism. In: Contemporary religions in Japan. International Institute for the Study of Religions; 1965. p. 1–41.
22. Curley MAM. Buddhism in modern Japan. In: The Wiley Blackwell companion to east and inner Asian Buddhism. John Wiley & Sons Inc.; 2014. p. 445–65.
23. Steinilber-Oberlin E. The Buddhist sects of Japan: their history, philosophical doctrines and sanctuaries, vol. 84. Routledge; 2010.
24. Van der Braak A. Zen spirituality in a secular age; Charles Taylor and Zen Buddhism in the west. Stud Spiritual. 2008;18:39–60.
25. Suzuki DT, Barrett W. Zen Buddhism: selected writings of DT Suzuki. Harmony; 1996.
26. Park P. Buddhism in Korea: decolonization, nationalism, and modernization. In: Buddhism in world cultures. ABC-CLIO; 2006. p. 195–218.
27. Park P. A Korean Buddhist response to modernity: the doctrinal underpinning of Han Yongun's (1879-1944) reformist thought. Seoul J Korean Stud. 2007;20(1):21–44.
28. Kyŏng-Hun P. Buddhism in modern Korea. Korea J. 1981;21(8):32–40.

29. Shim J-R. Buddhism and the modernization process in Korea. Social Compass. 2000;47(4):541–8.
30. Uttam J. Between Buddhist 'self-enlightenment' and 'artificial intelligence': South Korea emerging as a new balancer. Religions. 2023;14(2):150.
31. Khantipalo B. Buddhism explained: an introduction to the teachings of Lord Buddha with reference to the belief in and practice of those teachings and their realization. Thai Watana Panich Press; 1970.
32. Keyes CF. Buddhist politics and their revolutionary origins in Thailand. Int Polit Sci Rev. 1989;10(2):121–42.
33. McCargo D. Buddhism, democracy and identity in Thailand. Democratization. 2004;11(4):155–70.
34. Baker C, Baker CJ, Phongpaichit P. A history of Thailand. Cambridge University Press; 2022.
35. Cook J. Meditation in modern Buddhism: renunciation and change in Thai monastic life. Cambridge University Press; 2010.
36. Sihlé N. Buddhism in Tibet and Nepal. In: Buddhism in world cultures: comparative perspectives, vol. 245. ABC-CLIO; 2006.
37. Snellgrove, D., Indo-Tibetan Buddhism: Indian Buddhists and their Tibetan successors. 2003.
38. Powers J. Introduction to Tibetan Buddhism. Shambhala Publications; 2007.
39. Goldberg E. The re-orientation of Buddhism in North America! In: Method & theory in the study of religion, vol. 11(4). Brill; 1999. p. 340–56.
40. Glazier SD. Anthropology of religion: a handbook. Greenwood Press; 1999.
41. Goldberg ES. Buddhism in the west: transplantation and innovation. In: Buddhism in world cultures. ABC-CLIO; 2006. p. 285–310.
42. Ekman P, Friesen W. In: Calavia Balduz JM, López-Palop de Piquer B, Laita de Roda P, editors. Emotions revealed: recognizing faces and feelings to improve communication and emotional. Owl Books; 2007.
43. Kabat-Zinn J. Mindfulness-based interventions in context: past, present, and future. Clin Psychol Sci Pract. 2003;10(2):144–56.
44. Brady S, et al. The impact of mindfulness meditation in promoting a culture of safety on an acute psychiatric unit. Perspect Psychiatr Care. 2012;48(3):129–37.
45. Cohen-Katz J, et al. The effects of mindfulness-based stress reduction on nurse stress and burnout, part II: a quantitative and qualitative study. Holist Nurs Pract. 2005;19(1):26–35.
46. Ireland MJ, et al. A randomized controlled trial of mindfulness to reduce stress and burnout among intern medical practitioners. Med Teach. 2017;39(4):409–14.
47. Snyder G. Buddhist anarchism. Silent City Distro; 2018.
48. Gleig A. Engaged Buddhism. In: Oxford research encyclopedia of religion. Oxford University Press; 2021.
49. Gleig A. American dharma: Buddhism beyond modernity. Yale University Press; 2019.
50. Koné A. Zen in Europe: a survey of the territory. J Global Buddhism. 2001;2:139–61.
51. Das LS. Awakening the Buddha within: eight steps to enlightenment. Harmony; 1998.
52. Prebish CS. The Zen explosion in America: from before the pre-boomers to after the zoomers. In: The theory and practice of Zen Buddhism: a festschrift in honor of Steven Heine. Springer; 2022. p. 145–63.
53. Daniel M. Jung's affinity for Buddhism: misunderstandings and clarifications. Psychol Perspect. 2007;50(2):220–34.
54. Hayes SC, Follette VM, Linehan M. Mindfulness and acceptance: expanding the cognitive-behavioral tradition. Guilford Press; 2004.
55. Fung K. Acceptance and commitment therapy: Western adoption of Buddhist tenets? Transcult Psychiatry. 2015;52(4):561–76.
56. Fung KP-L, Wong JP-H. Acceptance and commitment therapy and Zen Buddhism. In: Handbook of Zen, mindfulness, and behavioral health. Springer; 2017. p. 271–88.
57. Fung K, Zhu Z-H. Acceptance and commitment therapy and Asian thought. In: Asian healing traditions in counseling and psychotherapy. SAGE Publications Inc.; 2017. p. 143.
58. Swart J. Applying Buddhist principles to mode deactivation theory and practice. Int J Behav Consult Ther. 2014;9(2):26.
59. Hayes SC, Strosahl KD, Wilson KG. Acceptance and commitment therapy: the process and practice of mindful change. Guilford Press; 2011.

Mental Health and Well-Being in Buddhism

Harold G. Koenig

Buddhists make up the world's fourth largest religion, with approximately 500 million adherents (7% of the world's population) [1]. The countries with the largest Buddhist populations are Cambodia (96.8%), Thailand (92.6%), Myanmar (79.8%), Bhutan (74.7%), Sri Lanka (68.6%), Laos (64.0%), Mongolia (54.5%), and Japan (33.2%). However, approximately half of all Buddhists in the world live in China (254 million, making up 18% of China's population) [2]. Buddhists comprise approximately 1% of the US population, two-thirds of whom are American-Asians.

Buddhism arose out of Hinduism in the fifth century BCE with the birth and teachings of Siddhartha Gautama (the Buddha or "awakened one"). Most scholars believe that the Buddha was a real person who lived near the India-Nepalese border and probably did not travel more than 200 miles from his home throughout his lifetime.

However, Gethin [3] indicates that we know very little about the historical Buddha with any degree of certainty, since written records only became available around the turn of the "Common Era" (year 0 in the Gregorian calendar).

According to Williams and colleagues [4], Siddhartha Gautama was the son of a local chieftain and grew up in an important aristocratic family. Wanting his son to pursue a career to replace him as the leader of the region, his father shielded him from religious teachings and any exposure to human suffering during his childhood and young adulthood [5]. At the age of 16, Siddhartha married his cousin who soon gave birth to a son. Until the age of 29, "prince" Siddhartha lived with his family in luxury not wanting for anything. However, as he approached the age of 30, he began to question his life. He began to go on outings to view how people lived in the surrounding community, finding that many residents were experiencing severe suffering, often struggling to survive because they were stricken by poverty, and dealing with painful illness, disability, old age, and inevitable death [3]. These observations caused him great distress, making him realize that all pleasures were only temporary, covering up the suffering that pervades all of life. Not being able to accept this, he thought that there

H. G. Koenig (✉)
Department of Psychiatry and Behavioral Sciences, Duke University Medical Center, Durham, NC, USA

Department of Medicine, Duke University Medical Center, Durham, NC, USA

Center for Spirituality, Theology and Health, Duke University Medical Center, Durham, NC, USA

Department of Medicine, King Abdulaziz University, Jeddah, Saudi Arabia

Department of Psychiatry, Shiraz University of Medical Sciences, Shiraz, Iran
e-mail: harold.koenig@duke.edu

H. S. Moffic et al. (eds.), *Eastern Religions, Spirituality, and Psychiatry*,
https://doi.org/10.1007/978-3-031-56744-5_11

must be a solution to suffering and left his family (wife and child) in search of that solution.

Leaving his home, he went away to live as a wandering homeless ascetic, begging for his food in the streets. Siddhartha sought mentorship under several Hindu teachers, who taught him to practice yoga and meditation, but this was not enough [6]. He tried asceticism and mortification and refused all food for a while, nearly starving to death. That too, however, was not the answer. However, after meditating continuously for 49 days, he reached a deep state of perfect equanimity and awareness when he awakened and attained Enlightenment [7]. He was aged 35 at that time, when he believed that he had found a solution to suffering. For the next 45 years until his death around age 80, he would teach his disciples what he learned at the moment of his Enlightenment, i.e., the Four Noble Truths: life is suffering, the cause of suffering is craving, the cessation of suffering is possible, and the way to end suffering is the Eightfold Path. These truths and the behaviors that resulted from them (summarized in the *Dhammapada*) [8] would then form the core beliefs and practices of Buddhism. For a more detailed history of the origins of Buddhism and the early life of the Buddha, see Koenig [9].

Major Beliefs in Buddhism

At the moment of Enlightenment, as noted above, the Buddha became aware of the Four Noble Truths. These are described briefly below.

Life is suffering. The Buddha realized that life mostly involves suffering, pain, dissatisfaction, misery, and lack of perfection. Separation from loved ones and attachment to those who do not love in return create pain. Therefore, this required action—something had to be done.

The cause of suffering is craving. To the Buddha, craving involved intense desire for what one does not have. The focus might be (a) seeking pleasure from food, sex, or intoxicants (drugs/ alcohol); (b) seeking to be loved or admired by someone; (c) seeking pleasure through taking a vacation or experiences; or (d) the desire to avoid unpleasant feelings, whether physical or emotional.

The cessation of suffering is possible. It is possible to achieve freedom, liberation from suffering. This is accomplished by the cessation of craving, i.e., the liberation from attachments of every kind. When reaching Enlightenment and arriving at Nirvana, one finds the true place of "refuge" from all suffering. Such a state exists and can be reached, but not without effort. First, however, comes belief in the Dhamma or the law which is a guide to the cessation of suffering.

The way to the cessation of suffering. It is by the Eightfold Path that one arrives at the cessation of suffering (see Dhammapada, verses 273–289). The Eightfold Path involves seeking right understanding, right intention, right action, right speech, right livelihood, right effort, right mindfulness, and right concentration.

Buddhist Practices

Traditional Buddhist practices follow from the Four Noble Truths above. In one way or another, Buddhist practices such as meditation and other actions to achieve the cessation of craving come from following the Eightfold Path. The first five paths (right understanding, intention, action, speech, and livelihood) comprise the ethics of Buddhism—the "five moral precepts." They form the foundation on which the remaining three paths rest. Ten "perfections" are said to result from the first five paths: generosity, morality, vigor, wisdom, patience, truthfulness, resolve, loving kindness, equanimity, and lack of desire. Diligently following the five moral precepts then prepares one to engage in the final three paths that lead to the awakened state [3].

1. *Right understanding* is the ability to distinguish right views from wrong views (those that do and do not lead to Enlightenment). An example of a wrong view is that lasting happi-

ness can be achieved through relationships, occupation, or any other activity, which is ignorance. In contrast, a right view is that everything is subject to constant change and therefore cannot be depended upon. Buddhists do not believe in "sin" per se, but rather attribute it to ignorance of what it means to be truly content and happy.

2. *Right intention* involves having a purpose in life that naturally follows from right understanding. This purpose is the intention to renounce all types of attachments; to stop clinging to pleasure, wealth, power, and fame; and to avoid hatred, violence, and cruelty to others (including animals).

3. *Right action* involves certain behaviors that are encouraged and other behaviors that are discouraged. One should not kill any living beings, but instead have compassion toward all. One should not cheat, steal, or otherwise gain possessions by dishonest means, but instead have respect for others and their possessions. One should not engage in any sexual misconduct such as adultery, rape, or other illicit sexual behaviors, but instead treat others with respect and honor.

4. *Right speech* involves speaking in a way that promotes peace and harmony with and between others. There should be no lying, gossip, slander, crude talk, or crude language. Right speech is speaking softly, gently, and affectionately, affirming the good in others.

5. *Right livelihood* is engaging in a profession or occupation that does not harm others or contribute to their suffering. Wrong livelihood, in contrast, would involve dealing in weapons or arms, drugs or intoxicants, human trafficking, prostitution, high-pressure sales, or trickery of any kind. For monks, as for the Buddha's disciples, this means seeking to possess only what is essential to sustain life, which might require begging for food.

The last three steps of the Eightfold Path deal with discipline, meditation, concentration, and control of the mind. These are grounded on the five moral precepts above.

6. *Right effort* emphasizes that people can improve themselves by personal effort. Such effort involves stopping whatever thoughts or actions that do not involve ethical or compassionate behavior. It also means letting go of greed, fear, hatred, or other negative states of mind that might interfere with or disrupt meditation or mindfulness.

7. *Right mindfulness* involves paying attention to whatever is happening in the present moment, both thoughts and actions. Right mindfulness discourages wandering thoughts about the past or the future that interrupt being present in the here and now. Remaining present-focused and open to whatever is occurring now is guided by having right views and right efforts during the course of daily living. The goal is to remain in the present moment throughout daily activities, including preparing for work, engaging in one's own job, and relating to friends, family, acquaintances, and coworkers. Mindfulness meditation is derived from this seventh step of the Eightfold Path.

8. *Right concentration* involves focusing the mind on a single object and excluding everything else from consciousness. The purpose is to unify the mind and bring conscious attention to a single point, a process that helps to train the mind and quiet the thoughts, thereby leading to deeper states of awareness and tranquility.

The Dhamma

The Dhamma (teachings of the Buddha that include the Four Noble Truths and Eightfold Path) is a central concept, perhaps THE most central concept, in Buddhism. According to Williams and colleagues [4], the original term for Buddhism was in fact *Dhamma* (p. 6). The Dhamma is considered to be "Ultimate Reality" or the "objective truth" of all things that exist. Following the Dhamma results in deliverance from all suffering, including the deliverance from the desire for deliverance itself, ultimately leading to Nirvana. When converting to Buddhism, the convert is instructed to say: "I take refuge in the Buddha. I take refuge in the Dhamma. I take refuge in the Sangha [Buddhist community]." Verses from the Dhammapada instruct:

> But who to the Buddha, Dhamma, and Sangha as refuge has gone, sees with full insight the Four Noble Truths;
> Misery, the arising of misery, and the transcending of misery, the Noble Eightfold Path leading to the allaying of misery.
> This, indeed, is a refuge secure. This is the highest refuge. Having come to this refuge, one is released from all misery [8] (verses 190–192).

According to Williams et al. [4], the Buddha intentionally chose a term (Dhamma) that indicated to others that he truly knew and taught how things finally *are* (p. 6). Those who disagreed with him, by definition, did not have the Dhamma but rather its opposite, the Adhamma. Therefore, when followed exactly in the way that its founder intended, Buddhism is an exclusive religion—it excludes other paths to Ultimate Reality (a conception of the Transcendent that comes very close to the notion of God in a religion that is largely considered nontheistic).

Not all Buddhist scholars, however, are in agreement with the above view of Buddhism as an exclusive religion. Others might argue that the Dhamma (or Dharma in Sanskrit) is a very complicated topic and there are many different yet valid ways of discussing this concept. Thich Nhat Hanh [10] says,

> Whenever the Four Noble Truths and Noble Eightfold Path are practiced, the living Dharma is there. There are said to be 84,000 Dharma doors … To take refuge in the Dharma is to choose the doors that are most appropriate for us … If you enjoy walking meditation, practice walking meditation. If you enjoy sitting meditation, practice sitting meditation. But preserve your Jewish, Christian, or Muslim roots. That is the best way to realize the Buddha's spirit. If you are cut off from your roots, you cannot be happy (pp. 164, 169).

Other Buddhist Practices

Besides mindfulness meditation (see below) and focused meditation, Buddhist practices may also involve "taking refuge" through rituals in a tem-

ple or at home. Buddhists may have a small shrine in their home, which may include a picture or statue of the Buddha. They may make offerings of clean water, flowers, or incense to the Buddha. This shows gratitude and respect. Buddhist practices that involve prayer and meditation either at a community temple or at home are not intended to be transactional as in the West, i.e., they are not typically done in order to "get something." In reality, though, Buddhists often meditate, pray, and worship in order to meet various human needs (financial, health, etc.). Furthermore, these worship practices are thought to have consequences in terms of karma that will ultimately benefit the worshiper.

Diversity of Beliefs and Practices in Buddhism

The three major branches or sects of Buddhism in East Asia are Theravada, Mahayana, and Vajrayana Buddhism. There is also a version of Buddhism practiced in the USA today, which varies to some extent from the three traditional branches.

Theravada Buddhism: Theravada Buddhism is the only branch of Buddhism that has survived almost continuously since early times. Most of its 100 million adherents live in Thailand, Myanmar, Sri Lanka, Laos, and Cambodia [11]. This branch of Buddhism coexists with other religions in Southeast Asia such as Hinduism, Christianity, Islam, and folk religions. The scripture on which all branches of Buddhism are based, particularly Theravadin Buddhism, is the Pali Canon. The Pali Canon includes the ancient teachings and practices of Buddhism from the early centuries Before the Common Era (BCE).

Mahayana Buddhism: Mahayana Buddhism is the largest branch of Buddhism, making up an estimated 350 million adherents. Most Mahayana Buddhists live in China, Japan, South Korea, and Vietnam [11]. Mahayana Buddhism, like Theravadin Buddhism, has coexisted in East Asia with many other endogenous religions such as Confucianism, Taoism, and Shintoism (Zen Buddhism is of the Mahayana tradition).

Vajrayana Buddhism: Vajrayana Buddhism, also called Tibetan Buddhism, has approximately 20 million adherents, most of whom live in Tibet, Nepal, Bhutan, and Mongolia [11]. Vajrayana Buddhism is an offshoot of Mahayana Buddhism. The Dalai Lama is a practitioner of Vajrayana Buddhism.

American Buddhism: The beliefs and practices of Buddhists in the USA differ from those of Buddhists in East Asia. Buddhist practices in the USA—such as mindfulness meditation— are often picked out as isolated practices to relieve stress while ignoring the five moral precepts on the Eightfold Path (e.g., right understanding, right action, right intention, right speech). This is particularly true for mental health professionals who are using mindfulness meditation as a secular mental health intervention (see below). As noted above, the first five steps on the Eightfold Path provide the framework on which mindfulness meditation (MM) is to be practiced. Ignoring that framework is unlikely to produce the results for which this practice was originally intended.

One of the most detailed reports on US Buddhists was based on a survey of 1237 American Buddhists, 72% of whom identified them- selves as practicing Buddhists, while the remaining 28% indicated that they believed in or practiced some aspects of Buddhism [12]. Of those who participated, 63% were converts to Buddhism and 4% were ordained Buddhist monks or nuns. The majority of respondents practiced Tibetan Buddhism or Zen Buddhism. When practicing Buddhists were examined (*n* = 886), 99% said that they meditated (66% daily or more often), 83% chanted or repeated a Buddhist mantra, 79% engaged in another form of Buddhist prayer, nearly half (47%) attended Buddhist gatherings on a regular basis (although only 16% attended services at a Buddhist temple "very often"), most (96%) read and studied Buddhist scriptures, and 76% agreed to acknowledging the "Three Refuges" (Buddha, Dhamma, Sangha) in the presence of other Buddhists [13]. With regard to under- standing and applying the steps of the Eightfold Path, 57% said that they sought right understanding, 58% said right thought, 63% said right speech, 66% said right action, and 74% said right livelihood. With regard to the final three steps, 60% agreed that they adhered to right effort, 60% practiced right mindfulness, and 53% engaged in right con- centration. Others (with the remaining per- centage for each group) indicated an understanding of these steps, but had difficulty applying them in their daily lives. Thus, in this select group of largely white non-Asian highly educated respondents, religious involvement was quite frequent.

Mindfulness Meditation

Mindfulness meditation (MM) and mindfulness- based stress reduction (MBSR) are used widely to treat a variety of psychological and physical health conditions in Western countries, making them relevant to providers from a range of clini- cal specialties including psychologists, counsel- ors, and healthcare and military chaplains [14]. MM/MBSR is now viewed by Western psycho- therapists as a secular practice (despite its deep roots in Buddhism) and is now being used in many different mental health treatments, includ- ing acceptance and commitment therapy, dialec- tical behavioral therapy, and mindfulness-based cognitive therapy. Despite the proposed secular nature of MM/MBSR, the core developers and promoters of this practice are almost all devout practicing Buddhists (Jon Kabat-Zinn, Thích Nhất Hạnh, Richard J. Davidson, Amishi Jha, etc.).

A number of meta-analyses of randomized controlled trials (RCTs) have now documented the benefits of MM/MBSR for the treatment of mental health problems and emotional disorders. Meta- analyses have now examined the effects of MM/ MBSR on depression (e.g., [15]), post-traumatic stress disorder (e.g., [16]), and substance use dis- orders (e.g., [17]). RCTs and meta-analyses of

RCTs have even examined the effects of MM/MBSR on physical health conditions such as chronic pain (e.g., [18]), rheumatoid arthritis (e.g., [19]), and high blood pressure (e.g., [20]), as well as on health behaviors such as smoking cessation (e.g., [21]) and weight loss (e.g., [22]).

Unfortunately, as noted earlier, mindfulness meditation has become divorced from its deep spiritual roots in Buddhism (and from the five moral precepts of the Eightfold Path). If practiced within the framework of the Eightfold Path, and the Buddhist moral precepts that underlie it, the benefits of MM/MBSR to mental health may be even greater.

God in Buddhism

Williams et al. [4] say that "Buddhists have no objection to the existence of the Hindu gods, although they deny completely the existence of God as spoken of in, e.g., orthodox Christianity, understood as the omnipotent, omniscient, all-good, and primordially existent creator deity, who can be thought of as in some sense a person" (p. 3, but also restated a second time on p. 5). The Buddha had a generally negative view toward the Hindu religion as practiced during his lifetime, and when his disciples asked him about a Supreme Being, the Buddha reportedly either remained silent or discouraged such questions [23].

Beliefs about God or a Supreme Being, and practices in this regard, today vary depending on the particular branch of Buddhism. Although Buddhists in the Theravada branch do not emphasize deities of any sort (at least theoretically), this is not necessarily true for Mahayana or Vajrayana Buddhism. In Mahayana Buddhism, there is belief in bodhisattvas or compassionate beings present at the highest levels of existence who serve to guard the world and come into the world to alleviate suffering. Mahayana Buddhists consider the Buddha to be an embodiment of the "cosmic dharmakaya," which has been described as "the body of reality itself, without specific, delimited form, wherein the Buddha is identified with the spiritually charged nature of everything that is" [24]. The cosmic dharmakaya, then,

resembles the notion of God in a pantheistic sense, as taught in Hinduism. As a result, Mahayana Buddhists may honor, pray to, and worship a divine-like being called Avalokiteśvara (translated literally "Lord who looks down"). Avalokiteśvara is a bodhisattva who embodies mercy, compassion, kindness, and love (very much like Jesus in Christianity). Despite being able to reach nirvana, Avalokiteśvara delays doing so in order to help humans on earth who are suffering [25]. Some of these characteristics sound quite similar to God as described in monotheistic Western religions.

However, this begs a question. What do traditional Buddhists today believe about God? This question has been asked in a systematic survey of Buddhists in the general population. The International Social Survey Program [26] examined the beliefs of 1226 Buddhists living in 40 countries around the world, most coming from Japan, Taiwan, and South Korea (primarily Buddhists from the Mahayana branch). Buddhists were compared to 45,438 non-Buddhists and 12,557 persons with no religious affiliation. The results were analyzed and presented in Koenig [9]. In summary, more than 80% of Buddhists in this sample indicated that they at least sometimes believed in the existence of God or a Higher Power, whereas only 18.6% said that they did not believe in God or did not know. When asked if they believed in God now or in the past, 69.0% said that they believed in God now. More specifically, 52.1% said that they believed in God now and in the past, whereas 16.9% said that they believed now but not in the past. Thus, when it comes to the views of many East Asian Buddhists today, belief in God is relatively common, despite traditional Buddhist teachings that tend to be nontheistic.

Buddhism, Life Satisfaction, and Mental Health

The relationship between Buddhism and mental health is comprehensively reviewed elsewhere [9], but will be briefly summarized here. In addition, analyses from three large random national and cross-national studies comparing Buddhists and non-Buddhists on life satisfaction will be reviewed here. Largely excluded here are studies of Western forms of mindfulness meditation that are not firmly grounded in traditional Buddhist beliefs.

In the first and second editions of the *Handbook of Religion and Health*, a total of 26 studies examining the relationship between Buddhism and mental health were systematically identified [27, 28]. These studies were categorized into those examining coping with stress, anxiety, depression, suicide, substance use/abuse, psychological well-being/life satisfaction, quality of life/self-rated health, personality traits, and intervention studies. Examples in each category are briefly reviewed below.

Coping with Stress

Holtz [29] compared 35 refugee Tibetan nuns (76%) and lay students (24%) arrested and tortured in Tibet because of their religious beliefs and compared them to 35 Tibetan controls who had not been tortured. Although anxiety symptoms were higher in those experiencing torture compared to controls (54% vs. 29%), there was no difference in depressive symptoms between the tortured and the controls. In trying to explain why Tibetan nuns experiencing torture did not have more depressive symptoms, investigators hypothesized (based on what they were told by participants) that Buddhism helped by providing an explanation for suffering that gave meaning to what they had experienced. By accepting and dealing with their situation in a proper manner and performing good works, they believed that this would provide positive karma that would improve their next lives. They believed that, as the Buddha taught, one's own suffering was little compared to the suffering of others and, in fact, could be used to reduce the suffering of others.

Anxiety/Worry

Tapanya and colleagues [30] surveyed 52 Christian elders (ages 65–90 years) in Canada and 52 Buddhist elders in northern Thailand (ages 65–89 years). This is one of the first studies (if not the first) to examine the relationship between *religiosity* and mental health in Buddhists. The words "church," "God," and "Bible" were modified for Buddhists in a Thai version of an extrinsic-intrinsic religiosity (ER-IR) scale. After controlling for gender, no difference was found in worry/anxiety between Christian and Buddhist elders. Buddhists scored significantly higher on ER than Christians, but there was little difference between groups on IR. A significant inverse relationship was found between IR and worry ($r = -0.24, p < 0.01$) in the combined sample. This was especially true in Buddhists ($r = -0.37, p < 0.01$). ER, on the other hand, was positively related to worry in Buddhists ($r = 0.29, p < 0.05$), but not in Christians. Investigators explained the positive relationship between ER and worry in Buddhists as possibly because interest in the extrinsic aspects of religion resulting from Buddhist beliefs might have created worry. While redemption and forgiveness for one's actions are possible in Christianity, the law of karma in Buddhism does not allow escape from the consequences of one's actions (i.e., there is no savior to help). Instead, Buddhists believe that only perseverance toward enlightenment will bring liberation and redemption from the cycle of death and rebirth. Thus, greater extrinsic religious behavior related to activities at church/temple among Buddhists might not alleviate responsibilities for their actions.

Depression

Limlomwongse and Liabsuetrakul [31] reported results from a prospective study of 610 pregnant Thai women (88.2% Buddhists) who were followed from prior to delivery until 6–8 weeks postpartum. The purpose was to predict the development of depressive symptoms. Participants were recruited from the University Hospital in South Thailand. The prevalence of significant depressive symptoms (assessed by a standard depression scale) was 20.5% during pregnancy and 16.8% at the postpartum follow-up. Predictors of change in depressive symptoms that were examined included demographics, obstetric history, previous psychological problems, planned/unplanned pregnancy, perception of pregnancy complications, and other attitudes toward pregnancy and delivery. After controlling for other predictors using logistic regression, non-Buddhists were over twice as likely as Buddhists to experience significant depressive symptoms on follow-up (OR = 2.1, 95% CI 1.0–4.0, $p = 0.03$). This effect emerged after controlling for negative attitudes toward pregnancy.

Suicide

In the first and second editions of the handbook, a total of four studies were identified on religion and suicide among Buddhist majority samples. Three of four found no association, and one reported a significantly higher rate of suicidal thoughts, attempts, or completions among those who were more religious. For example, Zhang and Xu [32] examined relationships between religious affiliation and self-rated religiosity and degree of suicide intent in a sample of suicide attempters. A Chinese version of the 8-item Beck Suicidal Intent Scale assessed suicidal intent. Suicidal intent in women was significantly higher among those who were more religious ($p = 0.02$), and a similar but weaker association was found in men ($p = 0.09$). However, after controlling for age, mental disorder, superstition, perceived gender inequality, and marital status, these differences became nonsignificant.

Substance Use/Abuse

Assanangkornchai et al. [33] examined differences in religious beliefs and practices between three groups: (1) 91 alcohol-dependent adults, (2) 77 hazardous/harmful drinkers, and (3) a control group of 144 nondrinkers or infrequent drinkers. These samples involved individuals living in Thailand who were recruited from inpatient and outpatient settings, as well as from hospital personnel, friends, and relatives. As noted earlier, Thailand is second only to Cambodia among

countries with the highest percentage of Buddhist affiliation (nearly 90%). Religious characteristics that were measured included whether the participant was raised in a religious family, religiosity of their parents, parent participation in religious activities, having religion forced on them as a child, and participation in religious activities as a child. No difference in these religious measures was found between the three groups. Men without alcohol problems, however, were more likely than hazardous/harmful or alcohol-dependent men to perceive themselves as moderately or strongly religious (86% vs. 74% and 75%, respectively), more likely to indicate that Thai men should observe the Fifth Precept (i.e., avoid distilled or fermented intoxicants) (28% vs. 8% and 14%, respectively), and more likely to say that one should always abstain from drinking on a holy day (35% vs. 13% and 9%, respectively). When analyses were adjusted for demographic characteristics, working status, social class, and area of residence, the strongest predictors of being a hazardous/harmful drinker or alcohol dependent were self-perception as moderately or strongly religious (OR = 0.41, 95% CI = 0.20–0.86, and OR = 0.48, 95% CI = 0.24–0.97, respectively), belief that religious teaching always influences daily life (OR = 0.30, 95% CI = 0.14–0.83, and OR = 0.50, 95% CI = 0.21–1.06, respectively), and interest in studying the Buddha's teachings (OR = 0.51, 95% CI = 0.28–0.93, and OR = 0.81, 95% CI = 0.47–1.41, respectively). Thus, among men, greater religious beliefs were found to be related to less alcohol abuse/dependence in this largely Buddhist sample.

Psychological Well-Being/Life Satisfaction

Yamaoka [34] analyzed data from a random sample of 8665 adults living in Japan, South Korea, Singapore, five cities in China, and Taiwan. The purpose was to examine relationships between religious faith and life satisfaction, somatic symptoms, and self-rated health. Religious faith (not described) was assessed with a single question that was dichotomized for analysis into "present" vs. "absent." Religious faith was present in 24–25% of participants in Japan, 7–27% in China, 26–41% in Hong Kong, 71–78% in Taiwan, 76–82% in Singapore, and 43–50% in South Korea. Logistic regression analyses indicated that the presence of religious faith was associated with a *higher number* of somatic symptoms (OR = 1.35, 95% CI 1.21–1.51) and *poorer* subjective health (OR = 1.14, 95% CI 1.01–1.29), but there was no relationship with life satisfaction (OR = 1.03, 95% CI 0.89–1.19).

Quality of Life

In a study that compared Buddhists and non-Buddhists on quality of life (QOL), Fazel and Young [35] examined 59 Tibetan refugees (Mahayana Buddhists) and 66 native Hindus living in Northern India. Results revealed that QOL (assessed by a standard scale) was significantly higher among Buddhist Tibetan refugees compared to native Hindus ($p < 0.001$, uncontrolled). Researchers concluded that "While both Hindus and Tibetans subscribe to the fatalistic attitude of Karma, the Tibetans report greater life satisfaction. If one looks beyond the superficial similarities in the concept of Karma, however, it becomes clear that Tibetans adopt a 'proactive' posture [emphasizing aspects of daily life that gave them positive karma] as opposed to the 'reactive' fatalism of the Hindus [finding reasons for their misfortunes in karma]" (p. 229).

Personality Traits

Saroglou and Dupuis [36] examined 105 Buddhists living in Belgium to determine the relationship between personality characteristics, cognitive structure, importance of values, and religiosity. Participants were obtained from Buddhist centers in Belgium belonging to the Tibetan Vajrayana tradition. Psychological characteristics assessed were need for closure (preference for order, predictability, decisiveness, discomfort from ambiguity, close mindedness),

agreeableness (kind, sympathetic, cooperative, warm, and considerate), and adherence to "values," all using standard measures of these constructs. Religiosity was assessed using a 14-item Investment in Buddhism Scale (IBS) developed by the authors that included frequency of practice (both collective and individual), self-identification as Buddhist, interest in Buddhism, finding a way of life through Buddhism, working on oneself through Buddhism, and willingness to share Buddhism with others and their children. Results indicated that "need for closure" and "close mindedness" were associated with lower scores on Buddhist collective religious practice. Buddhist "inner directedness" was associated with lower scores on preference for predictability. Overall IBS scores were associated with higher degrees of agreeableness and also tended to be positively associated with preference for tradition, conformity universalism, and benevolence. In contrast, higher IBS scores were associated with less need for security, power, achievement, and, especially, hedonism.

Intervention Studies

I focus here on interventions utilizing Buddhist beliefs and practices conducted in Buddhist populations, largely avoiding interventions using mindfulness meditation primarily because of the "huge differences between the Western and Eastern approaches" [37] (p. 23). That difference exists because Western mindfulness has largely been stripped of its religious components (i.e., the first five moral precepts of the Eightfold Path).

In the first study, Emavardhana and Tori [38] examined the effects of Vipassana meditation on psychological adjustment among two groups of 222 and 216 Thai persons (average age 18 years), compared to a young adult Thai control group ($n = 281$). Vipassana meditation is one of the oldest forms of Buddhist meditation developed within the Theravada tradition. Participants in the first two cohorts attended a 7-day Vipassana meditation retreat as part of activities supported by the Young Buddhist Association of Thailand.

Results indicated that compared to controls, meditators after the retreat scored higher on self-concept, positive ego defense mechanisms, maturity, tolerance of common stressors, and Buddhist beliefs and practices.

In another example of an intervention, Tori [39] compared the effects of attending a 3-day Roman Catholic retreat ($n = 102$), a 3-day Buddhist retreat ($n = 102$), or a control condition ($n = 102$) in 306 teenage Thai girls (average age 16 years). Thai girls in the Roman Catholic retreat group were from a large parochial high school; those attending the Buddhist retreat were part of the Young Buddhist Association of Thailand; and those in the control group attended government secondary schools in Bangkok. Results indicated that Thai girls attending the Buddhist retreat showed significantly greater change scores on emotional maturity and sympathetic warmth compared to Thai girls attending the Catholic retreat and those in the control condition.

In a third example, Rungreangkulkij and Wongtakee [40] examined the effects of Buddhist counseling in 21 persons with anxiety disorder in northeastern Thailand. Buddhist counseling was based on the "three universal natural laws": the law of impermanence (anicca), the law of suffering (dukka), and the law of selfishness or no self (detachment from the physical world and the ego) (anatta). Each session lasted 60–90 min and was organized into four stages: (1) developing rapport, active listening, and demonstrating compassion; (2) education using stories and explaining the universal natural laws; (3) practicing mindfulness meditation during the session (and at home); and (4) assessment of perceptions, beliefs, and understanding in the Buddhist tradition. By the end of 3 months of intervention, anxiety scores decreased significantly ($p < 0.001$). Also see Rungreangkulkij et al. [41] for an examination of Buddhist group therapy.

Summary

In the first and second editions of the handbook, a total of 22 observational studies and 4 clinical trials were identified. Five of the 22 observational studies were descriptive or qualitative, suggesting that Buddhist beliefs and practices are being used widely to cope with psychological stressors. Five quantitative studies compared Buddhists and non-Buddhists, with three finding that Buddhists had better mental health than non-Buddhists, one finding worse mental health, and one finding no difference. The remaining 12 studies examined the association between religiosity and mental health among Asian populations with a large proportion of Buddhists. Of those, one-third reported associations with better mental health or fewer suicidal tendencies, one-quarter reported associations with worse mental health, one study reported mixed results (positive for intrinsic religiosity, negative for extrinsic religiosity), and one-third found no association. Among studies since 2010 (see Reference 9, for review), two found better mental health in Buddhists, one found no difference between Buddhists and other religious affiliations, and one reported worse mental health. These studies suggest that (a) mental health of Buddhists is similar to (if not better than) that of non-Buddhists, (b) religious practices among Buddhists are sometimes but not always associated with better mental health and perceptions of health, and (c) Buddhist-based interventions are frequently effective in reducing distressing emotional symptoms in Buddhists compared to no treatment.

Recent Analyses

Koenig [9] analyzed data collected during three large random national and cross-national surveys. The first survey was the Spiritual Life Study of Chinese Residents [42] that examined a random sample of 7021 adults in mainland China. Analyses indicated that Buddhists ($n = 1168$) were equally as likely to say that they were "very happy" compared to those with no religious affiliation (33.2% vs. 33.2%), but were significantly less likely than members of other religious faiths (Christian, Muslim, and Taoist) to indicate that they were very happy (33.2% vs. 42.3%, $p < 0.05$). When the analyses were repeated in those who indicated that they were at least "somewhat religious," the findings were similar in that 33.0% of Buddhists indicated that they were very happy, compared to 42.5% of those affiliated with other religious groups. When asked to list the top three reasons for why they felt happy, Buddhists were less likely than members of other religious groups to include "my religious life."

In the second survey, Koenig [9] analyzed data from the 2008 *International Social Survey* Program (mentioned earlier) that involved a random sample of 59,063 persons aged 15–90 from 40 countries [26]. Most Buddhists ($n = 1224$) came from Japan (32.4%), Taiwan (31.9%), and South Korea (29.3%). The purpose was to first compare the happiness of Buddhists with the happiness of those from other religious denominations. Surprisingly, Buddhists were significantly less likely than those from other religious affiliations (primarily Christians and Muslims) to indicate that they were very happy (19.2% vs. 26.7, $p < 0.0001$). However, Buddhists were similar to members of other faith traditions in saying that religion helps people "find inner peace and happiness" (32.1% vs. 35.4%), although among those who were at least somewhat religious, Buddhists were less likely to report this (39.3% vs. 44.7%, $p < 0.05$). Buddhists were also significantly less likely to say that religion helps people "gain comfort in times of trouble or sorrow" compared with non-Buddhists (27.1% vs. 39.4%, $p < 0.0001$), with similar results among those who indicated that they were at least somewhat religious. Among Buddhists overall, self-rated religiosity was weakly but positively related to happiness ($r = 0.07$, $p = 0.02$, $n = 1194$).

In the third survey, Koenig [9] analyzed data from the 2005–2006 World Values Survey [43], which was a random cross-national survey of over 83,000 adults from 80 countries. In that study, Buddhists ($n = 3266$, primarily from Thailand, China, Japan, South Korea, Taiwan, and Hong Kong) were significantly more likely to report that they were "very happy" compared to members of other religious groups (primarily Christian and Muslim) (31.5% vs. 28.2%, $p < 0.0001$). The results were similar among

those indicating that religion was important in their lives. The positive findings, however, were largely from Buddhists in Thailand (a highly religious and largely Buddhist country). When Thai Buddhists were removed from the sample, the findings completely reversed (23.7% of non-Thai Buddhists indicated that they were very happy, compared to 28.2% of members of other religious faiths, $p < 0.0001$).

Conclusion

With regard to Buddhists vs. non-Buddhists, our systematic review of five studies published prior to 2010 found that three favored Buddhists over non-Buddhists, one found no difference, and one reported worse mental health in Buddhists; among studies published since 2010, two found better mental health in Buddhists, one found no difference, and one reported worse mental health. In three large random national and cross-national studies, one found better mental health in Buddhists (but only in Thai Buddhists), and the other two reported worse mental health in Buddhists compared to non-Buddhists. Thus, the findings are mixed, preventing any firm conclusions from being made. Although there is every reason to expect that Buddhists would have better mental health than non-Buddhists, based on the core Buddhist beliefs mentioned earlier, this is not always the case. With regard to the relationship between religiosity and mental health among Buddhists, nearly half of the observational studies found that greater religiosity was associated with better mental health, whereas about 10% found that it was associated with worse mental health and the remainder finding no association or showing mixed findings. Among interventional studies in Buddhists, however, all reported that treatments based on Buddhist beliefs/practices improved mental health (although adequacy of control groups was an issue). Thus, overall, the findings suggest that when Buddhists commit to and follow the core Buddhist principles outlined in the Eightfold Path, they usually experience good mental health.

Buddhist Interventions for Emotional Problems

If the Buddhist patient prefers a religiously integrated approach and the therapist is willing and qualified, cognitive behavioral therapy (CBT) from a Buddhist perspective should be considered. Resources exist that may help the therapist or Buddhist clergy in this regard. This includes a Buddhist CBT manual, along with therapist and patient workbooks, and an introductory video, all of which can be accessed through the Center for Spirituality, Theology and Health website without charge [44]. Religiously integrated CBT (RCBT), including that from a Buddhist perspective, is an evidence-based treatment that has documented effectiveness for the treatment for depression [45]. In Buddhist RCBT, maladaptive assumptions and dysfunctional cognitions are countered with verses from the Dhammapada (the Way of Truth as described by the Buddha). These scriptures facilitate cognitive restructuring that enables the person to engage in more positive, realistic, truth-based thinking that can help to relieve symptoms of depression or anxiety.

Therapists and pastoral counselors should also consider other evidence-based Buddhist treatments such as Vipassana meditation [38], 3-S therapy [46], Buddhist counseling [40], Buddhist group therapy [41], and mindfulness-based treatments [47] and might even recommend that the patient go on a Buddhist retreat [39] (see intervention studies mentioned earlier).

Summary and Conclusion

This chapter began with a brief history of Buddhism, reviewed the core religious beliefs of Buddhism (the Four Noble Truths), and discussed the practices that derive from those core beliefs (Eightfold Path), based on the Dhammapada. Beliefs about God in Buddhism were also examined, based on Buddhist teachings and on the actual beliefs of Buddhists in East Asia. Earlier and more recent research was then reviewed, first comparing the mental health and well-being of Buddhists with members of other religious affili-

ations and then examining the relationship between religiosity and psychological well-being in Buddhists (both observational studies and randomized controlled trials). The chapter concluded with a discussion of religiously integrated Buddhist interventions that may be utilized to address emotional problems in Buddhist patients.

References

1. World Population Review. Buddhist countries, 2022. 2022. https://worldpopulationreview.com/country-rankings/buddhist-countries. Accessed 26 Dec 22.
2. Starr KJ. 5 facts about Buddhists around the world. Pew Research Center; 2019. https://www.pewresearch.org/fact-tank/2019/04/05/5-facts-about-buddhists-around-the-world/. Accessed 26 Dec 22.
3. Gethin R. Foundations of Buddhism. New York: Oxford University Press; 1998. p. 9, 18, 20–1
4. Williams P, Tribe A, Wynne A. Buddhist thought: a complete introduction to the Indian tradition. 2nd ed. New York: Routledge; 2012. p. 21.
5. Thaper R. History of early India. From origins to AD1300. Berkeley: University of California Press; 2002. p. 137.
6. Narada MT. A manual of Buddhism, Buddha educational foundation. Kuala Lumpur: Buddhist Missionary Society; 1992. p. 14–20.
7. Conze E, translator. Buddhist scriptures. London: Penguin; 1959. p. 47–51.
8. Carter JR, Palihawadana M. The Dhammapada: the sayings of the Buddha, Oxford World's classics. Oxford: Oxford University Press; 2000.
9. Koenig HG. Buddhism and mental health: beliefs, research, and applications. Seattle, WA: CreateSpace Publishing; 2017.
10. Hanh TN. The heart of the Buddha's teaching. New York: Broadway Books; 1999. Hardcover edition originally published in 1998 by Parallax Press.
11. Johnson TM, Grim BJ, editors. World religion database. Leiden/Boston: Brill; 2022. May also access 2020 data from Association of Religion Data Archives, https://www.thearda.com/world-religion/national-profiles?u=220c.
12. Wiist WH, Sullivan BM, Wayment HA, Warren M. A web-based survey of the relationship between Buddhist religious practices, health, and psychological characteristics: research methods and preliminary results. J Relig Health. 2010;49(1):18–31.
13. Wiist WH, Sullivan BM, George DS, Wayment HA. Buddhists' religious and health practices. J Relig Health. 2012;51(1):132–47.
14. Koenig HG. Person-centered mindfulness: a culturally and spiritually sensitive approach to clinical practice. J Relig Health. 2023, forthcoming.

15. Reangsing C, Lauderman C, Schneider JK. Effects of mindfulness meditation intervention on depressive symptoms in emerging adults: a systematic review and meta-analysis. J Integr Complement Med. 2022;28(1):6–24.

16. Sun LN, Gu JW, Huang LJ, Shang ZL, Zhou YG, Wu LL, et al. Military-related posttraumatic stress disorder and mindfulness meditation: a systematic review and meta-analysis. Chin J Traumatol. 2021;24(04):221–30.

17. Li W, Howard MO, Garland EL, McGovern P, Lazar M. Mindfulness treatment for substance misuse: a systematic review and meta-analysis. J Subst Abus Treat. 2017;75:62–96.

18. Wielgosz J, Kral TR, Perlman DM, Mumford JA, Wager TD, Lutz A, Davidson RJ. Neural signatures of pain modulation in short-term and long-term mindfulness training: a randomized active-control trial. Am J Psychiatry. 2022;179:758. Available online at https://ajp.psychiatryonline.org/doi/full/10.1176/appi.ajp.21020145.

19. Zhou B, Wang G, Hong Y, Xu S, Wang J, Yu H, et al. Mindfulness interventions for rheumatoid arthritis: a systematic review and meta-analysis. Complement Ther Clin Pract. 2020;39:101088.

20. Intarakamhang U, Macaskill A, Prasittichok P. Mindfulness interventions reduce blood pressure in patients with non-communicable diseases: a systematic review and meta-analysis. Heliyon. 2020;6(4):e03834.

21. Maglione MA, Maher AR, Ewing B, Colaiaco B, Newberry S, Kandrack R, et al. Efficacy of mindfulness meditation for smoking cessation: a systematic review and meta-analysis. Addict Behav. 2017;69:27–34.

22. Carrière K, Khoury B, Günak MM, Knäuper B. Mindfulness-based interventions for weight loss: a systematic review and meta-analysis. Obes Rev. 2018;19(2):164–77.

23. Jayaram, V. (2016). The Buddha on God. http://www.hinduwebsite.com/buddhism/buddhaongod.asp. Accessed 27 Dec 22.

24. Ray R. Secret of the Vajra world. Boston: Shambhala Meditation Center; 2001. p. 13.

25. Leighton TD. Bodhisattva archetypes: classic Buddhist guides to awakening and their modern expression. New York: Penguin Arkana; 1998. p. 158–205.

26. International Social Survey Program (ISSP) (2008). Dataset downloaded from the Association of Religion Data Archives (ARDA), and were collected by Dr. Max Haller and his team at the Institut für Soziologie, Universität Graz, Austria. https://www.thearda.com/data-archive/browse-categories. Accessed 29 Dec 22.

27. Koenig HG, Larson DB, McCullough ME. Handbook of religion and health. 1st ed. New York: Oxford University Press; 2001.

28. Koenig HG, King DE, Carson VB. Handbook of religion and health. 2nd ed. New York: Oxford University Press; 2012.

29. Holtz TH. Refugee trauma versus torture trauma: a retrospective controlled cohort study of Tibetan refugees. J Nerv Ment Dis. 1998;186(1):24–34.

30. Tapanya S, Nicki R, Jarusawad O. Worry and intrinsic/extrinsic religious orientation among Buddhist (Thai) and Christian (Canadian) elderly persons. Int J Aging Hum Dev. 1997;44:73–83.

31. Limlomwongse N, Liabsuetrakul T. Cohort study of depressive moods in Thai women during late pregnancy and 6-8 weeks of postpartum using the Edinburgh postnatal depression scale (EPDS). Arch Womens Ment Health. 2006;9(3):131–8.

32. Zhang J, Xu H. The effects of religion, superstition, and perceived gender inequality on the degree of suicide intent: a study of serious attempters in China. Omega. 2007;55(3):185–97.

33. Assanangkornchai S, Sam-Angsri N, Rerngpongpan S, Lertnakorn A. Patterns of alcohol consumption in the Thai population: results of the National Household Survey of 2007. Alcohol Alcohol. 2010;45(3):278–85.

34. Yamaoka K. Social capital and health and well-being in East Asia: a population-based study. Soc Sci Med. 2008;66(4):885–99.

35. Fazel MK, Young DM. Life quality of Tibetans and Hindus: a function of religion. J Sci Study Relig. 1988;27:229–42.

36. Saroglou V, Dupuis J. Being Buddhist in Western Europe: cognitive needs, prosocial character, and values. Int J Psychol Relig. 2006;16(3):163–79.

37. Schmidt S. Mindfulness in east and west–is it the same? In: Walach H, Schmdit S, Jonas WB, editors. Neuroscience, consciousness and spirituality. Dordrecht: Springer; 2011. p. 23–38.

38. Emavardhana T, Tori CD. Changes in self-concept, ego defense mechanisms, and religiosity following seven-day Vipassana meditation retreats. J Sci Study Relig. 1997;36(2):194–206.

39. Tori CD. Change on psychological scales following Buddhist and Roman Catholic retreats. Psychol Rep. 1999;84(1):125–6.

40. Rungreangkulkij S, Wongtakee W. The psychological impact of Buddhist counseling for patients suffering from symptoms of anxiety. Arch Psychiatr Nurs. 2008;22(3):127–34.

41. Rungreangkulkij S, Wongtakee W, Thongyot S. Buddhist group therapy for diabetes patients with depressive symptoms. Arch Psychiatr Nurs. 2011;25(3):195–205.

42. Spiritual Life Study of Chinese Residents. Association of Religion Data Archives (ARDA). Collected by Dr. Anna Sun and her research team and was funded by the John Templeton Foundation. 2007. https://www.thearda.com/data-archive/browse-categories. Accessed 29 Dec 22.

43. World Values Survey (WVS). Dataset was downloaded from the World Values Survey. World Values Survey Wave 5: 2005–2008. Official Aggregate v.20140429. 2005–2006. World Values Survey Association. Aggregate File Producer: Asep/JDS,

Madrid, Spain. http://www.worldvaluessurvey.org/WVSDocumentationWV5.jsp. Accessed 11-7-16.

44. CSTH. Religious cognitive behavioral therapy: Buddhist version. Durham, NC: Duke University Center for Spirituality, Theology and Health; 2014. https://spiritualityandhealth.duke.edu/index.php/religious-cbt-study/therapy-manuals/. Accessed 29 Dec 22.

45. Koenig HG, Pearce MJ, Nelson B, Shaw SF, Robins CJ, Daher N, Cohen HJ, Berk LS, Bellinger D, Pargament KI, Rosmarin DH, Vasegh S, Kristeller J, Juthani N, Nies D, King MB. Religious vs. conventional cognitive-behavioral therapy for major depression in persons with chronic medical illness. J Nerv Ment Dis. 2015;203(4):243–51.

46. Margolin A, Beitel M, Schuman-Olivier Z, Avants SK. A controlled study of a spiritually-focused intervention for increasing motivation for HIV prevention among drug users. AIDS Educ Prev. 2006;18(4):311–22.

47. Chen Y, Yang X, Wang L, Zhang X. A randomized controlled trial of the effects of brief mindfulness meditation on anxiety symptoms and systolic blood pressure in Chinese nursing students. Nurse Educ Today. 2013;33(10):1166–72.

Deeper Understanding of Self and Psychiatry: Personal Insights from a Tribal Buddhist in North India

12

Rajesh K. Mehta

This chapter has afforded me the opportunity to embark on a profound journey of self-discovery within the context of Buddhist practice. These reflections are organized into sections that examine the influence of Buddhist principles on these experiences. Additionally, I explore the potential integration of these elements into the fields of mental health and psychiatry, recognizing their capacity to enrich and deepen our comprehension of well-being and psychological health.

Nurtured by Buddhism: A Journey of Spiritual Growth and Tradition

Growing up in a Buddhist family was a unique and enriching experience. It allowed me the freedom to discuss noble practices, life, death, monastic life, karma, and the importance of family values with my nun aunt, affectionately known as "Jomo Aane," and her spiritual mentor, His Holiness Choegon Rinpoche Tenzin Chokyi Gyatso. As a child, I fondly remember attending a winter school near "Tashi Choeling," Gonpa, alongside other kids my age. During this time, I memorized various Buddhist mantras and prayers, which I continue to chant with my family to foster a spiritual connection. The intricately illustrated temples in my village, initially daunting, gradually transformed into sources of knowledge, wisdom, and a deeper understanding of Buddhism. Even in the United States, Buddhism remains an integral part of my life. Chanting Buddhist mantras, meditating, and praying together at home and in our local Buddhist temple keep me grounded. One remarkable aspect of our practice is the use of the "Mani wheel," a cylindrical wheel made from materials like metal, wood, or stone, adorned with intricate designs. These prayer wheels aid in meditation and accumulate wisdom and good karma. Spinning the wheel is akin to reciting prayers orally, and it serves to set aside negative energy and bad karma. The inner section of the wheelhouse is tightly scrolled with paper or other materials inscribed with mantras. For me, Mani is an inseparable part of Tibetan and Buddhist traditions. We also keep a handheld prayer wheel in our home for daily prayers. Buddhists carry these prayer wheels for hours and even during long pilgrimages, rotating them clockwise whenever they have a free hand.

R. K. Mehta (✉)
Department of Psychiatry, Case Western Reserve University, Cleveland, OH, USA

Psychiatry Residency Program, MetroHealth Medical Center, Cleveland, OH, USA

Association of Family Psychiatrist, Cleveland, OH, USA

Northeast Ohio Society of Child, and Adolescent Psychiatry, Washington, DC, USA

Family Committee, Group for the Advancement of Psychiatry, Dallas, TX, USA
e-mail: https://www.familypsychiatrists.org

At monasteries and temples, you will often find prayer wheels at the entrance gates, and devotees spin them before passing through. Another tradition we uphold is offering water, known as "Yonchap," in seven bowls each morning as a way to accumulate merit and virtue. Besides water, these bowls can be filled with flowers, salt, incense, grains, food, and fruits. I have learned that in Buddhism, water symbolizes purity, clarity, calmness, and life-giving qualities. It is readily available to all, does not harm others, and carries profound spiritual significance.

Buddhism and Life in the Village of Spillow

Nestled in the tranquil landscapes of Himachal Pradesh, India, Spillow emerges as a small village in the heart of Kinnaur District, within Pooh Tehsil. It stands 10 miles east of the district headquarters, Reckong Peo, and 104 miles from the state capital, Shimla. Spillow finds its place in the "Shumso" Valley, gracing the national highway 22, perched at an elevation of 2360 m above sea level. Kinnaur, a land where Hinduism and Buddhism coalesce, paints a unique cultural canvas. Each Kinnauri village bears the mark of this fusion—a pre-Buddhist-era Hindu temple and a Buddhist Gompa stand side by side, embodying the Indo-Tibetan traditions. It is a testament to the harmonious coexistence of two ancient faiths. Flowing through this picturesque village with gentle grace, the Sutlej River enters and exits the embracing mountain valley, etching its indelible mark on the serene landscape. In Spillow, the practice of the Drukpa Kagyu Tibetan Buddhism lineage flourishes. Nuns and monks, adorned in distinctive red robes, lead monastic lives. An annual ritual, known as "Vajra Sattva Prayer," lasting 5–7 days unfolds in August or September at the nunnery. Under the guidance of His Holiness Choegon Rinpoche Tenzin Chokyi Gyatso, nuns and monks unite in prayer, seeking the well-being of all beings. Chanting, rituals, and prayers play a pivotal role in this form of Buddhism. During the Vajra Sattva ceremony, the Om Vajra Sattva Hum mantra resonates, elevating the spirits of both the listener and the entire village. It is believed that repeating this mantra and seeking Vajra Sattva's blessings purifies and instills gratitude. During Vajra Sattva, my family and I chanted the mantra while commuting, at work, and during evening family time, collectively accumulating 30–60 min each day. This cumulative chanting involves the entire village, fostering a sense of unity and spirituality. The "Dechen Choeling" nunnery in Spillow stands as one of the oldest nunneries in Himachal Pradesh. It is where my aunt and her 15 nun companions received their education and knowledge of Buddhism. To me, the nunnery represents a beacon of equality in the practice of Buddhism. I witnessed the transformation in their practice, knowledge, and education when they were guided by a guru. Nuns in my village, once primarily seen as aides in farming and chores, underwent a metamorphosis as they embraced their Buddhist knowledge. They were encouraged to reside in the monastery, leading a celibate life and abstaining from actions that harm any living beings. This evolution highlights the profound impact of Buddhism on their lives and the importance of spiritual education in Spillow.

Lessons from Lama Maime: Wisdom, Compassion, and the Path of Buddhism

My earliest memory of my grandfather, whom we affectionately called "Lama Maime," is etched in the image of him donning a crimson robe, clutching a handheld prayer wheel known as "Mani." In every corner he ventured, I witnessed the reverence bestowed upon him by my parents and fellow villagers. He was revered for his wisdom, compassion, and the tribulations he had faced throughout his life. As far as I comprehend, Lama Maime chose the path of renunciation and became a Buddhist monk following his wife's passing in the early 1980s. He received teachings from various lamas, but his principal guru was a nun named "Ani Dontok Dolma" from the Spillow village. My father recounted that he had undertaken a Buddhist meditation retreat known as "Thap" twice, enduring 4 months each time. I have dim memories of celebrating his retreat completion with joy and shared achievements within the family. Before the loss of his wife, Lama Maime had been a devoted family man who practiced Buddhism amid the trials and tribulations of a typical family life. His journey was marked by early nomadic living, familial conflicts, family deaths, illnesses, and financial setbacks. Reflecting upon his life and his contributions to our village and the spiritual blessings he bestowed upon our family fills me with profound affection and pride. Lama Maime was instrumental in constructing the "Dayoongur" temple, which he later gifted to the villagers. Presently, the villagers take turns lighting prayer candles there every evening. During full moons, I have joined the villagers in chanting, circumambulating, and illuminating candles, forging a deep connection to the spiritual traditions of my community.

Two incidents involving Lama Maime have left an indelible mark on me, serving as my inspiration to delve deeper into Buddhism and its practices. The first incident occurred when I was a 16-year-old boarding school student recovering from a hairline ankle fracture sustained during a soccer match. During that respite, Lama Maime frequently visited our home to spend time with me. We would sit in the sun, engrossed in lengthy conversations. I soon discovered his penchant for sharing his life stories with me, and I cherished every moment of our time together. One afternoon, as he sat beside me, tears welled up in his eyes while recounting his upbringing, family life, karma, samsara, maya, and the story of Buddha's life, including his own journey to becoming a monk. By the end of our conversation, I felt profoundly connected to the essence of life, as if his experiences were echoes of Buddha's teachings, reaffirming the Four Noble Truths. The second incident pertains to Lama Maime's passage from this world. By then, I had formed certain assumptions about the lives of monks and nuns, believing that they attained salvation upon death, achieving samadhi and liberating themselves from the cycle of rebirth. In 2000, when I was in my first year of medical school, Lama Maime

suffered a stroke. The news was a profound shock, and I grappled with questions about how such a fate could befall a monk, especially my grandfather. His departure unfolded differently from what I had anticipated. Bedridden for 2 years, his gradual decline was both perplexing and sorrowful. It was during this period that I began to fathom the significance of our present and past karma, realizing that life's circumstances are a culmination of these karmic threads. Lama Maime's journey inspired me to explore the intricacies of life, death, rebirth, and the "Bardo," the intermediate state between one life and the next. It taught me the art of embracing life and death with equanimity while comprehending the universal impermanence that governs all aspects of existence. Unfortunately, I was unable to attend his cremation process due to my medical school commitments. However, I vividly recall a dream in which Lama Maime appeared as a radiant, healthy monk, smiling warmly at me. I shared this dream with my parents, and they explained it as his way of bidding farewell. Although he has not visited my dreams since, his memories continue to bring me solace and smiles, for which I feel eternally blessed.

A Journey of Healing: Psychiatry, Buddhism, and Empathy

My boarding school trips were always made special by a visit to "Tso-Pema" Rewalsar, a quaint Buddhist pilgrimage village nestled in Mandi District, Himachal Pradesh. Whether I embarked on "kora" pilgrimage paths alone or with my parents, spun prayer wheels etched with "Om Mani Padme Hum"—meaning "jewel in the lotus," fed the fish in Rewalsar lake, or contemplated the ever-changing waves symbolizing the impermanence of time, these experiences left me refreshed and spiritually enriched. As I journeyed through life, I encountered uncertainties, responsibilities, career decisions, and experience of death and loss. In the face of these challenges, self-reflection, unwavering support of my family, guidance from mentors, and my deep-rooted Buddhist practice became instrumental in helping me navigate the complexities of both my professional and personal life. My path to becoming a psychiatrist unfolded during my medical school journey, illuminating my true calling in mental health care. This realization filled me with contentment, and I could vividly envision my professional journey ahead. When I shared my aspirations with my parents and Jomo Aane, their happiness mirrored my own. The reward of understanding and treating mental illness deeply resonated with me.

I firmly believe that within every individual lies the potential to attain a state akin to Buddha's enlightenment, to comprehend suffering, and then extend compassionate help to humanity. Providing the necessary care to my patients and their families brought me profound satisfaction. The moment I was accepted into the Psychiatry Residency program at St. Louis University School of Medicine in St. Louis, Missouri, remains etched in my memory as a source of relief and contentment. My subsequent fellowship in child and adolescent psychiatry at the Institute of Living in Hartford, Connecticut, expanded my clinical knowledge of child development. It also provided answers to my own existential questions about life, delving deeper into developmental and psychological theories. This journey illuminated the complexity of individuals, acknowledging both their strengths and weaknesses and recognizing their potential for positive transformation. Moreover, it underscored the profound interconnectedness of family members. My unwavering belief in the inherent capacity of every human being to achieve a Buddha-like state led me to explore mindfulness and meditation practices.

I have embarked on vipassana courses twice in my life, with the anticipation of more to come. In my family, I am not alone in this pursuit, as several practitioners of vipassana meditation have delved deeper into the understanding of the mind, impermanence, and practice of being "in the present." Over time, I shed my misconception that practicing Buddhism shields one from life's setbacks. My grasp of the Four Noble Truths, their practical application, and a profound analy-

sis of their spiritual significance made me more accepting of life's realities. This spiritual journey has transformed me into a more empathetic and understanding individual, capable of perceiving various perspectives when addressing complex situations and problems. I have recognized striking similarities between Buddhist teachings—the refuge of Buddha, Buddhism, sangha, and the teacher—and psychotherapy. Both involve learning from supervisors, grasping techniques, receiving support and guidance from peers, and gaining profound knowledge through practice. I firmly believe that my practices find their foundation in my upbringing and understanding of Buddhism through my family and personal experiences.

Nurturing Professional Connections: Psychiatry and Beyond

Being a Buddhist practitioner has allowed me to forge deeper connections with patients and their families, regardless of their religious beliefs. The shared aspects of religious devotion have been a personal resource, notably contributing to positive therapeutic improvements in patient care. I can recall working with patients from diverse religious backgrounds, including Islam, Hinduism, Judaism, Christianity, and Jehovah's Witnesses. My profound respect and reverence for the diversity of religious beliefs and traditions, and intermittently but appropriately disclosing my religious background, have consistently played a crucial role in advancing our treatment progress. One particularly vivid memory involves a grandmother who was curious about my own religious background. She shared extensively about how she faithfully took her grandchild to church every Sunday, and I was deeply impressed by their commitment and devotion to Christianity. They expressed a sense of uniqueness in receiving treatment from a Buddhist psychiatrist, which made them feel special. This experience highlighted to me that Buddhism is often perceived as a neutral and positive perspective in such contexts, and it also made me realize that I was seeing some similarities between my own religious beliefs and theirs.

I actively participate in several prominent psychiatric associations, cultivating a vast network of colleagues and mentors who span regional, national, and international levels. My involvement encompasses the Ohio Psychiatric Physician Association at the regional level, the American Psychiatric Association at the national level, and esteemed international organizations, such as the Indo-American Psychiatric Association, the World Social Psychiatry Association, and the International Child and Adolescent Psychiatrist and Allied Professions. Furthermore, I hold the position of secretary within the Association of Family Psychiatrists and play an active role within the Group for the Advancement of Psychiatry Family Committee. These affiliations collectively form what I consider my professional "sangha." Just as a sangha in Buddhism represents a community of practitioners who support and inspire each other in their spiritual journey, these associations provide a similar nurturing environment in my psychiatric career. They serve as invaluable sources of inspiration, guidance, and camaraderie, enriching my professional path.

Conclusion

As a result of my journey, I have grown to be more empathetic, understanding, and adept at seeing diverse perspectives when addressing various situations and challenges effectively. I have noticed striking parallels between Buddhist teachings—the refuge of Buddha, Buddhism, sangha, and the teacher—and psychotherapy, where I have learned from supervisors, grasped therapeutic techniques, received guidance from peers and supporters, and honed my practice. I firmly believe that my practices are rooted in this upbringing and my understanding of Buddhism, shaped by my family and personal experiences. Cultural and national variations influence how Buddhism is practiced worldwide. In this chapter, I provide insight into the practice of Buddhism in Spillow, Kinnaur, Himachal Pradesh, India, where a rich tapestry of culture, religion, and Tibetan influences converge. Two books which inspired me, and I refer for Buddhist practice guidance, are "The Tibetan Book of Living and Dying" by Sogyal Rinpoche and "The World of Tibetan Buddhism," translated, edited, and annotated by Geshe Thupten Jinpa. Sogyal Rinpoche's insights into life, death, and human experience have deeply resonated with me, inspiring me to cultivate empathy and a compassionate understanding of others. The teachings of the Dalai Lama, as elucidated by Geshe Thupten Jinpa, have provided me with valuable wisdom on Tibetan Buddhism, which has enriched my therapeutic practice and my ability to connect with patients and their families. To me, geographical location matters little, as a shared faith, common understanding of family and cultural values, and Buddhist practice instill in me a profound sense of connection with the people in my village and with humanity through Buddhist practices. We each have unique life experiences and have interpreted life in our own ways. My comprehension of patients and their families is enriched by my own religious practices. I feel most at ease and fully present when I am with patients and their families, actively listening to their concerns and contributing to their overall well-being.

Sikh Tenets and Experiences That Relate to Mental Health and Well-Being

13

Narpinder K. Malhi, Shawn Singh Sidhu, Ravinderpal Singh, and Manpreet Kaur Singh

Introduction

Sikhism originated in the Punjab region of the Indian subcontinent around the end of the fifteenth century CE [1]. It is the fifth largest religion worldwide with ~20–30 million followers [2]. The word Sikhism is an extension of the word "Sikh," pronounced sik-kh ("kh" should be pronounced as in Mikhail), not seek or seekh. The word "Sikh" comes from the Sanskrit root śiṣya, which means learner or śikṣa, meaning "instruction." Thus, Sikhs consider themselves lifelong spiritual learners and are encouraged by the tenets of the faith [3]. Sikhism is a monotheistic faith; however, its definition of the higher power can differ from other monotheistic faiths, and this description will follow. In addition to being spiritual seekers, Sikhs believe unequivocally in equality, service to others, hard work, and earning an honest living. Sikhs refer to their faith as "Gurmat" (Guru's doctrine) or "Sikh Dharma" and refer to

their path as "Sikhi" or "Gursikhi." The term "Panth" refers to their way of life and to their community as a collective [3]. People who identify as Sikh define themselves in a multitude of ways but as per the *Sikh Rehat Maryada* [4], the Sikh Code of Conduct, in which a Sikh is defined as any human being who faithfully believes in:

- One immortal higher power
- The historical teachings of Ten Gurus, from Guru Nanak Dev Ji (1469) to Guru Gobind Singh Ji (1708)
- The current Guru, otherwise known as the *Guru Granth Sahib*
- The baptism bequeathed by the tenth Guru, Guru Gobind Singh Ji
- Who does not owe allegiance to any other religion

Sikhs have routinely represented a visible minority throughout history. They have also not had a sovereign or independent Sikh state, and many live in a global diaspora. Sikhs have been exposed to generations of historical trauma and oppression by many rulers and for a variety of reasons, the principle of which relates to their inherent instinct to defend the rights and freedoms of others who are oppressed. If healthcare professionals appreciate the historical context that shapes Sikh identity, experiences, and inclinations, it can go a long way to build trust with Sikh patients and their families, especially in vulnerable health-related circumstances.

N. K. Malhi (✉)
Department of Behavioral Health, ChristianaCare, Wilmington, DE, USA

S. S. Sidhu
University of California San Diego, San Diego, CA, USA

R. Singh
Innova Kellar Center, Fairfax, VA, USA

M. K. Singh
Stanford University, Stanford, CA, USA
e-mail: mksingh@stanford.edu

The aim of this chapter on Sikhism is to introduce various Sikh tenets to provide a basic understanding of its theology as it pertains to a clinical context. Importantly, individual Sikh practices vary widely, as with any group. This chapter attempts to provide a descriptive framework for understanding a range of attitudes, behaviors, life views, values, and core beliefs of most observant Sikhs, acknowledging potential exceptions to these norms.

History and Origin of Sikhism

Sikhism originated from the spiritual teachings of Guru Nanak Dev Ji (henceforth referred to as Guru Nanak, 1469–1539), the first Guru and originator of the faith. Guru Nanak Dev was born in 1469 in Talwandi, a town 55 miles west of Lahore (currently in Pakistan). He was subsequently succeeded by nine Sikh Gurus. The term "Guru" comes from the Sanskrit word *gurū*, which literally translates to "out of the darkness (gu) and into the light (ru)" and effectively means to mentor, guide, or master as an expert in a corpus of knowledge or field. Around the age of 30, Guru Nanak had a mystical experience from which he emerged stating, "there is no such thing as a Hindu, there is no such thing as a Muslim, there is just humanity and oneness." From that point forth, he gave up all his possessions and started spreading his spiritual teachings by traveling by foot to different parts of India and even as far as modern-day Iraq. He was accompanied on this journey by Hindus and Muslims alike who resonated with his message of unity [5]. At the time, India was structured around a rigid caste system, in which people's lives and upward mobility were determined based on their status at birth. Guru Nanak openly challenged this notion, asserting that all are equal, and he included scriptures from so-called low-caste sages of the time to demonstrate that their wisdom was just as important to understanding the human condition as Guru Nanak's teachings. Guru Nanak also wrote several scriptures on gender equality in praise of women, which was also avant-garde for the time and region.

Guru Nanak communicated through the power of spoken word and used music to enhance the emotional experience of the lyrical word. Consequently, scriptures in Sikhism are composed in a variety of musical scales. In fact, Sikhism is the only major world religion in which the entire holy book is written with guidance on how to adapt the words to music.

Guru Nanak Dev Ji's first and most influential contribution to the Sikh faith is known as the *Mool Mantar* (or *Mūl Mantar*), in which he provides the Sikh definition of the higher power:

੧ਓ ਸਤਿ ਨਾਮੁ ਕਰਤਾ ਪੁਰਖੁ ਨਿਰਭਉ ਨਿਰਵੈਰੁ ਅਕਾਲ ਮੂਰਤਿ ਅਜੂਨੀ ਸੈਭੰ ਗੁਰ ਪਰੁਸਾਦਿ ॥ (Jap) *ikk ōankār sat(i)-nām(u) karatā purakh(u) nirabha'u niravair(u) akāl(a) mūrat(i) ajūnī saibhan gur(a) prasād(i).* — GGS[a] (seventeenth c.), p. 1	"There is one ultimate higher power, a oneness, that is the eternal reality and truth throughout all creation and throughout all time. This power is without fear and without hate and animosity. It is immortal, never incarnated, self-existent, and known by grace through the true Guru. Meditate on this."

[a] *Guru Granth Sahib* (*GGS*), henceforth referenced with corresponding page number [6]

The *Mool Mantar* was revolutionary when conceived because it deviated significantly from depictions of God as having a human form, or likely residing in the sky or heaven, or who issues judgment, or responds to conditional rituals or sacrifices. Guru Nanak's description of the higher power is a loving, nonjudgmental, compassionate essence that is felt as minutely as every cell in the human body, yet as vastly as the entire universe. The greatest task, then, for a Sikh, is to connect to this essence through meditation and awareness and to see this essence in humans, animals, plants, and all of life itself.

The history of Sikhs is closely associated with the sociopolitical environment in the northwest Indian subcontinent in the seventeenth century. At the time of Guru Nanak's life, India was invaded by the Mughal Empire [7], which sought to rule its subjects with fear and intimidation. The second Guru, Guru Angad Dev Ji, developed and formalized the written alphabet of the Sikhs called Gurmukhi, which made possible the elaboration of oral teachings into written scripture and spread the message of unity by creating community kitchens ("*langar*") where, even today, all are welcome and fed. The third Guru, Guru Amardas Ji, dedicated himself to a lifetime of selfless service, institutionalizing langar through a collection of community resources (*dasvandh*), and innovated distinct Sikh ceremonies (e.g., weddings), pilgrimages, festivals, temples, and rituals. The fourth Guru, Guru Ram Das Ji, expanded and created Sikh "Gurdwaras" (places of worship) and built the Harmandir Sahib, or Golden Temple. The fifth Guru, Guru Arjan Dev Ji, was the most prolific Sikh writer in history and compiled all the hymns of the Gurus. He was burned alive by the Mughal Empire for challenging the norms and beliefs of the time. The sixth Guru, Guru Hargobind Ji, created the principles of "*miri and piri*," meaning that all Sikhs have a duty to be saint-soldiers, attending to both their political or communal lives with others ("*miri*") and their spiritual lives ("*piri*"). He was also the first Sikh Guru who established a Sikh military for self-defense. The seventh Guru, Guru Har Rai Ji, was a healer who created hospitals and grew medicinal herbs for the ill. The eighth guru, Guru Har Krishan Ji, was a mere boy at the time he was named Guru. Selecting a child Guru demonstrated to all Sikhs that wisdom and love are values that are beyond the limitations of age. He died at a very young age while caring for those who were suffering from smallpox. The ninth Guru, Guru Tegh Bahadur Ji, was a scholar and a saintly individual and was beheaded by a Mughal Emperor for advocating for the rights of religious minorities.

Guru Gobind Singh Ji was the tenth Guru, born in 1666. He was a magnificent leader, poet, and warrior. He created the largest Sikh army in history to function principally in defending justice and freedom for all. He also created the first Sikh baptism ceremony ("*amrit*"), which, in some ways, is akin to a rebirth or a fresh start.

When Sikhs take *amrit*, they part ways with their former selves and pledge to make their spiritual life their highest priority with daily spiritual practice. All Sikhs are given the last name of Singh for men or Kaur for women, leaving behind old caste systems or notions of status in society and symbolizing that men and women are equal. A major difference in Sikh baptism, when compared to that of other faiths, is that it is typically a commitment that a Sikh chooses to make rather than a universal rite expected in childhood. We highlight here the importance of volitional choice to being a Sikh because it contrasts with the common misperception particularly by individuals who resent being born into Sikhism that they must remain a Sikh without agency.

The Sikh baptism ceremony, or *amrit*, gives practicing Sikhs an outwardly recognizable physical identity. Guru Gobind Singh Ji wanted Sikhs to be easily recognizable beacons in their community and to be people who would be seen as helpful by the public. These characteristics of the Khalsa Panth, or collective Sikh community, include adopting "five Ks:" *kes* or *kesh* (uncut hair, representing saintliness and spirituality), *kangha* (comb for cleanliness), *kachha* (short trousers for chastity), *kara* (steel bracelet to encourage righteous actions and behavior), and *kirpan* (a sword defending justice) [5].

The Current Guru (Scripture) of Sikhism

The last human (tenth) Sikh Guru, Gobind Singh (1666–1708), passed on permanent spiritual authority to the *Guru Granth Sahib* after him. Thus, the *Guru Granth Sahib* is not seen as a holy book, but rather the physical embodiment of all the wisdom in Sikhism. It is instructive to mention that the scripture contains contributions from the first through fifth and ninth Gurus, as well as compositions of Hindu bhaktas, Muslim divines, and Sufi poets of the time. The *Guru Granth Sahib* is comprised of 1430 pages (known as *angs*, or literally "parts of the body"), and 6000 hymns or verses called *Shabads*. Through metaphor and concrete instruction, the *Guru Granth Sahib* outlines strategies to improve one's thoughts, feelings, and connectedness. The language used is *Gurmukhi* that was evolved during the medieval period and is leavened with expressions from Sanskrit, Persian, and Arabic, with the accompanying alphabet developed by the second Guru, Guru Angad Dev Ji. Meditation, humility, and acceptance are viewed as essential to cultivating a meaningful relationship with God [8].

The *Guru Granth Sahib* is divinely inspired and covers topics related to religion, morality, and self-identity. Scriptural recitation and reading may occur throughout the day. The Sikh place of collective worship and gathering is called a Gurudwara. While Sikhs believe that people can connect to the Divine anywhere, Gurdwaras are the epicenters of Sikh communities and always house the *Guru Granth Sahib*. Of note, many Sikhs also keep the *Guru Granth Sahib* in their individual homes but doing so requires adherence to norms of respectful care of the sacred text. Gurdwaras also serve as common places for worship, sharing a community kitchen to prepare and serve food for all and providing shelter to all who are in need. Sikhs turn to Gurdwaras in periods of joy and sorrow, and Gurdwaras are expected to help immediately when faced with local calamities and atrocities. Sikhs have also established globally mobile charitable organizations such as Khalsa Aid International, which aims to provide support around the world to victims of disasters such as floods, earthquakes, famine, and war. Sikhs seek guidance through a daily *Hukamnama* ("command"), which is a randomly selected reading from the *Guru Granth Sahib*. Although the sanctity of the *Guru Granth Sahib* may prohibit its presence in traditional hospital prayer rooms, copies of an abridged Gutka (a small book containing the essential verses from the holy scripture) may be made available for Sikhs [9].

Fundamental Principles of Sikhism

Sikhs believe that there is only one, universal, formless, timeless higher power for all people, who is also the creator of this universe and all living beings. The Divine is considered equally present among all people, and thus there is no theological ground to discriminate against people based on gender, caste, race, or ethnicity. Sikhs live by three daily principles: meditating on the higher power through "mantra" or a repetitive meditation of the name of the Divine, earning a living by honest means, and sharing good fortunes with the needy and through selfless service to humanity. Sikhs yearn to live in accordance with *Hukam* (god's will/Supreme command) and believe that everything happens in accordance with that which is predestined.

Sikhs also believe in reincarnation and in Karma, which refers to the sum of a person's actions that determine future states of existence. The Sikh scripture explains Karma as follows:

> *The body is the field of karma in this age; whatever you plant, you shall harvest* (GGS 78).

All incarnations are said to have pain and suffering at their core, except the human life, which has the unique opportunity to connect mindfully to the Divine (GGS 631). Prioritizing progression along a spiritual path can release one from the cycle of rebirths or *Mukti* (GGS 434), translating to states of bliss, freedom, and liberation. This liberation (*Mukti*) is obtained by meeting the guru through *naam simran* (remembering the name) [10]. *Naam simran* means repetitive chanting of the word of the higher power, "*Waheguru*"

(Wondrous Lord), the effect of which can be enhanced in a congregation of other religious people called *sangat*. Reciting *naam simran* can cultivate an anxiety- and stress-free life [11].

According to the *Guru Granth Sahib*, *Gurmukhs* (those who turn their face towards the Guru/light) are individuals who are guided by the Divine and have overcome their base desires and ego, whereas *manmukhs* (those who turn their face towards themselves) are stuck in their own individualistic egos. Sikhism opposes egocentrism. The ideal balance of a Sikh's life is implied in the principles of *grihasti* (married life rather than asceticism), *seva* (selfless service), *simran* (remembrance of God), abiding *miri-piri* (temporal and spiritual power), and embodying a *sant-sipahi* (saint-soldier or saint-warrior) persona, combining spiritual power with a readiness to engage in courageous acts [9].

The scripture warns Sikhs of the five major weaknesses of the human condition that may be at odds with its spiritual essence. These five vices are lust (*kaam*), anger (*Krodh*), greed (*maya*), attachment to temporal things (*moh*), and pride (*ahankar*). Sikh philosophy compares the physical body as a robe influenced by one's Karma [8]. Sikhism resonates with other philosophies that emphasize that genetic, environmental, and personal factors contribute to preserving physical and mental health [8].

Articles of Faith (Five Ks)

A Sikh who has taken part in a baptism (*amrit*) ceremony or initiation into the Khalsa is called an *amritdari* Sikh and follows the code of discipline, the Sikh *Rehat Maryada*. *Kes-dharis* or "hair-bearing" Sikhs have adopted parts of Khalsa but not the full discipline. Religious beliefs and identity impact medical care and how intervention risks and benefits are received [12, 13]. Amritdari Sikhs always wear their five articles (five Ks) of faith that form a Sikh's external identity and commitment to the Sikh way of life [14].

The five Ks (Articles of Faith) are as follows:

1. Uncut hair (*Kesh*) signifies saintliness and spirituality with appreciation to the Divine for the natural form creating in the human body. To an observant Sikh, hair is as much a part of the body as an arm or a leg, and thus cutting one's hair can be traumatic.
2. A wooden comb (*Kangha*) is worn in the hair and reminds practicing Sikhs to maintain order, tidiness, and cleanliness of their bodies.
3. A steel bracelet (*Kara*) represents self-restraint and gentility. The circular shape of Kara is a reminder of oneness, infinity, righteous actions, and the higher power. It reminds the Sikhs to use their hands to carry out only good deeds.
4. A small sheathed sword (*Kirpan*) is also worn as an emblem of courage and commitment to truth and justice. The sword is used only in defense of the vulnerable, or to seek justice and readiness to fight oppression.
5. A type of underwear knickers (*Kachhehra*) represents purity of moral character and serves as a marker of readiness and agility, functionally permitting unrestricted free movement.

Although these articles of faith are always worn by observant and baptized Sikhs, daily practical use among Sikhs is variable. Some Sikhs grow their hair and wear turbans and may not be baptized, while others who are clean-shaven may express their devotion in other ways.

Articles of Faith and Healthcare

Understanding the significance of the five Ks can help healthcare professionals approach them with sensitivity. No article of faith should be removed from a Sikh patient without first obtaining consent except in an acute emergency when consent or healthcare proxy consent cannot be obtained.

Addressing concerns and discussing how the articles of faith will be handled can signal respect and build trust. This includes using clean hands and placing them in respectable spaces (i.e., not on floors, not with shoes or near anyone's feet, not with dirty laundry) [15]. Refer to image 1, which highlights the physical appearance of five Ks.

We would like to expand briefly on the kirpan and kes in a healthcare setting. The kirpan resembles a small knife or sword, with the dull blades usually ranging in size from 2 to 6 in. Kirpans are always sheathed and worn with a *gatra* (a strap) underneath a Sikh's clothing [16]. There can be a perception that a Kirpan is a dangerous and intentionally concealed weapon; however, instances of violence with kirpans are exceptionally rare, if not nonexistent. Healthcare staff and hospital security should be educated about kirpans so that they can openly discuss religious rights in a culturally sensitive manner with patients and caregivers.

Many Sikhs believe in keeping their long and uncut hair (Kes) as a way to accept the Divine will. If the hair must be removed for any medical indications or procedures, patients or family members should be advised in advance to make an informed decision, with careful consideration of risks, benefits, and alternatives. During COVID-19 pandemic, many healthcare professionals from the Sikh faith felt under pressure to remove their facial hair to conform to the personal protective equipment (PPE) requirements necessary for frontline workers. Due to critical shortages of PPE including powered air-purifying respirators (PAPRs) during the pandemic, many Sikh professionals made attempts to design novel ways to use PPE, which worked around beards and turbans. These examples illustrate the need for increased awareness of the integral role that unshorn hair plays in Sikh life and of the importance of maintaining their religious code of conduct under any circumstance [17].

Turban

Among Sikhs, the turban, also known as the *Dastar*, is a religious head covering that signifies many virtues including equality, fighting for injustice, self-respect, courage, piety, and honor. After the inception of the *Khalsa*, uncut hair and the turban covering it became an integral part of the Sikh identity. As such, the turban is held in very high regard by Sikhs, worn even by unbaptized and unobservant Sikhs for major life events such as weddings or funerals to show respect to the community [18]. Sikh females commonly braid their hair or tie it back and may cover their hair with head coverings called *chunni or dupatta* [19] or choose to wear a turban. All Sikhs cover their heads in religious places—a requirement in the presence of the *Guru Granth Sahib* [19]. Although many ethnic minority groups are subjected to discrimination due to their appearance, Sikhs are particularly vulnerable to discrimination as they wear distinct head coverings [20].

Since September 11, 2001, many turban-wearing images of terrorists have circulated the media, creating negative conscious and unconscious biases towards Sikhs worldwide [18]. This has led to acts of discrimination and hate crimes. These include verbal and physical assaults, attacks on the community, Gurdwaras, and multiple mass shootings and murders (most notably in Oak Creek, Wisconsin, in 2012). There has also been a significant rise in racial and religious profiling [21]. Although the decision to tie a turban is very personal, family and community input and support play important roles in providing guidance about value formation, beliefs, and religious practices [22]. Sikhs have reported a decrease in the wearing of the five Ks and other identifiable articles of faith in the context of discrimination and the rising influence of Islamophobia [23]. These oppressive acts towards the Sikh identity could have long-term implications for physical and mental health [20] (Fig. 13.1).

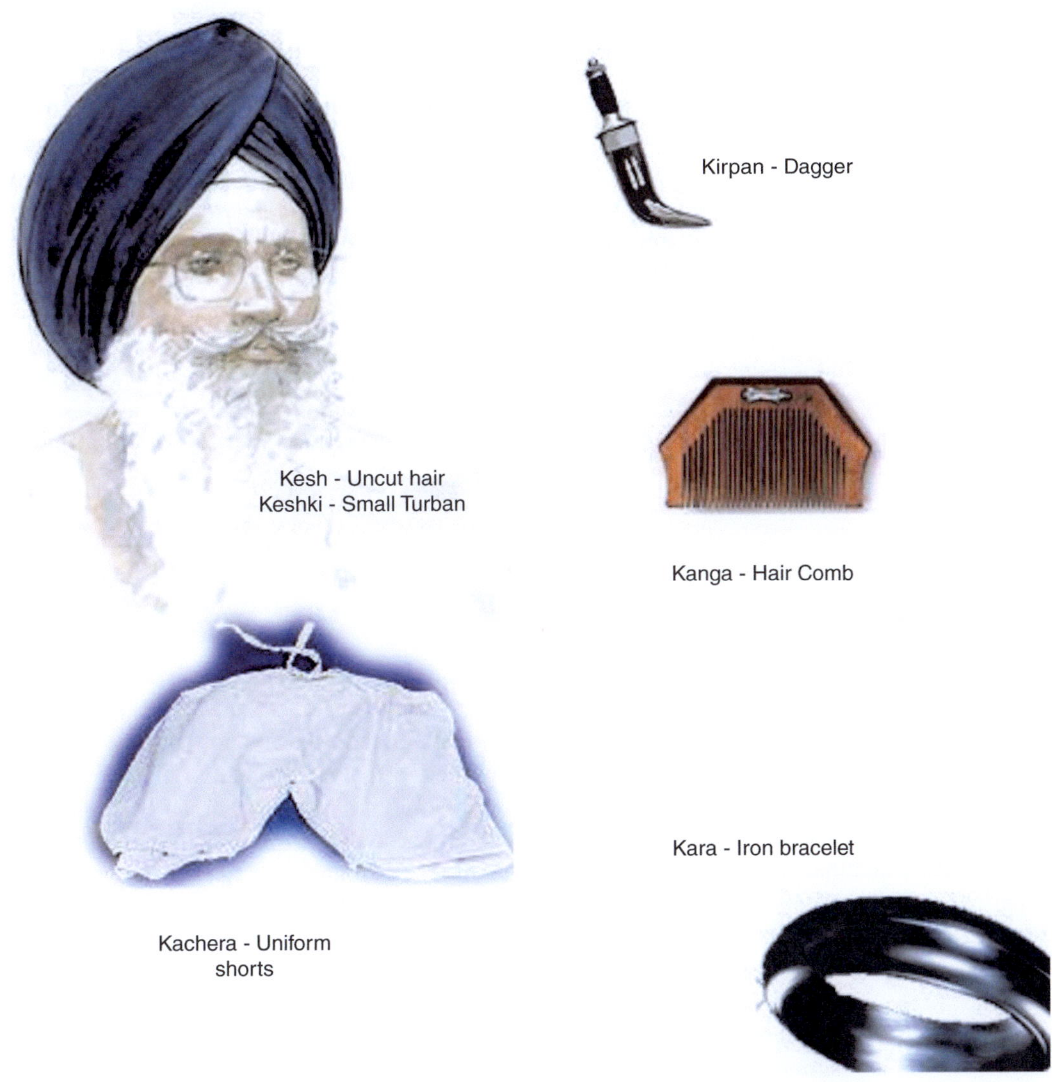

Fig. 13.1 Image of five Ks in Sikhism. (Source: http://sikhguru.org.uk/sikhsim/sikh-identity/the-5-ks/)

The Holy Sikh Scripture, *The Guru Granth Sahib*, and Mental Health

The holy *Guru Granth Sahib* is a focal point for Sikh teachings, experience, and faith (Kalra 2013). The text references sadness (*dukh*) and happiness (*sukh*), which are both part of a unified concept of creation (GGS 125). The term *dukh* refers to mental, emotional, spiritual, and existential suffering and encompasses depression, anxiety, severe mental illness, developmental concerns, and so on. One commonly held view in Sikhism is that pain and suffering come from egocentrism and separation from a connection with the Divine (GGS 59). Conversely, immeasurable peace, satisfaction, acceptance, and love come from a connection to the Divine (GGS 813). In this verse from the *Guru Granth Sahib*, "*Nanak dukhia sabh sansar*" (GGS 954), everyone is described as having sadness in their lives such that the world is overflowing with pain and suffering (GGS 767). This passage provides the real-world (versus theoretical) perspective that all of humanity experiences ego-centric "conditional happiness," in which satisfaction only comes when certain outcomes are obtained [8]. *Dukh*, or pain, can sometimes be seen as a Divine gift for Sikhs, in the sense that painful experiences can fuel and inspire critical changes, awareness, help-seeking behavior, and appreciation for what people have in life. However, when pain does not fuel such changes, it only triggers a cycle of endless and inescapable suffering [8]. Another explanation for sadness comes from bad *Karma*, which may cause suffering (GGS 15), whereas good *Karma* helps a person resist pain (*dukh*), disease (*rog*), and fear (*bhau*) (GGS 184) [8]. An important distinction between Sikhism and other Eastern religions is that Sikhs believe that Karma can be changed actively, moment by moment, by good deeds and connection with the Divine, rather than being destined to self-determinism. The text also mentions other factors which can cause depression such as unfulfilled desire (*kaam*), anger (*krodh*), egotism (*ahankaar*) (GGS 51), or love or greed for materialistic things (*maya*) (GGS 909). Although described hundreds of years ago, these factors remain salient today and will likely continue to be a part of the human experience. The concepts of pain and suffering serve as a reminder for Sikhs to remain aware of humanity and the realities associated with human existence [24].

The *Guru Granth Sahib* provides a metaphor for depression and suffering that compares sadness and agony to a deer being caught in a trap (*fahi fathey mirag*), causing individuals to continually cry out in pain (GGS, 23). There is mention of decreased interest or pleasure in activities (GGS 179) and self-neglect (GGS 225). Weeping (*rona*) (GGS 316) and loss of sleep (*neend*) and appetite have been mentioned as symptoms of sadness observed with separation from the Divine (GGS 244), as is a heaviness on the head (*sir aavey bhaar*) (GGS 222) [8].

To manage depression and find happiness, the text suggests meditating (*naam simran*) (GGS 1421) and selfless service of others (*seva*) (GGS 110). Meditation can be done 24 h a day (*aath pahar*) (GGS 901) buffering against depression [8]. *Sarab rog ka aukhad nam* in the text equates the Lord's name to medicine and remedy to cure all ills (GGS 274). The text also emphasizes Sikhs to come and join together in the *Sangat* or holy congregation to dispel the sense of duality and to relieve sorrow and achieve satisfaction (*Hoe eikathr milieu maerae bhaaee, dhubidhhaa dhoor karahu liv laae*, GGS 1184). *Sangat* is the modern-day version of therapy in the form of peer support available for Sikhs if they want to seek and can serve as a therapeutic resource for mental illness. In contrast, *ninda*, or negative gossip towards others, is listed as a factor that increases depression, anxiety, and suffering while judging others.

Historical Events and Sikh Identity in India

Punjab is an important Indian state for the Sikh community due to its indistinguishable ties to the origins of the Sikh religion and the history that ensued after its founding. Consequently, the northern Indian state of Punjab continues to have the highest concentration of Sikhs in the world. Amritsar is a holy city in Punjab where in 1577 the *Harmandir Sahib*, or Golden Temple, was constructed. Although Sikhs do not believe in pilgrimages, the Golden Temple is the most sacred space for Sikhs globally and has housed the *Guru Granth Sahib* in its inner sanctuary since 1604 [25]. As the popularity of Sikhism grew in the region of Punjab, it posed a threat to the Mughal Empire, which used to force subjects to convert and accept Islam. When the fifth Guru refused to make changes in the holy text and the ninth Guru refused to accept Islam, it led to their executions in 1606 and 1675, respectively. The Sikh community responded to these traumatic attacks on religious leadership by militarizing to protect themselves and the freedom of any religion. For a very brief period in history, Sikhs did have an independent homeland known as the *Khalsa Raj*. With the decline of the Mughal Empire, one warrior named Maharaja Ranjit Singh, won control of Punjab completely around 1800 and then came to threaten British control over India. After

Maharaja Ranjit Singh's death in 1839, Punjab descended into chaos, and following two wars with the British, the state was finally annexed in 1849 to become part of British India [5].

It is impossible to speak about the Sikh identity in contemporary India without acknowledging the impact of the India-Pakistan partition in 1947. The cost was what is called by later generations as "ethnic cleansing," involving the displacement of 12 million people who were mainly Sikhs, the deaths of another 500,000, as well as the loss of ~140 Sikh Gurdwaras to Pakistan [3]. Sikhs were left devastated, seeing their homeland, Punjab, divided into two states: the secular state of India with a Hindu majority and a newly created Islamic state of Pakistan, without an independent homeland of their own. Almost all Sikhs residing in western Punjab at that time migrated to be on the Indian side of the partition. Through persistent political efforts by the Sikhs, the Indian central government finally issued orders in 1966 to redraw the boundaries of Punjab to embrace those whose first language was Punjabi and to acknowledge that Sikhs constituted a majority in the new state of Punjab [6].

In 1984, the Indian Army attacked the Golden Temple on one of the busiest holidays of the year to curb advocacy movements for Sikhs in their homeland. The attack, known as Operation Blue Star, caused major damage to the complex's building and the death of approximately 1600 Sikh men, women, and children. Numerous human rights violations including sexual assault of women and desecration of the holy site followed, including the death of approximately 3000 Indian soldiers. Later in the year, Indira Gandhi, the Prime Minister of India, was assassinated by two Sikh bodyguards. This, in turn, prompted an organized government and police-sponsored response against innocent Sikh citizens, particularly in the Delhi area, resulting in mob violence and revenge killings of approximately 15,000–30,000 Sikhs. These incidents were followed by a state of internal civil war within Punjab between Sikh freedom fighters and police that lasted until 1992 [6]. These events have highlighted the influence of nonideological influences, political history, and tension in the formation of a newfound Punjabi Sikh identity [25]. In the research study by Seagall (2020), Punjabi Sikh survivors' accounts of violence in 1984 reveal the concrete ways that trauma influences collective memory and identity. Through their accounts, interviewees demonstrated a sense of helplessness and awareness of the dangers that the Sikh identity poses as well as the threats of their visible articles of faith.

Although Sikhs have emerged as a distinct socioreligious community, they have continued to face various socio-economic challenges in modern-day Indian Punjab. These include access to education, health services, substance use treatment, and unbalanced sex ratios (despite the Sikh teachings of gender equality). Shifting the workforce from farming to non-farming sectors and towards more productive employment pathways is another challenge for the Punjabi Sikh community [26]. These challenges have resulted in despair leading to increasing rates of suicide, particularly among farmers [27, 28]. In the fall of 2020, farmers from many states including Punjab traveled to the outskirts of India's capital to protest three farm acts that would have been detrimental to existing poor ecological and economic conditions for farmers. These protests were dismissed by the Indian government, which further strained relations between the Indian government and many marginalized communities in India who were predominantly Sikhs.

Sikh Diaspora

The term diaspora refers to the Greek term used for Jewish dispersal, which has been adapted to any faith communities living in countries other than their historical homeland and independent of their emigration and settlement due to traumatic events [3]. Sikhs remain concentrated in South Asia, with about 22 million adherents in India and 20,000 in Pakistan. The next largest Sikh communities around the world are in Canada (650,000), the USA (500,000), and the UK (450,000), with smaller numbers in Southeast Asia (175,000) and East Africa (50,000–100,000). Within North America, the largest communities are concentrated in California, New York, and New Jersey in the USA and in Vancouver and Ontario in Canada. There are nearly 300 Sikh places of worship (Gurdwaras) in the United States, the first of which was founded in 1912 in Stockton, California [29]. Migration of Sikhs from British India to North America happened in the early twentieth century. Some reasons for migration include worsening economic conditions in Punjab under British colonial land policies and heavy recruitment of Sikhs into British armies around the world. The roots of the Sikh settlement in North America can be traced to the celebration of Queen Victoria's Diamond Jubilee in 1897, when a Sikh regiment based in India was sent to London to attend the rituals [30]. In 1970, the US census reclassified people "having origins in the Indian subcontinent" as white, which led Association of Indians in America (AIA) to oppose the ruling. It was in 1980, amid pressures within the Indian community for recognition, that the census created an "Asian Indian" category when Indian Americans were a recognized minority. Sikhs were consequently acknowledged as Asians from 1980 onwards [31].

Sikhs and the Impact of 9/11

As above, Sikhs experienced a turning point on September 11, 2001, when they became the target of hate crimes in the Unites States. Since 9/11, there has been increased prejudice and discrimination against Muslims which have been generalized to anyone who might bear similarities to Muslims in appearance [32]. Many Sikhs became targets of hate crimes ranging from verbal attacks to physical harm because they were mistaken for Muslims by their long beards and turbans. Sikhs do not condone the targeting of Muslims under any circumstance. Nevertheless, negative stereotyping of Arabs and Muslims and their false equivalence with terrorism, including in significant pop culture and media references, have also caused Sikhs to be the target of these attacks due to lack of cultural competence by those unfamiliar with Sikhs [32]. The first fatality of such hate crimes was a Sikh, Balbir Singh

Sodhi, who was killed on September 15th, 2001, by a man who thought he was a Muslim. Sikhs are also placed in a very difficult position regarding Islamophobia. Sikhs view Muslims as equal brothers and sisters in the pursuit of spirituality. When being mislabeled as a Muslim extremist or terrorist, there can be a suggestion from others that Sikhs should simply state that they are not Muslim. However, this does not resolve the unwarranted attacks towards Muslims, which is antithetical to the Sikh concepts of oneness, humanity, justice, and defending others who are vulnerable in society. 67% of Sikh children experience bullying in schools. This is especially the case for Sikh boys for their unique turbaned identity [33].

The following case example highlights this dilemma for Sikhs:

At a clinic at the VA medical center in Omaha, Nebraska, a trainee Sikh physician who wears a turban and grows his beard just started his third-year outpatient psychiatry clinic rotation. He is an international medical graduate from India and speaks with an accent. A Caucasian male veteran in his 60 s who served in Operation Enduring Freedom (OEF) enters the office for his appointment with his wife. The patient has been diagnosed with PTSD and major depressive disorder. As the trainee physician introduced himself as "Dr. Singh," the patient looked at him and asked, "Are you a Muslim? Where are you from?" Dr. Singh delayed answering the question, feeling uncertain about not wanting to contribute to defaming Muslims by insisting that there is a difference between Muslims and Sikhs. The patient then becomes impatient and asks again, "Well? Are you a Muslim? Are you from the Middle East?" Dr. Singh then stammers, "Sir, my role is to provide you and your family with high-quality and compassionate care, and I would love to focus on how I can be of service to you." The patient then angrily replies, "Go back to your own country," and storms out of the office without finishing the appointment.

Racial and religious profiling of Sikhs due to their mistaken identity occurs in a variety of places, such as airports, workplaces, and restaurants. According to the Federal Bureau of

Investigation (FBI), between 2020 and 2021, anti-Sikh hate crimes increased by 140%, from 89 to 214. Despite the prevalence of such incidents in the United States, there is little research on the psychological distress experienced by the Sikh community after 9/11. National Sikh advocacy organizations such as SALDEF (Sikh American Legal Defense and Education Fund) and Sikh Coalition have taken the initiative to educate the wider public about Sikhs, mobilize around their civil and religious rights, and draw attention to hate crimes [30].

Sikhs and Intersectionality

Sikhs and other South Asian Americans encounter a triple quandary in that they must navigate their Sikh identity, the pressures of being a model minority, and the challenges of a disembodied marginalized identity [34]. In the United States, Sikhs are a racial, ethnic, and religious minority group. Sikhs, like any other minority group, also have their collective experiences of historical and intergenerational trauma and shared cultural experiences as explained above in the text (1947 India partition, 1984 genocide) [35]. The concept of intersectionality was developed by the scholar Kimberlé Williams Crenshaw in the late 1980s to understand the legal and epistemological frameworks for people who are at the intersection of multiple oppressions, which since then has grown across many public contexts [36], and to understand the entangled nature of multiple identities [37]. Bowleg et al. demonstrated the challenges faced by individuals who occupy a minority status within more than one identity category, which has multiplicative effects on levels of stress [38]. The relation between self-reported discrimination and mental and physical health (self-reported physical health conditions and direct, physiologic measures [BMI, waist-to-hip ratio, and blood pressure]) has been well described among Sikh Asian Indians. Outcomes of this study showed that discrimination was significantly associated with poorer self-reported mental ($B = -0.53$, $p < 0.001$) and physical health ($B = -0.16$, $p = 0.04$) while controlling for socioeconomic,

acculturation, and social support factors [20]. The concept of intersectionality Sikhism merits further exploration as Sikhs are at the intersection of multiple forces of oppression, predominantly religious and racial majoritarianism in India and globally [35].

Sikhs and Mental Health

Culture refers to a system in which words, behaviors, events, and symbols have ascribed meanings that is agreed upon by members within a given cultural group [39] and affects how people conceptualize their distress. Although the *Guru Granth Sahib* denounces any belief in witchcraft or spirit possession, many South Asian cultures believe that mental illness is caused by an evil eye or possession by a demon [40]. The sharing of these beliefs by Sikhs is more of a cultural concept rather than a religious interpretation of mental health. The prevalence of mental health-associated morbidity in Punjab is 13.41%, which is higher than the national average (10.6%). There is a higher prevalence of alcohol (7.9%) and substance abuse (2.4%) in Punjab compared to other states, which contributes to higher morbidity. In addition, rural Punjab observes higher mental health morbidity as compared to other states where it is seen in urban areas. These differences may be due to crop failure, rising debt, higher cost of cultivation, and unemployment in rural Punjab [41].

Punjabi people are more likely to be diagnosed as having subclinical and physical and somatic disorders as compared to Western patients and other South Asian subgroups [42, 43]. Women of Punjabi origin have been more likely to present with "sinking heart," using phrases like "weight on my heart/mind" preferentially to describe emotional distress [44]. One-third of young people in India display poor knowledge of mental health problems and hold negative attitudes towards people with mental health problems, and one in five young people in India experiences actual/intended stigmatizing behavior [45]. Young people are unable to recognize the causes and symptoms of mental health problems and commonly believe that recovery is unlikely [45].

Mental health service-seeking behavior among Asian immigrants (AIs) is hampered by cultural stigma, lack of awareness of services available, and poor understanding of mental health issues [46, 47]. Additional barriers include a lack of culturally and linguistically available resources, the high cost of mental health services, the desire to avoid worrying family members, and, for adolescents and young adults, the perception of parents' lack of knowledge regarding mental health issues [48]. In a US population sample of adult male and female Sikh immigrant participants ($N = 350$), language preference for Punjabi rather than English to complete the survey pointed to a subgroup with higher levels of depression and lower life satisfaction. Depression was largely underreported suggesting a reluctance to discuss mental health challenges. While multiple sociocultural variables have been associated with depression, negative religious coping and anxiety may be important predictors [48]. Similarly, Asian patients in the UK are more likely to attribute psychotic symptoms to supernatural causes during the first-episode psychosis and more likely to seek help from faith-based organizations [49]. No relation was found between expressed emotion and parental burden in UK Sikh parents who instead exhibit emotional over-involvement characterized by self-sacrificing and overprotective behavior [50].

In another ethnographic study in the UK which explored the contemporary Sikh views ($N = 50$) on mental illness from a religious perspective, older Sikhs tended not to see the origin of mental illness from a biomedical point of view but rather ascribed mental illness to external factors such as a lack of faith or a result of bad "Karma" [11]. Karma introduces the notion that current illness is a consequence of bad deeds in previous births, which raises concerns about stigma, prejudice, and discrimination within the community. Consider this example:

A recently retired female Punjabi Sikh patient in her early 60 s with a history of hypertension, diabetes mellitus type 2, and rheumatoid arthritis was referred by primary care for evaluation of her ongoing depression symptoms. She migrated to the USA in her 30s. During her appointment with the psychiatrist, she reported feeling sad with decreased appetite, poor sleep, and nonadherence with her medications. She also reported feeling guilty as she is not able to support her husband who is suffering from multiple medical issues. Her psychiatrist who was a Caucasian-American recommended to start medications and psychotherapy to address her symptoms. The patient showed her reluctance to start treatment and questioned how it will address her symptoms. She blamed her Karma and expressed her desire to do more *seva* and *simran* for relief of her symptoms. After a couple of sessions, the patient was lost to follow-up.

A misunderstanding of the concept of Karma could lead some Sikhs to believe that mental health symptoms are a result of something they did in a previous life, thus signaling that they have brought this upon themselves and deserve to suffer. Sikhs have also had to be incredibly stoic throughout centuries of oppression to maintain their independence and identity. All these factors can lead some Sikh patients to delay seeking mental health treatment, or not seek it at all. For Sikhs, faith and spirituality play an important role in treatment. Sikhs have also turned to relaxation techniques such as meditation and Kundalini yoga and physical exercise such as Sikh martial arts (*Gatka*) to balance their mind and emotions. On the other hand, young Sikhs, based on their level of acculturation in the diaspora, may be more accepting of mental health diagnoses and seeking professional help [11].

Sikhism and Spirituality

Religion is generally organized by consensus and involves beliefs, practices, and rituals related to the sacred. In contrast, spirituality is considered more personal, something people define for themselves that is largely free of the rules, regulations, and responsibilities associated with organized religion [51]. Religion and spirituality have generally been shown to be beneficial for the mental health of many patients and have been associated with greater well-being, higher quality of life, and lower rates of depression, anxiety, and suicide [52]. To live a Sikh way of life, it is important to give up *Haumai* (egocentrism and overt individuality to the extent of selfishness) and accept humility. Spiritual meditation is done by chanting *"Waheguru"* repetitively to achieve a superconscious and blissful state along with relaxation of the body and mind. The feeling of spirituality in which Sikhs are encouraged to accept God's will (*Hukam*) rather than blame themselves for their circumstance has remained a core value of Sikhism and helps foster resilience [35].

Sikhism promotes these five virtues to live a happy and spiritual life.

- *Sat* (Truth): The higher power is true, and all awakened souls practice truth and reflect upon the word of the higher power. O Nanak, through the Name, I have obtained salvation and understanding; this alone is my wealth (GGS, p. 600).
- *Santokh* (Contentment): Practice truth, contentment, and kindness. One who is so blessed by the higher power renounces selfishness and becomes the humble dust of all (GGS, p. 51).
- *Daya* (Kindness): Be kind to all beings—this is more meritorious than bathing in the 68 sacred shrines of pilgrimage or giving of charity (GGS, p. 136).
- *Nimarata* (Humility): God-consciousness is steeped in humility (GGS, p. 273).
- *Pyaar* (Love): Let the awe of the creator be your feet and let the creator's love be your hands; let the creator's understanding be your eyes (GGS, p. 139).

Singh (2008) also provides a six-step hexagonal Sikh spiritual model useful in counseling. After psychoeducation, a therapist works with Sikh patients' self-realizations to strengthen five virtues and control five vices, followed by spiritual meditation [40]. An awareness of Sikh religious and spiritual beliefs can enable integration of traditional healing practices to provide culturally adapted psychotherapeutic interventions [53].

Recommendations for Clinicians

Clinicians working with Sikhs can effectively foster the well-being of this intersectional community. Cultural competence is defined as a set of congruent behaviors, attitudes, and policies that come together in a system or agency or among professionals and enable that system, agency, or those professionals to work effectively in cross-cultural situations [54]. When clinicians examine their own identities and attitudes, they create a safe place where people from diverse cultural backgrounds can thrive spiritually, socially, emotionally, and physically. The therapeutic holding environment affirms individual identities and needs [55]. Clinicians who self-reflect and co-learn with patients create a practice and narrative of cultural humility, encouraging patients to attend to their stories, keenly seeking to understand the social and historical context in which marginalized communities emerge [55]. It is important for clinicians to acknowledge the complex issues surrounding the ethnic difference in mental health care in minority communities. Clinicians may strive to provide services that promote shared decision-making, pay attention to cultural differences, and focus on therapeutic engagement [56]. The lack of mental health awareness and the culture of stigma and shame, along with the complexity of the Sikh cultural history, highlight why cultural competence among clinicians is so critical while caring for Sikh patients.

There is sparse research to guide culturally competent care for Sikhs. Clinicians are advised to gain knowledge and understanding of Sikh religious beliefs, values, and history, which can help facilitate the development of trust in the therapeutic relationship. It is vital to understand visible religious articles of faith such as the five Ks and the turban and their role in Sikh life while simultaneously recognizing within-group differences. Clinicians who have an appreciation of the historical events that have caused centuries of intergenerational trauma can better understand the evolution of a Sikh's identity and potential threats to self-esteem. As with any patient, it is important to ask questions about family history, historical dates and events, and intergenerational acculturation to understand the patient holistically [35].

Collectivist cultural values in Sikhs include family interdependence, collaboration, communalism, and conformity to social roles and norms. Most Sikhs will turn to their family, faith, and community (*sangat*) prior to seeking out mental health services [32]. Turning to Sikh scripture, persistent belief in *Hukam* (God's will) and Karma, *naam simran* (remembering God), and *seva* (community service) are central to Sikhism and are utilized by Sikhs often as coping skills during periods of distress.

The "saint-soldier" or "warrior-saint" identity is actively sought by many Sikhs as an ideal state of psychological well-being. Through intergenerational storytelling and fighting for social justice, this identity has been ingrained in Sikh core religious and cultural values [35]. Clinicians might explore when this theme is adaptive versus maladaptive (e.g., "strong and stoic" and help-rejecting) to understand where they stand in terms of willingness to ask for help and willingness to change.

Clinicians can also participate in community outreach, which can provide an opportunity to get to know more about the Sikh community. Collaboration to participate in community events can enhance alliance and trust with mental health professionals. Other interventions include providing psychoeducation on mental health topics, educational outreach to schools to offer lessons on Sikh history, and participation in online forums on religion to raise awareness. Clinicians can also participate in advocating at a policy level to protect the civil rights of Sikhs who currently experience discrimination in a prevailing politically divisive global context.

Conclusion

This chapter introduced readers to the basic principles of Sikhism and explored mental health perspectives among Sikhs. Sikh values are defined based on the Sikh code of conduct. The history and genesis of Sikhism provide foundations for practices that define Sikh ways of life. Although theological principles relating to mental health and well-being have evolved and have been extensively described in the scripture, there remain gaps in research exploring experiences related to mental health among Sikhs. We then provided some examples of views of mental illness as described in the Sikh scripture, followed by an exploration of the theme of mental health from a cultural perspective. We further examined different social, political, and religious factors that have come to shape Sikh identity. We also discussed Sikhs' religious beliefs, values, and discrimination faced due to their visible identity and explored how Sikhs capitalize on religion and a sense of community to promote psychological well-being. Finally, we concluded by exploring spirituality within the context of Sikhism and described interventions that clinicians can utilize to provide culturally competent care for Sikh patients.

References

1. Singh G. A history of the Sikh people (1469–1988). New Delhi: Allied Publishers; 1998.
2. United Sikhs. About Sikhs. https://unitedsikhs.org/. Accessed 04-08-2022.
3. Nesbitt E. Sikhism a very short introduction. 2nd ed. Oxford University; 2016.
4. Sikh Rehat Maryada. https://gurunanakdarbar.net/. Accessed 04-08-2022.
5. Singh P, Fenech L. The Oxford handbook of Sikh studies. Oxford University; 2014.
6. Sri Granth. https://www.srigranth.org/. Accessed 04-08-2023.
7. Sikhism. https://www.britannica.com/topic/Sikhism/guru-nanak. Accessed 04-08-2023.
8. Kalra G, Bhui K, Bhugra D. Does Guru Granth Sahib describe depression? Indian J Psychiatry. 2013;55(Suppl 2):S195–200.
9. Nesbitt E. Sikhism. In: Cobb M, Puchlaski CM, Rumbold B, editors. Oxford textbook of spirituality and healthcare. 1st ed. Oxford University; 2012. p. 89–96.
10. Kalra G, Bhui K, Bhugra D. Sikhism, spirituality and psychiatry. Asian J Psychiatry. 2012;5(4):339–43. https://doi.org/10.1016/j.ajp.2012.08.011.
11. Jhutti-Johal J. Sikhism and mental illness: negotiating competing cultures. In: Cave D, Norris RS, editors. Religion and the body: modern science and the con-

struction of religious meaning. Brill; 2011. p. 235–56. http://www.jstor.org/stable/10.1163/j.ctv2gjx03h.15.

12. Sidhu M, Griffith L, Jolly K, Gill P, Marshall T, Gale N. Long-term conditions, self-management and systems of support: an exploration of health beliefs and practices within the Sikh community, Birmingham, UK. Ethnicity Health. 2016;21(5):498–514. https://doi.org/10.1080/13557858.2015.1126560.

13. Kristiansen M, Irshad T, Worth A, Bhopal R, Lawton J, Sheikh A. The practice of hope: a longitudinal, multi-perspective qualitative study among South Asian Sikhs and Muslims with life-limiting illness in Scotland. Ethnicity Health. 2014;19(1):1–19. https://doi.org/10.1080/13557858.2013.858108.

14. The British Library. Origins and development of Sikh faith: the Gurus. In: Smarthistory. 11 Mar 2021. https://smarthistory.org/origins-and-development-of-sikh-faith-the-gurus/. Accessed 19 Jan 2023.

15. Sikhism-Healthcare-Guide. https://www.sikhcoalition.org/wp-content/uploads/2021/10/Sikhism-Healthcare-Guide-Electronic.pdf.

16. Kirpan Factsheet. https://www.sikhcoalition.org/wp-content/uploads/2016/12/kirpan-factsheet-aug2018.pdf. Accessed 04-08-2023.

17. Singh R, Grewal B. Your hair or your service: an issue of faith for Sikh healthcare professionals during the COVID-19 pandemic. Ann Work Exposures Health. 2021:1–4. https://doi.org/10.1093/annweh/wxab009.

18. Klein W. Responding to bullying: language socialization and religious identification in classes for Sikh youth. J Lang Identity Educ. 2015;14:19–35.

19. Ahluwalia MK, Nadrich T, Ahluwalia IS. Sikh youth coming of age: reflections on the decision to tie a turban. Counsel Values. 2019;64(1):20–34. https://doi.org/10.1002/cvj.12092.

20. Nadimpalli SB, Cleland CM, Hutchinson KM, Islam N, Barnes LL, Van Devanter N. The association between discrimination and the health of Sikh Asian Indians. Health Psychol. 2016;35:351–5.

21. Ahluwalia MK. "What's under there?" The questioning of civil rights for Sikh men. J Soc Action Counsel Psychol. 2013;5:50–8.

22. Ahluwalia MK, Flores Locke A, Hylton S. Sikhism and positive psychology. In: Kim-Prieto C, editor. Cross-cultural advancements in positive psychology, Religion and spirituality across cultures, vol. 9. New York: Springer; 2014. p. 125–36.

23. Singh B. The five symbols of Sikhism. Sikh Formations Relig Cult Theory. 2014;10:105–72. https://doi.org/10.1080/17448727.2014.882181.

24. Valetta V. Mental health in the Guru Granth Sahib: disparities between theology and society. Sikh Res J. 2020;5:2.

25. Segall HD. 1984 and Film: trauma and the evolution of the Punjabi Sikh identity. Undergraduate thesis, Oberlin College. OhioLINK Electronic Theses and Dissertations Center. 2020. http://rave.ohiolink.edu/etdc/view?acc_num=oberlin1589802152696357.

26. Ghuman R. The Sikh community in Indian Punjab: some socio-economic challenges. Int J Punjab Stud. 2012;19(1):87–109.

27. Gill A, Singh L. Farmers' suicides and response of public policy: evidence, diagnosis and alternatives from Punjab. Econ Polit Wkly. 2006;41(26):2762–8.

28. Singh S, Kaur M, Kingra HS. Farmer suicides in Punjab. Incidence, causes, and policy suggestions. Econ Polit Wkly. 2022;57(25):13–7.

29. Sikhism reporters guide. 2021. https://www.sikhcoalition.org/wp-content/uploads/2018/01/sikhism-reporters-guide%2D%2Delectronic.pdf. Accessed 04-08-2023.

30. Kurien P. Shifting U.S. racial and ethnic identities and Sikh American activism. The Russell Sage Foundation. J Soc Sci. 2018;4(5):81–98.

31. Dutta M. Asian Indian Americans: search for an economic profile. In: Chandrasekhar S, editor. From India to America: a brief history of immigration, problems of discrimination, admission and assimilation, vol. 25. La Jolla, CA: Population Review Publications; 1981. p. 76–85.

32. Ahluwalia M, Pellettiere L. Sikh men post-9/11: misidentification, discrimination, and coping. Asian Am J Psychol. 2010;1(4):303–14.

33. Preventing and addressing school bullying. https://www.sikhcoalition.org/our-work/creating-safe-schools/preventing-and-ending/school-bullying/. Accessed 01-29-2023.

34. Roopra HK. The effects of racialization on Sikhs in America: an intersectional approach. Senior theses. 2020. p. 383. https://scholarcommons.sc.edu/senior_theses/383.

35. Ahluwalia MK, Alimchandani A. A call to integrate religious communities into practice: The case of Sikhs. Counsel Psychol. 2013;41(6):931–56. https://doi.org/10.1177/0011000012458808.

36. Ratti M. Intersectionality, Sikhism and Black feminist theory: reconceptualizing Sikh precarity and minoritization in the US and India. Sikh Formations. 2019;15(4):1–29. https://doi.org/10.1080/17448727.209.1565307.

37. Crenshaw K. Demarginalizing the intersection of race and sex: a Black feminist critique of antidiscrimination doctrine, feminist theory and antiracist politics. Univ Chicago Legal Forum. 1989;1989:139–67.

38. Bowleg L, Huang J, Brooks K, Black A, Burkholder G. Triple jeopardy and beyond: multiple minority stress and resilience among Black lesbians. J Lesbian Stud. 2003;7(4):87–108.

39. Gaw AC. Concise guide to cross-cultural psychiatry. 1st ed. American Psychiatric Publishing Inc.; 2001.

40. Singh K. The Sikh spiritual model of counseling. Spiritual Health Int. 2008;9:32–43.

41. Chavan BS, Das S, Garg R, Puri S, Banavaram A. Prevalence of mental disorders in Punjab: findings from National Mental Health Survey. Indian J Psychiatry. 2018;60(1):121–6.

42. Bhui K, Bhugra D, Goldberg D, Dunn G, Desai M. Cultural influences on the prevalence of common

mental disorder, general practitioners' assessments and help-seeking among Punjabi and English people visiting their general practitioner. Psychol Med. 2001;31:815–25.

43. Bhui K, Bhugra D, Goldberg D, Sauer J, Tylee A. Assessing the prevalence of depression in Punjabi and English primary care attenders: the role of culture, physical illness and somatic symptoms. Transcult Psychiatry. 2004;41:307–22.

44. Bhugra D, Baldwin D, Desai M. Focus group: implications for primary and cross-cultural psychiatry. Primary Care Psychiatry. 1997;3:45–50.

45. Gaiha SM, Taylor Salisbury T, Koschorke M, Raman U, Pattricrew M. Stigma associated with mental health problems among young people in India: a systematic review of magnitude, manifestations and recommendations. BMC Psychiatry. 2020;20:538. https://doi.org/10.1186/s12888-020-02937-x.

46. Leung P, Cheung M, Tsu V. Asian Indians and depressive symptoms: reframing mental health help-seeking behavior. Int Soc Work. 2011;55(1):53–70.

47. Rastogi M. Coping with transitions in Asian Indian families: systemic clinical interventions with immigrants. J Syst Ther. 2007;26(2):55–67.

48. Roberts LR, Mann SK, Montgomery SB. Mental health and sociocultural determinants in an Asian Indian community. Fam Community Health. 2016;39(1):31–9. https://doi.org/10.1097/FCH.0000000000000087.

49. Singh SP, Brown L, Winsper C, Gajwani R, Islam Z, Jasani R, Parsons H, Rabbie-Khan F, Birchwood M. Ethnicity and pathways to care during first episode psychosis: the role of cultural illness attribu-

tions. BMC Psychiatry. 2015;15:287. https://doi.org/10.1186/s12888-015-0665-9.

50. Lloyd H, Singh P, Merritt R, Shetty A, Singh S, Burns T. Sources of parental burden in a UK sample of first-generation North Indian Punjabi Sikhs and their white British counterparts. Int J Soc Psychiatry. 2011;59(2):147–56. https://doi.org/10.1177/0020764011427241.

51. Koenig HG. Research on religion, spirituality, and mental health: a review. Can J Psychiatry. 2009;54(5):283–91. https://doi.org/10.1177/070674370905400502.

52. Weber SR, Pargament KI. The role of religion and spirituality in mental health. Curr Opin Psychiatry. 2014;27(5):358–63. https://doi.org/10.1097/YCO.0000000000000080.

53. Currie LN, Bedi RP. Integrating traditional healing methods into counselling and psychotherapy with Punjabi and Sikh individuals. In: Proceedings from the 2018 Canadian counselling psychology conference; 2019. p. 1–14.

54. Cross T, Bazron B, Dennis K, Isaacs M. Towards a culturally competent system of care, vol. I. Washington, DC: Georgetown University Child Development Center, CASSP Technical Assistance Center; 1989.

55. Hansen H, Riano N, Meadows T, Mangurian C. Alleviating the mental health burden of structural discrimination and hate crimes: the role of psychiatrists. Am J Psychiatry. Published online 1 Oct 2018. 2018; https://doi.org/10.1176/appi.ajp.2018.17080891.

56. Singh S. How to serve our ethnic minority communities better. Lancet Psychiatry. 2019;6(4):P275–7.

Pu Cheng

Brief Tao Bio

My family name, Cheng, can be traced back over 3000 years ago, stemming from the position of Shaman serving as a channel between men and the sky. My given name, Pu, means "uncut jade" that just preserves its natural characteristic. This example of myself reflects Taoism's presence in Chinese culture. I was born, raised, and educated in China; then immigrated to the USA along with my family; and then worked my way to become a practicing psychiatrist here. Later, I will talk more about Taoism from my personal perspective.

Introduction

As one of the world's oldest countries and civilizations, with documented over 4000-year history, China has developed its unique philosophy and religion. Taoism, by consensus, is the most important native Chinese philosophical and spiritual tradition, based on the ideology of the ancient Chinese philosopher Lao Tzu (Tzu is the traditional Chinese honorable title for sage).

"Tao," which means "way/path" in Chinese, is the central idea in Taoism. It points toward a path to achieve the ultimate harmony, peaceful coexistence, and acceptance of human and nature, thereby achieving inner peace and longevity.

History of Taoism

Lao Tzu, who lived around sixth century BCE, wrote the foundational text Tao Te Ching. Another ancient Chinese philosopher Zhuangzi (third century BCE) further expanded the ideology by his thoughts on the nature of reality and nonintervention.

During the Han dynasty (202 BCE–220 CE), Taoism gained widespread popularity as officially endorsed by the emperor, with the development of practices such as meditation, alchemy, and religious practices.

In the Tang dynasty (618–907 CE), Taoism reached a peak of influence and cultural significance under central government promotion and started the spread of Taoist practices to other countries, such as Japan and Korea.

Starting in the seventeenth century, Taoism was introduced to Europe and eventually all over the world in the next few centuries.

In modern times, Taoism has experienced a resurgence of interest both within China and around the world, as people seek spiritual and philosophical guidance in a rapidly changing

P. Cheng (✉)
Elevance Health-Carelon Behavioral Health, Indianapolis, IN, USA

Meridian Health Services, Muncie, IN, USA

world. Today, Taoism continues to be practiced by millions of people, both as a religious tradition and as a philosophical and spiritual path.

Basic Principles of Taoism

We have briefly noted the concepts of Taoism and will now explore more details of Taoism, which is quite different from, if not opposite to, Western philosophy.

Tao, or "the way/path," is the most fundamental principle of Taoism. However, it is a bit difficult to precisely articulate the meaning of Tao, as Tao Te Ching (the "Holy Scripture" of Taoism) says, "The Tao that can be told is not the eternal Tao"—meaning that the Tao as an intangible and elusive force that cannot be fully understood or grasped, but can only be experienced and lived. A close approximation found in the Merriam-Webster dictionary is: "Tao is the unconditional and unknowable source and guiding principle of all reality as conceived by Taoists." Although this sounds very vague, it reflects Taoist's ultimate respect for the natural rule.

Compared to Tao, the concept of Yin and Yang is much clearer, more tangible, and better accepted. But instead of being simply superficially dichotomous, the actual meaning of Yin and Yang is much deeper and more fluid. While Yin represents light, warmth, and activity, Yang represents darkness, coldness, and passivity. Yin and Yang are not simply against each other, but mutually contribute to each other to create a dynamic and sophisticated balance, which ensures the harmony of the universe.

Tao Te Ching also emphasizes the importance of living a simple and natural life, by letting go of unnecessary possessions and desires, by avoiding excessive materialism and self-centeredness, by embracing the natural rhythms of life, and by being attuned to the cycles of the seasons and the elements, so to achieve the goal of inner peace and harmony with Mother Nature. This coincides with the modern concept of environmental preservation. It is amazing that our ancestors thought about this more than 2000 years ago.

Another important principle of Taoism is Wu-Wei, which means "nonintervention." This refers to the idea that one should not resist the natural flow of events, but instead should go with the flow and act in a spontaneous and natural way. This concept might appear to be "foreign" to Western viewers, but a good analogy might be the holistic approach in medicine, which considers the whole person instead of only targeting the disease. It can be utilized as a political approach, as it was during the Han dynasty when the central government policy helped enormously in the recovery of society after a brutal civil war, which caused the fall of Qin Dynasty.

Lastly, Taoism teaches the importance of humility and nonattachment to the ego. By letting go of pride and self-centeredness, one can cultivate a spirit of compassion and empathy towards others and attain a greater sense of inner peace and contentment. This also contributes to the collectivist culture in Chinese and some other Asian cultures subject to Taoist influence.

Overall, one can easily tell the difference between Western philosophy, which emphasizes changing the environment to achieve individual's goals, and Taoism, which promotes the integration of human and nature, considering mankind as an inseparable part of an interrelated universe.

Taoism and Chinese Culture

Taoism, both as a religion and philosophy, through thousands of years of time, has deeply shaped Chinese traditions. As a major native religion in China, it has its own temples, priests, and religious practices and still plays a significant part of modern Chinese religious culture, along with Confucianism, Buddhism, Christianity, Islam, and other faiths.

As a major philosophy, Taoism's concepts such as Yin and Yang have shaped Chinese ethics, metaphysics, and epistemology. For example, Chinese believe that the female is represented by Yin and male by Yang and that each enhances and supports the other; if one gets sick, it means Yin-Yang homeostasis has been interrupted.

Taoism also has significant influence on Chinese art and literature. Examples include calligraphy, painting, sculpture, music, poetry, and many more. Taoist themes and motifs, such as images of mountains, rivers, and immortals, have been a common feature of traditional Chinese art for centuries and are still part of the tradition, especially in holidays such as Spring Festival.

Taoism is also fundamental to the theory and concepts of traditional Chinese medicine. As mentioned earlier, traditional Chinese medicine believes that disruption of Yin-Yang homeostasis is the etiology of illnesses and that by carefully choosing different herbal medications that represent Yin-Yang, along with acupuncture to dredge the invisible channels inside of the body called Jing-Luo to improve the circulation of Yin-Yang, one can reestablish the homeostasis and health.

Taoism and Asian Culture

Taoism has had a significant impact on many other Asian cultures beyond China, including that of Japan, Korea, Vietnam, and others. These countries absorbed Taoism, which blended with their own unique traditions to create diverse cultures.

Taoism has influenced major religions in many parts of Asia, particularly in Japan and Vietnam. An example of the way Taoist beliefs and practices have been incorporated into the religious diversity of Asia is Vietnamese Tam Giao, an amalgam of religious and philosophical Taoism, Buddhism, and Confucianism.

Taoism has also influenced many other Asian philosophical traditions, such as Zen Buddhism in Japan and Confucianism in Korea. Many of the concepts and principles of Taoism, such as Wu Wei and Yin-Yang, have been integrated into these philosophical systems.

Taoism has also had an impact on the art and literature of many other Asian cultures, such as in Japan, Korea, and Vietnam, and is an essential part of their marvelous history and cultures.

Taoism and Western Culture

Taoism was introduced to the Western world long before the Wu-Tang Clan established it (Wu-Tang mountain is one of the sacred places for Taoism). Since around seventeenth century, it has had a significant impact on Western culture, particularly in philosophy, spirituality, and arts.

Taoism influenced several prominent Western philosophers, including Friedrich Nietzsche, Martin Heidegger, and Alan Watts, among others. They were interested in Taoist concepts such as the interconnectedness of human and nature, importance of naturalness and spontaneity, integration of the spiritual and material, and limitations of human knowledge and understanding of nature.

Taoism has also influenced Western spirituality, particularly in the form of Taoist meditation, tai chi, and qigong practices. These practices have become popular in the West as a way of promoting physical and mental health, reducing stress, and cultivating inner peace.

Taoism's cosmological idealism of the individual as a celestial being and the universe as a single vital organism with its interconnectedness may have also influenced Western environmentalism, particularly in ecology movement. This movement emphasizes the importance of protecting and preserving the natural world and recognizes that human beings are only one part of a larger ecological system. This fits into Taoism's concept of harmonious cosmic unity.

Taoism World Influence

I was walking down the street in Chicago and saw a Tao restaurant that made me smile. Although I did not check to see if it served genuine Chinese food, it was an example of Taoism's world influence.

Another popular example is martial arts, such as tai chi, qigong, and kung fu. Many of the principles of Taoism, such as naturalness, balance, and harmony, have been integrated into these practices, popularized by movie stars such as

Bruce Lee, Jackie Chen, Jet Li, and, of course, the famous Kung Fu Panda.

Famous Tao People

There are many famous individuals who have served as significant figures in Taoism's development and evolvement and prosper around the world. Lao Tzu (sixth century BCE) was the legendary founder of Taoism and author of Tao Te Ching. Zhuangzi (third century BCE), a philosopher in the era of Warring States period in China, further expanded the ideology and established several important concepts such as Wu-Wei. Zhang Daoling, who lived in Han dynasty (1st–second century), established Taoism as the main native religion in China. And Alan Watts, a British-American philosopher, helped introduce Taoism concepts into the Western world. In psychology, Carl Jung and Abraham Maslow played a significant role in introducing Taoist concepts into mental health practices.

Famous Taoist Quotes

Taoism has many famous quotes reflecting its deep insight and wisdom.

"The Tao that can be told is not the eternal Tao. The name that can be named is not the eternal name."—Tao Te Ching, Chapter 1. This quote might be the most well-known one, although some find its meaning ambiguous and hard to grasp. It emphasizes the ineffability of the Tao, or the ultimate reality, and suggests that words and concepts cannot fully capture its essence, as it is something known rather than thought.

"Nature does not hurry, yet everything is accomplished."—Tao Te Ching, Chapter 14. This quote illustrates the concept of "Wu-Wei" or "nonintervention," emphasizes the importance of naturalness and spontaneity, and suggests that by aligning oneself with the rhythms of nature, one can achieve great things without undue effort.

"The journey of a thousand miles begins with one step."—Tao Te Ching, Chapter 64. This quote emphasizes that everything has a starting point and is a process of accumulation.

"He who knows does not speak. He who speaks does not know."—Tao Te Ching, Chapter 56. This quote suggests that true wisdom about the Tao knows that it cannot be described with words. It has been extended to mean that knowledgeable people do not feel the need to talk all the time, while those who are ignorant offer an opinion on everything.

Taoism's Applications to Modern Society

Taoism has many practical applications to modern society in areas such as social justice, personal development, and environmental sustainability, to name a few.

One can gain deep insight and self-awareness, and therefore develop inner peace, eventually achieving body-mind harmony, by practicing Taoism through meditation, qigong, or tai chi. Especially in today's world, with its increasing demands of technology, productivity, and other life stressors, learning how to forgo control, desire, and anxiety can help one find greater peace and the ability to thrive.

Taoism emphasizes traditional family values, compassion, humility, and Wu-Wei, which can enhance positive relationships between people within society, thereby helping us become more empathetic and understanding of each other and eventually achieve social harmony. This is even more important in today's world, which is more chaotic and challenging than ever, and in which it is essential for world leaders to solve issues via communication and mutual understanding, instead of by confrontation and war.

With the advance of technology comes more demand of resources, so that many are worrying how much our earth can handle. Taoism's emphasis on naturalness and harmony with nature can help mankind recognize the interconnectedness of human and nature, have more insight into the importance of environmental sustainability, and put real effort into protecting and preserving it for future generations.

Taoism and Chinese Traditional Medicine

Traditional Chinese medicine originates from the Taoism philosophy regarding one's relationship with the universe. In contrast to the Western concept of body-mind duality, eastern philosophies of Taoism adopt a holistic conceptualization of an individual and environment, by which health is perceived as a harmonious equilibrium that exists between the interplay of "Yin" and "Yang." While Western thought divides the body, mind, cognition, emotions, and behavior into discrete entities, Eastern philosophy regards the physical and spiritual as indivisible yet two distinctly different aspects of the same reality, with the body serving as the root for the blossom of the mind. One's physical, emotional, and spiritual well-being are taken as an integrated whole, underlying a systemic conception of the equilibrium of human existence. In Western philosophy, patients are taught to fight their illness, while in Eastern philosophy, they are encouraged to regard disease as symptomatic of the patient's bodily dysfunction and inner disharmony; the treatment therefore focuses on strengthening the patient's entire body system and restoring inner balance, instead of tackling only the physical manifestation of the illness [1].

Religion and Mental Health

Although the relationship between psychology and religion has historically been tumultuous, over the years, the attitudes of mental health professionals towards religion have become more positive as research has generally found a positive relationship between religiosity and positive physical and mental health. Several studies have found integrating religion/spirituality into therapy with medication and CBT to be potentially effective in treating certain psychiatric conditions including schizophrenia, depression, and eating disorders [2].

While some current studies and evidence support the efficacy of religion/spirituality therapy, further study is needed, and the decision to use such therapy involves issues of client preference and therapist comfort [3].

Taoism, the Mind and Mental Health

Taoism has a unique view of the mind and its role in shaping our perception and experiences of the world, which generates some overlap between the principles of Taoism and psychiatry. Both aim to promote mental health well-being and balance in individuals, although Taoism focuses on holistic ideology and psychiatry primarily focuses on biological and psychological aspects.

Taoism's view is non-dualistic, emphasizing the interconnectedness of all things and considering the world as a dynamic balance between opposing forces (Yin-Yang). While this perspective applies to the mind and mental health, including conditions such as depression, it encourages individuals to accept their emotions without judgment, to help them cultivate a more compassionate and accepting relationship with themselves. The concept of Yin and Yang helps individuals understand and balance their own emotions and behavior. By recognizing that different emotions and behaviors are complementary aspects of the same whole, individuals can work towards finding a sense of balance and harmony in their lives, so as to help alleviate symptoms of depression. This is similar to the CBT concept of avoiding cognitive distortions such as dichotomous thinking, as well as to some concepts of existential therapy.

Taoist practice also involves cultivating the inner self, including the mind, through meditation, mindfulness, and other techniques such as tai chi. One can achieve the goal of developing a sense of inner calm and clarity by becoming more aware of one's thoughts, emotions, and physical sensations. These practices are similar to certain therapeutic approaches in psychiatry, such as breathing techniques and meditation that can help reduce symptoms of depression by reducing stress, improving mood, and promoting relaxation.

Wu-Wei is a key Taoist concept that translates to "nonintervention." It involves learning to act in accordance with the natural flow of the universe and trusting one's intuition rather than forcing outcomes through excessive effort or control. The idea is to encourage individuals to avoid excessive or unnecessary effort and to allow events to unfold naturally, as one would in a holistic approach. This principle could be useful in the treatment of anxiety symptoms by encouraging individuals to let go of excessive control and to trust the process of healing and personal growth.

The Taoist emphasis on simplicity and acceptance can be applied in clinical practice by encouraging individuals to focus on the present moment and to let go of worries and fears about the future or regrets about the past, which are common stressors leading to mental health issues such as depression and anxiety. This can help individuals to develop a greater sense of peace and well-being, thereby regaining mental health and homeostasis.

Certain principles of Taoism are used as the basis of specific counseling techniques. Carl Jung used the Taoist concept that an individual's conscious and unconscious mind can work together to create balance and self-healing for neurosis. In his book "The Secret of the Golden Flower: A Chinese Book of Life," he wrote that psychic process of intuition could be obtained by the Taoist practice of Wu-Wei [4]. Abraham Maslow frequently wrote about the Taoist "let be" attitude and recommended nonactive, noninterfering contemplation rather than an analytical premature approach, as he believed that Taoist healing was a natural process by which individuals could experience events with less ego involvement and less psychological intensity through accepting their psychological pain [5].

Overall, Taoism views the mind, body, and spirit as interconnected and emphasizes the importance of taking care of all aspects of one's well-being. This holistic approach can be integrated into clinical practice by considering the individual's physical, emotional, and spiritual well-being when developing a treatment plan. Although this seems unlikely to replace the current psychiatric approach to mental illness, it can serve as a valuable adjunctive treatment option and provide additional benefit to those who are suffering.

Review of Case Studies of Taoist Applications in Mental Health

For the Chinese, traditional Taoism still has strong relevance to mental health, as Taoistic concepts of mental health stress the transcendence from self and secularity, dynamic revertism of nature (the philosophy of the balance of opposites), integration with nature, and pursuit of the infinite. Compared to Western concepts of mental health, Taoism advocates self-transcendence, integration with the law of nature, inaction and an infinite frame of reference instead of social attainment, self-development, progressive endeavor, and personal interpretation. In a multicultural environment, culturally sensitive and competent approaches are essential [6].

As mentioned above, Yin-Yang is the most fundamental concept of Taoism. Contrary to an individually centered mental health model based on Western culture, the Yin-Yang model focuses on eliminating or transforming individual desire to promote the unity of mankind with nature and society [7].

There are other applications of Taoism to mental health.

Taoist cognitive therapy based on the philosophy of Taoism to conform to natural laws by letting go of excessive control so as to regulate negative affect and correct maladaptive behavior can help to change modes of thinking and coping, in combination with medication [8].

A study in Taiwan indicates that schizophrenic patients believed that their long-term hospitalization and diagnosis of schizophrenia have impacted their spiritual life, specifically by expressing the feeling of a confused sense of fate; of being punished by a higher being; and of being deprived of life development, hope, and connection with family and society. By applying Taoist principles, nurses could help these patients with their spiritual journey by remaining aspirational and encouraging renewal and revival [9].

Taoist concepts have also been applied to other Asian populations. In a recent Vietnamese study, Tam Giao, which is a coexistence of religious and philosophical Taoism, Buddhism, and Confucianism through cultural additivity, provided a unique mindset with psychological resilience against COVID-19 pandemic-related psychological outcomes, as its ethical values and philosophies may have aided with health literacy, community solidarity, and positive outlook and in relieving some of the psychological impacts of the pandemic, such as post-traumatic stress, depression, anxiety, and other symptoms [10].

Taoist concepts have also been applied within Western mental health practice for many years. Besides Jung's and Maslow's practice, Bolen explored the relationship of Taoism and synchronicity [11], while Price applied the Taoism concept in family therapy [12].

Random Thoughts About Taoism and Western Culture from an Immigrant's Perspective

Immigration brought the change around the globe, from population and culture to technology and religion. It has profound impact on the countries and on the individual's life.

We often talk about culture shock to describe the emotion we experience when facing a different culture. But it is more a slow process than an instant reaction. We immerse ourselves into this mixture, absorb its nutrient, while struggle to stay afloat.

It is interesting to look back and realize that my internal motivation to immigrate was the opposite to Taoism's "go with the flow." But wasn't I answering the call from my heart and following my nature? As I immigrated to the states, and have been working hard to build my root here, so my children can thrive here and pursue their dreams, eventually settle down, and consider here as our home, I was able to find my inner peace and finish my Taoism circle, just like Yin and Yang.

My children, as second-generation immigrant, will also face a lot of challenges, not only the conflict between two cultures, but also between generations. I serve as a major barrier in this regard, possibly due to the traditional Chinese style that parents are in a dominant authoritarian role, which, obviously, is not well accepted by my American-minded children. Taoism concept might help me out, by applying the "Wu-Wei" mentality, to let children follow their nature, expanding boundary, or even learn from failure of course to a tolerable degree. Overall, I just want them to thrive and enjoy life, instead of being a copy of myself, let alone a hero to save the mankind.

Life is full of stress, in a realistic way instead of pessimistic way, and Taoism might facilitate resilience and let us to look into our inner self, accept who we are, recognize the limitation or imperfection, and continue to go on with our lives. It is not an altitude of giving up, but more to let go something we cannot control and focus onto something more meaningful or operable, as we only have limited lifespan and are able to achieve limited goals.

To my understanding, Taoism is not a doctrine that one needs to follow to the exact word. Just like Lao-Tzu said in Tao Te Ching, "The Tao that can be told is not the eternal Tao." Everyone can have his/her own understanding and interpretation of Taoism, as everyone has different nature, and everyone is a unique individual. Therefore, Taoism can have different meaning and application for each one based on his/her nature while following the same general principles.

From a religious-alike perspective, Taoism is somewhat similar to the "higher power" mentioned in 12-step program. It might or might not be referred to as God. It lets you do your thing and follow your nature, but at the same time is omnipotent and omnipresent. Maybe we might be more easily able to sense it, while recognizing our insignificance, such as on the apex of Mountain Everest, or witnessing polar light, or looking into the starry sky like Kant, etc.

In summary, in my eyes, just like swimming, Taoism helps me to immerse and adapt to the secular life, but occasionally pull my head above the water, look around, and find my path to the destination.

Future Applications of Taoism

What other future applications might Taoism have? This has been a subject of research in various fields including philosophy, religion, psychology, and cultural studies. As clinicians, we might continue to explore possible ways of utilizing its wisdom in mental health practice; artists and historians might study its cross-cultural impact and create more varieties of art and literatures; scientists might be able to utilize Taoist principles to find sustainable ways of advancing technology and human life while preserving nature; world leaders and activists might utilize the ideology to make this world a more inclusive and peaceful place for everyone; and all of us can hope to find inner peace using Taoist concepts.

References

1. Chan CLW, Ho PSY, Chow EO. A body-mind-Spirit model in health. Soc Work Health Care. 2002;34(3–4):261–82. https://doi.org/10.1300/j010v34n03_02.
2. Azhar MZ, Varma S. Religious psychotherapy in depressive patients. Psychother Psychosom. 1995;63(3–4):165–8. https://doi.org/10.1159/000288954.
3. Hook JN, Worthington EL, Davis DE, Jennings D, Gartner AL, Hook JP. Empirically supported religious and spiritual therapies. J Clin Psychol. 2009;66:46. https://doi.org/10.1002/jclp.20626.
4. Lü D, Wilhelm R, Jung CG. The secret of the golden flower: a Chinese book of life. Mansfield, CT: Mansfield Centre; 2014. ISBN: 978-1-61427-729-3.
5. Moss RC, Perryman KL. East meets west: integration of Taoism into Western therapy. In: Ideas and research you can use: VISTAS 2012, vol. 1; 2012. p. 33.
6. Yip K. Taoism and its impact on mental health of the Chinese communities. Int J Soc Psychiatry. 2004;50(1):25–42. https://doi.org/10.1177/0020764004038758.
7. Wang K. The Yin–Yang definition model of mental health: the mental health definition in Chinese culture. Front Psychol. 2022;13 https://doi.org/10.3389/fpsyg.2022.832076.
8. Zhang Y, Young D, Lee S, Zhang H, Xiao Z, Hao W, Feng Y, Zhou H, Chang DF. Chinese Taoist cognitive psychotherapy in the treatment of generalized anxiety disorder in contemporary China. Transcult Psychiatry. 2002;39(1):115–29. https://doi.org/10.1177/136346150203900105.
9. Yang C, Narayanasamy A, Chang S. Transcultural spirituality: the spiritual journey of hospitalized patients with schizophrenia in Taiwan. J Adv Nurs. 2012;68(2):358–67. https://doi.org/10.1111/j.1365-2648.2011.05747.x.
10. Small S, Blanc J. Mental health during COVID-19: Tam Giao and Vietnam's response. Front Psychiatry. 2021;11 https://doi.org/10.3389/fpsyt.2020.589618.
11. Bolen JS. The Tao of psychology: synchronicity and the self. New York: Harper Collins Publishers; 1979.
12. Price JA. The Tao in family therapy. J Syst Ther. 1994;13(3):53–63. https://doi.org/10.1521/jsyt.1994.13.3.53.

Zoroastrian Religion: Zoroaster— The First Prophet

G. Pirooz Sholevar

Prologue

The fundamental goal of a religion is to provide a guide to a purposeful and virtuous life. It is to help its followers to interact and relate well to others and the community. They should sustain a viable social and physical environment for everyone and a promising future for humans, animals, and their habitat.

The core tenets of the religion cannot be based only on the contemporary beliefs and observations prevailing at the time, which can dramatically change with the advance of knowledge. Religiously based belief that the world is flat and stationary, and torture everyone who does not think so, would lose its legitimacy with the discovery that the world is like a globe and is in constant motion in a lawful manner.

Legitimacy of a religion increases when their core emphasis remains equally valid thousands of years after its inception. A religion that emphasizes responsible interaction with the soil, water, air, and fire and keeps them unpolluted is refreshingly up to date and in harmony with today's knowledge. Tolerance and respect for the religious beliefs of other people are an ideal view at

any time and obligatory today. Insistence on hegemony of one religion at the expense of demeaning and invalidating other people's beliefs is not tolerable. Many enlightened ideas have been sacrificed to the violent and authoritarian demands of people with the sword.

The moral and ethical emphasis of a religion may be the best guide to its legitimacy rather than the number of its practitioners. The Samaritan religion is highly respected with the name of "good Samaritan" adorning many hospitals, schools, churches, and charity organizations bearing their name. The words of "good Samaritan" are incorporated almost in any language and culture. It does not lose its immense meaning and value because the Samaritan people have dwindled down to only 750 people [1]. They have been invited throughout history by many nations including Romans, Israelites, and Palestinians as an ally.

Jesus Christ glorified them, and many people mistakenly thought of Christ as a Samaritan due to his tender regard for them.

Introduction to Zoroastrianism

The Ancient Persian Religion

Zoroastrianism is an ancient Iranian/Persian religion and one of the world's oldest organized faiths, based on the teachings of the first prophet

G. P. Sholevar (✉)
Division of Child, Adolescent and Family Psychiatry, Jefferson Medical College, Thomas Jefferson University, Philadelphia, PA, USA

Nueva Vida Behavioral Health Center, Philadelphia, PA, USA

Zoroaster. The Indo-Iranian religions had a common origin but divergent trajectory. Zoroastrianism is arguably the first monotheistic religion in the world, and it includes a dualistic cosmology of good and evil within its monotheistic ontology. This has given rise to some misunderstanding about its monotheistic nature. Zoroastrians worship an uncreated and benevolent God with the name of Ahura Mazda ("Lord of Wisdom"). Ahura Mazda is the Supreme Being, uncreated, and has no equals [2].

Ahura Mazda is opposed by a destructive force, Ahriman who is commonly known as Devil or Satan (Angra Mainyu) [3].

The origin of Zoroastrianism dates back to the second Millennium BCE, 1800 or 1500–1200 BCE, which is estimated to be the time attributed to legendary Moses. The oldest historical document between Hittites and Indo-Iranians in 1480 BCE mentions five Indo-Iranian Gods [4, 5]. Zoroastrianism entered the recorded history around the middle of the sixth century BCE. It became the state religion of the ancient Iranian/Persian empires for more than a millennium from 600 BCE to 650 CE. Its influence as well as the numbers of its followers declined, after the invasion of the Persian Empire by Arabs/Muslims. The religion encountered its second destructive suppression, and its members were forced to convert, be killed, suffer extreme punitive financial taxation, or run away (the first destructive assault was by Alexander of Macedonia) [6, 7]. As a result, a sizeable number of remaining Zoroastrians fled to India and formed a distinct group called "Parsis," their names being based on their Persian origin. The Parsis are the most numerous group of Zoroastrians in the world now followed by the people of Iran/Persia, the USA, England, Canada, Tajikistan, Australia, New Zealand, Turkmenistan, Pakistan, and Armenia [8, 9]. Their number of Zoroastrians declined significantly due to brutal oppression by an invading enemy in the seventh century. The hostile forces against them still continue to force coercive conversions through economical and legal means.

Zoroaster claimed that he was a prophet from the God: Ahura Mazda who is the creator of the world and everything in it. Ahura Mazda first created "Asha" which is the life force and present in all creation and development. The force for creations is opposed by the destructive and evil force (Angra Mainyu), which opposes creation by death, illness, sorrow, pollution, and most importantly darkness to eliminate light. The ceaseless struggle and war between these two forces had given rise to the misunderstanding that Zoroastrian is a dualistic and not a monotheistic religion because it highlights the substantial struggles between good/right, life, and light on one side and evil, falsehood (Druj), destructiveness, and death in the opposition. However, the eventual victory of life, light, and goodness over destructive force, Druj, and darkness is expected. Zoroastrianism is an exceptionally optimistic religion [10–12].

This religion is founded on the principle of free will, which is the capacity to choose between the principles prescribed by the Wise Lord; his principal helpers, namely the Bounteous Seven immortals; humans; and animals. The destructive force has chosen to promote falsehood and destruction in distinction from his "twin" who chose the right spirit. Some animals chose to assist humans. Three animals, namely ox/cow, dog, and horse, particularly serve humans.

Zoroaster entered the recorded history between 600 BC and 700 BC, which is considered the age of sages. He overlapped with two great Persian Emperors Cyrus the Great and Darius the Great.

Zoroaster and Other Religions

Zoroastrian is an Indo-Iranian religion, and their Gods have many common but also different characteristics. Zoroastrianism has highly influenced the religions of Judaism, Christianity, and Islam. The concepts of heaven and hell, final judgment, and angels were introduced by Zoroastrianism. Satan/devil was introduced into Judaism to replace the serpent as the principal source of evil. Anticipation of Messiah and final judgment were introduced by Zoroaster and adopted by Judaism, Christianity, and the Shia branch of Islam. The Zoroastrian too prays five times/day based on sunrise, noon, and sunset, and two additional times were later adopted by Islam.

Plato's concept of the completeness and perfection of "forms" is based on Zoroastrianism as well as the Socratic inquiries into "virtuous" life. [7–12].

The God: Ahura Mazda

The Wise Lord

Ahura Mazda's and Zoroastrianism's most familiar image is his many engraved profiles in stone as a bearded flying man on two wings extending forward and backward representing the past and the future. The depiction is known as Faravahar [4, 13].

Ahura Mazda is the Wise Lord who has created everything in the universe. He is all wise, bounteous, and undeceiving. He remains changeless although his teachings remain flexible and adaptive. He has no equal, and no one can take the heaven from him. He is the creator of everything good. He is just and truthful and endorses proper deeds. He is all powerful with mythical energy on cosmic scale. He first created "Asha" which represents light, truth, creativity, and goodness. The three "paths" of Asha are spreading happiness through (1) good thoughts (spiritual quality), (2) good words, and (3) good deeds (charity).

Ahura Mazda was first witnessed by the prophet Zoroaster when fetching some water from a lake for morning holy rituals. One of the Amesha Spentas led him to Ahura Mazda who taught him about the principles of the religion. To overcome Zoroaster's initial strong disbelief, Ahura Mazda took him to the beginning of the time and let him see that Ahura Mazda has been there from the beginning and has created Asha and all the goodness through it. Ahura Mazda wanted Zoroaster to teach people to enhance happiness through good deeds and charity and protect the purity of the basic elements in the world.

The Bounteous Immortals

Amesha Spenta

The seven bounteous immortals are to serve people to achieve the goals of Ahura Mazda, good mind, truth, and righteousness (Asha). They have been referred to as sons (wives in old Avestan language) of Ahura Mazda and are his emanations. Some are male, and some are females. They are each represented with a month of the year and a day of the week. Prime among them is the right-mindedness. They are assisted by a large number of lower deities who are also "worthy of worship" [4, 13–15].

Deity	Tasks	Month
Ahura Mazda:	Creator wise lord	Farvardin/March
Spenta Mainyu:	Wisdom, goodness, light, protector of everything (sky, water, earth, plants, children yet unborn, cattle)	
Asha:	Best truth, justice, righteousness, correctness	
	Made of fire (God's Sevenfold Fire)	Ordibehesht/April
Vohu Manah:	Good thought: good deeds	
Hvar Khshaeta:	Sun	
Mithra/Mehr	Contracts (sanctity of), love	
Haurvatat/ Khordad	Wholeness, water, integrity, health	
Amertat:	Immortality, growing plants, multiplying sheep	
Spenta Armaiti:	Holy devotion, growing plants, multiplying sheep	
Kshathra Vairya:	Desirable dominion, protection of metals, power as embodiment of a warrior	
Armaiti:	Piety, devotion, green earth, fertility, and childbirth	

Zoroaster

The First Prophet

Zoroaster is a Greek rendering of the name Zarathustra, which is the original name in the sacred book of Avesta. He is also known as Zartusht/Zardosht in Persian and Zaratosh in Gujarati. He is the founder of the religion of Zoroastrianism [14, 15].

The Zoroaster as described in the recorded history was born in the sixth to seventh century BCE: in 628 BCE. He lived 77 years and died in 551 BCE. His life coincided with the beginning of the Persian Empire and the two prominent Persian rulers Cyrus (569–530 BCE) and Darius I (529–486 BCE). Zoroaster was a priest and from the priestly caste before initiating the new religion. He stated that he has encountered a vision of the Lord Ahura Mazda, the "Lord of Wisdom," who appeared to him and instructed him on the principles of Zoroastrianism, including the history of how he created the world, free will, and Asha [10, 13].

The universe is considered the contested ground between [13] Asha, light, and rightness, in contrast to [4] the destructive force, which promotes falsehood, lie, and destruction of life by decay (Druj). The battle between the truth and falsehood is ongoing throughout life. Ahura Mazda is expected to win the battle and end falsehood and decay. The people and the animals have the free will to join either camp. Ahura Mazda has set the example by choosing the light and rightness and expects people to choose the same virtuous path. They should be prepared to battle with the actions manifesting the destructive force in the form of disease, death, decay, and destruction of life. Ahura Mazda created a fertile earth covered with green and vegetation. The destructive force named Ahriman has created mountains and valleys to impose hardship on people and animals and made deserts and barren lands [16].

The heaven is named "The House of Songs," or "Abode of Light," and houses the virtuous and their family after they reunite in the afterlife. The followers of falsehood and lie would end up in the "house of sorrow" and encounter torments and regrets until their souls are purified [17, 18].

The Origin of the Universe

Cosmology

In order to vanquish Ahriman, Ahura Mazda/Ohrmazd created the world as a battlefield to be limited in time to 9000 years. He offered the timeframe to Ahriman as a pact, and it was mutually accepted. Ahriman then created a range of opposing creatures. Ahriman attacked Ohrmazd first to destroy his creations, but Ohrmazd defeated him with the help of a sacred Zoroastrian prayer (Ahuna Vara). There was a period of no action for 3000 years. In the second of a total of four battles, Ahriman was assisted by the prostitute (primal woman) to attack the material universe. He killed the primal bull. The marrow of the primal bull gave birth to the plants. His semen was collected and purified in the moon to produce the useful and friendly animals. Ahriman then killed Gayomart, the primal man, whose body produced the metals and whose semen was preserved and purified in the sun. Part of the semen produced the plant rhubarb from which the first human couple would be born [4, 13].

Ahriman tried to pervert the first human couples, and it was only with the advent of Zarathustra after 3 years that Ahriman's supremacy ended. This alliance allows Ohrmazd and Ahriman to fight on equal terms until the end of the last 3000 years when Ohrmazd is predestined to triumph.

Humans As a result of actions of Ahriman, men are mortal but they do not die totally. Six immortal parts of humans survive which are:

- Life (Ahu)
- Religion (Daena)
- Knowledge (Baodah)
- Soul (Urvan)

- Preexistent souls (Fravashi)
- The preexisting, spiritual, "heroic" part of soul (Manes and Pitarah) which has a protective defensive power that continues even after death

Following death and during afterlife, the person crosses a bridge (Requiter bridge), which is guarded by two dogs. The people with virtuous and just life are assisted by a beautiful damsel, which is the person's religion (Daena). The people who have lived unvirtuous lives will be accompanied by a hideous hag, and the bridge will narrow to the point of a razor thinness, and they would fall off the bridge into the hell. The good souls proceed to paradise and the bad ones to hell. The souls whose actions are equally balanced between virtuous and evil actions will go to an intermediate place for purification.

Creation

Cosmogony

In the beginning of the world, there was *Ahura Mazda* "the wise lord" who was self-created. He and *Angra Mainyu* have always existed separately. Angra Mainyu/Ahriman (a vector) is a destructive counterforce, who is a force of negation and opposed to creation and the welfare of what has been created by Ahura Mazda. It appears that the two forces have existed from the beginning. Ahura Mazda could not be the creator of the destructive force (Angra Mainyu) because his creations are all good and pure. There is a variation that the destructive force, *Ahriman*, and the righteous thoughts/spirit were created a set of "twins," but Angra Mainyu chose the path of evil and destructiveness. In a different variation by Zurvanism, the twins were created by Zurvan (time).

Ahura Mazda constituted the sky and was separated by a layer of "void" from Angra Mainyu. This coexistence lasted for 3000 years. Ahura Mazda then created Asha, which was infinite light in the form of a fire. The fire was bright, white, round, and visible from afar. From Asha, everything was born subsequently, 3000 years later. Ohrmazd then created Gayomart, the primal man, who was conceived as spherical in the image of the sky. Ohrmazd, the lord of all things, produced him from infinite light and the form of fire, whose nature was that of Ohrmazd and whose light was that of fire [4, 13].

Man's Helping Animal Friends

Three animals have special positions in Zoroastrianism, namely cow/ox, dog, and horse, because they have chosen to be devoted friends and helpers to humans in multiple ways [4, 13].

The cow provides people with milk and milk products. Ox/cow can be sacrificed to God and can strengthen the bond between the God and men. There are approximately 1 million milk cows providing milk products to 400 million people in the USA.

The preferred way of nourishment is the consumption of water, milk, and plant products. The consumption of meat is clearly the less desirable source of nourishment because it involves the slaughter of the cow and ox. The ox labors heavily to till the ground to grow wheat. The cow provides milk and milk products. The slaughter of cow and ox should be an act of worship by burning the fat of the animal on the altar of God and giving the hind legs to the priest.

The horse has been the major agent of transportation carrying people over very long distances and at a very high speed. They have been equally useful in carrying loads for long distances. They have provided means of communication between long distances. They became more useful in transportation after the invention of wheel, which resulted in the production of carts and carriages.

Horses were faithful and courageous partners on battleground and in the warfare. They carried soldiers on their back, making the cavalry a formidable force in warfare. The use of chariots first for transportation but subsequently as a weapon was a major intervention invented by Persian Empire. The horses were as likely as the soldiers, or more likely, to be killed as demonstrated in the "charge of the light brigade." The battle cry of Richard III giving his "kingdom for a horse" highlights the importance of this partner.

The dogs have had a status similar to that of the human beings in the Zoroastrianism. They guarded the soul of the dead person for 3 days by sitting by him and protecting him from evil spirits. Mistreatment of the dogs was sternly punishable and strictly forbidden. The person who mistreats the dog should submit to a long list of 18 lines of punitive actions to make up for his sin. The soul of a person who kills a dog will be hauling constantly in hell for his action.

When the dog dies, an announcement is sent out to the community, under the name of Ahura Mazda that "The soul has taken to the road" to the eternal bliss. The dog is dressed up as a Zoroastrian person in Zoroastrian human attire, with the shoulder cover (sadre) and a girdle (kusti) around his waist. For 3 days, the dog's favorite food is left by him for consumption by his soul. He will then be transported to the tower of silence in the same way that a dead man's body is transferred. After the vultures have picked the bones clean of the soft tissues, there is a disposition of the bones in a way similar to human bones.

Conceptual Beliefs

The conceptual structure of life is the fundamental characteristic of Zoroastrian religion. Friedrich *Goethe*, the German Philosopher, has named Zoroastrianism as the first and the foundational religion which established morality. He expounded his view brilliantly in his book "Thus Speaks Zarathustra." Goethe's impact on *Richard Strauss* the celebrated musician inspired "A Fanfare" for Zarathustra, which was further popularized when it was used as the opening musical theme for the movie "A 2001 Odyssey."

Ahura Mazda, the Wise Lord, is omniscient but not omnipotent. He will prevail over the destructive forces at the end and redeem everyone including those who have previously chosen the path of lie and falsehood. Bounteous/holy immortals, (Amesha Spenta), are the emanations of Ahura Mazda and are representatives and guardians of different aspects of creation and the ideal personalities. They are assisted by a league of countless divinities called Yazatas, meaning people who are "worthy of worship." They take care of both moral and physical aspects of creation.

Ahura Mazda will ultimately prevail over evil, and at that point, the reality and the world will undergo a cosmic renovation called Frashokereti. The time would become limitless, and the souls of the dead people, even those who were initially banished into darkness, will be reunited with "the best dominion." They will be surrounded by immortality.

Zoroastrian theology includes foremost the importance of a threefold path to Asha. They revolve around (1) good thoughts, (2) good words, and (3) good deeds. All three of them place heavy emphasis on spreading happiness through charity. They respect the spiritual equality and duties of both men and women.

There is a strong emphasis on the protection and renovation of nature and its elements, which has made Zoroastrianism entitled as "The First Ecological Religion." There is renovation and protection of water, earth, fire, and air, which are the foundations of purity and purification. The main representatives of Ahura Mazda, the creative spirit mentality, are entitled Amesha Spenta. Ahura Mazda interacts with creation through his own emanations, Amesha Spenta: bounteous holy immortals.

The concept of free will and active participation in life is fundamental to Zoroastrian religion. Even the animals chose to be on the side of goodness and righteousness or on the opposite side. Ahura Mazda himself has chosen the side of light, rightness, and virtue.

The foundational concept of Zoroastrianism is the presence of Asha created by the Wise Lord. It is the creative and sustaining force of the universe. Opposed to Asha is its antithesis, which is chaos, falsehood, lies, destruction of life, and humanity. The destructive agents are created by Angra Mainyu, which later was named "Ahriman." The actions of the destructive force are named "Druj," which represents the falsehood, sickness, darkness, destruction, and death.

Both good and evil were born as a set of twins, which were equal to each other. One of the two forces, namely the destructive one, or Angra Mainyu, chose the path of destructiveness, while the other one chose the path of righteousness.

Other fundamental concepts of Zoroastrianism are:

1. Rightness, righteousness versus *falsehood (Druj)*
2. Freedom of choice
3. Good thoughts
4. Good words
5. Good deeds
6. Active participation in the battle between truth and falsehood by any creatures, particularly human beings and animals
7. Humans and all creatures are the partners of Ahura Mazda and essential to victory

- *Rightness*

    There is a constant battle between doing the right things, which is morally and ethically correct, and it benefits people, animals, plants, and the primary elements. The primary elements are water, wind, air, earth, and fire. It is a falsehood to believe that one can act injuriously toward others without damaging the larger number of innocent creatures.

    The maintenance of purity is essential! One cannot pollute the elements and the materials without negative consequences.

    The light is the foundation of the truth and rightness.

    Falsehood and darkness are where the destruction begins.

- *Free Choice*

    Humans and animals have a freedom of choice to act in a righteous fashion, which maintains the life force, creativity, and service

to others. In the beginning of time, many animals chose to be on the side of righteousness and reject falsehood. Many animals, particularly the cow/ox, dog, and horses, chose to champion righteousness. Many other animals, including insects, chose to be on the side of destructiveness. *Snake* is universally considered an agent of Ahriman and interchangeable with him.

The concept of Satan did not exist in Hebrew Torah (The Five Books of Pentateuch). The serpent was held responsible for misleading Eve and Adam.

The concept of Satan was borrowed from Zoroastrian religion during the Babylonian exile and emerged very prominently and subsequently in the books of JOB and Daniel.

- *Good Thoughts*

    Good thoughts are extremely broad and encompassing. It is similar to the concept of "Word" in the gospel of John that states that "in the beginning there was 'Word' and the Word was with God." The concept of thought is more encompassing than the concept of the Word in the gospel. The thoughts are the underlying and fundamental cognitive and affective processes/forces, which perceives and evaluates the environment, the needs of everyone in the environment, and the significance of everyone. It then "thinks" and constructs a course of action, which would be most protective of everyone based on the principles of righteousness and protection of purity of basic elements and environment and least detrimental to others. It then collaborates with "good word" for a method of articulation with high fidelity to the "good thought." The thinking and cognitive processing may be different in different situations and have to be determined in the most effective and productive fashions.

    The principles of avoidance of harm to other people, purity of the elements, and protecting oneself from corruption are the guidelines for the thoughts. Many thoughts which have appeared to be desirable at the time may prove to have detrimental consequences. For example, the leading physicists concluded at the end that they would not have enlisted in the development of nuclear weapons if they knew of the manner of its use and consequences.

The good thoughts are conscious of the outcome to make sure that ones' thoughts, comments, and actions do not lead to destruction.

- *Good Words*

  Good words are dictated by the good thoughts with the adherence to the principle of rightness and avoidance of falsehood. It does not have any resemblance to the pleasant social comments, which may falsely represent the person's thinking and lead the other person into wrong conclusions.

  Good thoughts have to be based on telling the truth and righteousness with the full evaluation of the environment. Making a comment which is substantially true, but can be misused and eventually used against other people or the speaker, does not qualify as good words.

- *Good Deeds*

  The good deeds are the deeds which are motivated and energized by good thoughts and good relationship with others. The role of the consensus or its desirability should be considered. The short-term and long-term consequences to self and other people and the collective discussion and decision-making may be desirable. One may decide to refrain from doing the right thing if the potential for misuse and destructive action against other people, including the person himself, is highly likely.

Note The collective deeds of many people in the world have resulted in the deterioration of the environment, including impure air, polluted waters, and toxic soils in a deteriorating environment. The destructive forest fires may be the result of the pollution of many elements in the environment, which has given rise to global warming. This is obviously a debatable issue according to people's orientation, but could be an example of collective misdeed of many people in the world and particularly the more powerful people at the expense of the most powerless and vulnerable people

Avesta

Central Religious Text

The Avesta, the religious book of Zoroastrians, is written in the Old Persian dialect of Avestan and is a collection of several religious texts [19–25]. The history of Avesta has been the subject of speculation in many Pahlavi texts with varying degrees of authority. The current version of Avesta dates back to the period of Sasanian Empire. According to this version, Ahura Mazda created the 21 Nasks of original Avesta, which Zoroaster brought to King Vishtaspa. Each copy was written on 1200 ox hides and was kept in the Imperial Treasury until it was burned by Alexander of Macedonia. Sections of a second copy of the book were sent to Greece and dispersed among them. This statement, although controversial, has been affirmed in Pahlavi sources of Denkart and Tansar-Nama. During the Sasanian Empire, Ardeshir ordered Tansar, his high priest, to complete the search of locating the original texts of Avesta, which were in possession of the Greeks. Shapur the Second and Khosrow revised the collections and ensured its Orthodox character and translation into Pahlavi.

The compilation of the Avesta can be authoritatively traced to the Sasanian Empire, of which only fractions survive today in the Middle Persian language. The later manuscripts date subsequent to the fall of the Sasanian Empire: the latest being from 1288: 590 years after the fall of the Sasanian Empire. The texts that remain today are the Gathas, Yasna, Visperad, and the Vendidad, of which the latter's inclusion is disputed within the faith. Along with these texts is the individual, communal, and ceremonial prayer book called the Khordeh Avesta, which contains the Yashts and other important hymns, prayers, and rituals. The rest of the material from the Avesta is called "Avestan Fragments," in that they are written in Avestan, incomplete, and generally of unknown provenance. Other Middle Persian and Pahlavi books include Denkard, Bundahishn, Menog-i Khrad, Epistles of Manushchihr, and Dadestan i Denig. The collection of texts was compiled in successive stages until it was completed under the Sasanians. It was then four times larger than what has survived. Summary of its 21 books, or Nasks, is given in one of the main texts written during the brief Zoroastrian Renaissance in the ninth century: The Denkard, "The Acts of Religion." It is written in Pahlavi, the language of the Sasanians.

Significant progress was made when it was discovered that the old Avesta language was closer to Sanskrit than the Pahlavi language. A three-volume translation of Avesta was published as part of Max Muller's Sacred Books of The East, which also included five volumes of translations from the later Pahlavi literature of Zoroastrianism.

Gathas [19] are the 17 oldest hymns in Avesta and attributed to Zoroaster himself. The language is somewhat cryptic, and the theology is unfamiliar. The 17 hymns of the Gathas are organized into five sections. In the first part, Zoroaster praises Ahura Mazda and the six bounteous immortals (Amesha Spenta). He then pleads to the soul of ox for help against the cruelty of the wicked. Ahura Mazda appoints Zoroaster as the ox's guardian; however, the ox's soul complains that Zoroaster is powerless. Zoroaster then pleads for aid in fulfilling his assignment and asks for divine knowledge.

The hymns describe the dualistic world, "The primal spirit is paired with their opposite destructive forces, with Ahura Mazda and Angra Mainyu each being independent in their actions." One represents good thoughts, good words, and good deeds, which summarizes Zoroastrianism ethics. Angra Mainyu chose evil thoughts, evil words, and evil deeds.

Many of the Gathas consist of dialogues between Zoroaster and Ahura Mazda. They remain abstract and spiritual in their presentation. In later texts, the concept of a bridge over which souls must cross to enter the world of the dead was added. The hymns of Gathas are in various meters and are a dialect different from the rest of Avesta, except for the seven chapters. They are chiefly in prose. They appear to have been composed shortly after the prophets' demise. All these texts are imbedded in Yasna, which is one of the main divisions of Avesta and recited during

the ceremony of the same name, which means "sacrifice." The Visperad (all the judges) is a Yasna augmented by additional imbrications and offering to the lords (Ratus). Videvdat or Vendidad ("Law Rejecting the Daevas") consists of two introductory sections, including 18 sections of rules.

The Yashts [20] (hymns) are each addressed to one of the 21 deities, Mithra and Anahita. Verethragna section describes the fate of the soul after death. The small Avesta (Khurda Avesta) [23] is made up of minor texts and is used as a book of prayers.

The Avesta is a collection of texts compiled in successive stages until it was completed under Sasanian Empire. It was four times larger than what has survived. Of summary of his 21 books, or Nasks, only one is preserved in Videvdat.

Other works in Pahlavi include Bundahishn, "Primal Creation," a cosmology. Most of the Pahlavi books are anonymous, such as Menog i Khrad, "The Spirit of Wisdom," an elusive summary of a doctrine based on reason, and the book of Artay Vraf, which describes Vraf's descent into the Netherlands, as well as heaven and hell, and the pleasures and pains awaiting the virtuous and the wicked [26].

The Pahlavi books are not considered the scripture. Nevertheless, they are sacred literature and some of the major sources for understandings of Zoroastrianism.

Death and Disposition of Body

Death of a person indicates that the physical life has been invaded by the destructive force of Ahriman. It is no longer pure. Any contact with the body is a source of impurity [4, 13, 27–31].

The dead body cannot be buried or burned in funeral pyre. The earth and fire are sacred, and the contact of the body will pollute them. Therefore, the body is carried after 3 days to a "tower of silence" (Dakhma) and left on the ground naked. The vultures and ravens pick and eat the skin and organs and leave the bones clean of any soft tissues quickly and in a couple of days.

The bones are gathered subsequently and placed in the special well in the bottom of the tower between a layer of charcoal and Lyme. The bones disintegrate slowly and gradually thereafter.

The prayer sessions and ceremonies are offered prior to the transfer of the body to the tower of silence and at the time of transfer of the bones.

In Zoroastrian religion, there is no prohibition against exploration or dissection of a dead body due to an illness or natural causes, which can obviously enhance the knowledge of disease process, treatment, or anatomy. Such prohibitions by the three of the major religions, namely Christianity, Islam, and Judaism, have impeded medical progress for centuries.

A dog will stay for 3 days with the dead body to protect the soul from evil spirits. The favorite meal of the dead person is provided next to the body for the nourishment of the soul. The preferred type of dog for this function is what is called a "four-eyed dog," which is a dog with two black spots over the two eyes. Such dogs are reputed to be more detective of the evil spirits and ward them off.

The disposition of the body in towers of silence has been voluntarily altered in Iran in the past few decades for public health reasons as well as due to the scarcity of vultures in some areas. A modification of the practices has taken place, and the dead body is placed on a slap of stone or concrete, and a second slap of concrete is placed on the top.

The disposition of the body of a dog will follow the same steps as it will be described separately.

The soul of a dead person begins its journey after death. The soul of both virtuous and nonvirtuous people travels to a bridge for determination of their destiny. The virtuous people are met by a fair maiden who leads them to the "house of light and songs" (paradise). The bridge widens significantly and becomes very welcoming.

The soul of a nonvirtuous person is met by miserable looking hag. The bridge narrows down and becomes like a razor, and the person would fall down in a pit of misery, sorrow, and regret. There is no fire in the dungeon because fire is a sacred element and should be protected from contamination by impurity.

The suffering of nonvirtuous souls is temporary and nonpermanent. They proceed through the process of purification from their deeds and then join the company of souls of virtuous people. The family congregates together, and the children, parents, grandparents, and previous generations stay together in paradise. The reunion with family and social network exemplifies the emphasis of the Zoroastrian religion on the social context of life.

A river of molten metals will flow on the earth on the final day of judgment when the Savior (Saoshyans) arrives. The Moulton mental will be like warm milk for the virtuous people but will be tormenting toward the wicked. The first group will be carried to the paradise and the second one to the dungeon of misery and hell.

Ahriman will also have the choice of repentance from his evil, to become purified and join the virtuous people in paradise. If he chooses otherwise, he will be contained, neutralized, and excluded.

The Molten River will fill the valleys and flatten the mountains, and the earth becomes flat, smooth, productive, and generous. "Everyone will live on level grounds."

Gender Roles and Marriage

The preferred marriage has been between the cousins and members of close families. This was an assurance against marrying someone who is not fully known and may be nonvirtuous in his beliefs and practices. The consanguinity may enhance the risk of some diseases such as diabetes as a result of inbreeding. Therefore, the marriage among second-level cousins reduces risks. The marriage between uncles and aunts, and nephews and nieces, is forbidden. Marriage to nonzoroastrians is not favored, and the children of such marriages are not recognized as Zoroastrian by the conservative groups.

The status of men and women is considered to be equal [29]. Men and women have equal rights to decide to join or terminate their marriage, unlike some other religions where man has higher privileges. Polygamy and having more than one spouse are not allowed (although the nobilities and some religious people have abused their power in the past). The second marriages are not favored. The divorce is not favored, but it can be initiated by a woman or a man alike. The male children are not favored or receive any preferential treatment. In case of the death of a parent without a formal and written will, the male and female offspring receive an equal share of the inheritance. The women were to be excluded from the household interactions during their menstrual period or after childbirth. A portion of the house, such as one-fifth or one-third of the house, would be left to the menstruating woman or the woman who had just given birth. The household duties were performed by the husband while the woman was menstruating and the food would be taken to her. There was a distance of 3 feet for delivery of the food and 12 feet for other activities. The women were expected to stay away from fire and water by 12 feet in order to prevent contamination of these two elements.

There are extensive teachings about affectionate and responsible interaction between men and women. The practice of good deeds and good thoughts was particularly emphasized. This is particularly interesting in view of the new research that the husband, wife, and the members of the family tend to be most antagonistic and degrading and demeaning toward each other in comparison to interactions among nonfamily members.

Fire Temples: Atashkada

Zoroastrians did not have any temples as a place of worship in their religion. The idea of a temple entered Zoroastrianism when Cyrus conquered Babylon in 539. Babylonians were very active in establishing and constructing temples. The emphasis of temples was also brought in by the Jews, who were taken to Babylon during the captivity. The emphasis of the old Egyptians in making religious sacrifices came with the Hebrews to Babylon [30].

Fire was a strong representative of light, which is the principle factor in the Zoroastrian religion. It represents vitality, warmth, procreation, and transformative power of fire, symbolizing the same aspects of the divine force. It stands against the forces of darkness and evil and corruption [25]. Fire was first misrepresented by Greeks stating that Zoroastrians were fire worshipers, and it was subsequently used maliciously by the Muslim invaders in order to deny and obscure the Monoteistic nature of Zoroastrians, which was arguably the first Monoteistic religion in the world [31–34].

Fire temples were an extension of the hearth fire at homes, which represented the same forces. It was elevated to be used as a temple in the worship of God. In the beginning of Zoroastrian religion between years 1500 and 1000 BCE, the fires at temple were displayed under the open sky. Atashkada represents the most sacred part of the temple when the fire was being burned on a constant basis. Maintaining the purity of the fire was essential. Therefore, the priests covered their face from below the eyes to lower neck with a cloth so that the droplets of saliva do not accidentally spray on the fire and make it profane. Only the most devout Zoroastrians were allowed to the close proximity of the fire, but it is still a fair distance away. The less devout people have had to maintain a higher level of distance.

After the Arab invasions in 651 CE, the Muslims converted the fire temples to Mosques. Today, there are approximately 245 fire temples in existence in the world; 45 of them exist in Mumbai and another questionable 85 in the rest of India. There are approximately over 100 more Atashkadas remaining throughout the world. The number of active Atashkadas in Iran are probably around nine [5]. The fire has been kept burning constantly in places of worship, as well as inside of the houses, during the first few centuries of Zoroastrian predominance in Persia. They represented and symbolized the same factors but in different situations.

Having light in a place of worship in most likelihood is a remnant of Zoroastrianism. It was further transformed to having a light in a temple and a church representing the presence of the God. Some people feel that the presence of light in a place of worship may have predated all the above religions.

Zoroastrianism

Festivals and Holidays

The Zoroastrian religion has six designated holidays, which coincide with the beginning of the four seasons and other occasions [29, 30]. The dates of these holidays have been a source of confusion between the Zoroastrian calendar in Persia and the one used by Parsis in India. Furthermore, the year was 360 days and did not account for intercalations so the differences are reconciled. Three or four of the above festivals are particularly important, although their importance is different in different countries and different locations [31–36].

Spring Solstice: Nowruz

Nowruz, the first day of spring, is the beginning of the new Zoroastrian year. The word means New Day and is spelled in several slightly different but very similar ways. It celebrates the spring equinox on March 21st (it can change between March 20th and 22nd based on the year). It is celebrated by 300 million people in the world, which is significantly more than the number of Persians and Zoroastrians. The Nowruz celebrates that the days are becoming progressively longer with more light in the world and the nights shorter. The families go through extended spring housecleaning and getting rid of the old leftovers from winter. The old clothes from winter are washed and preferably given to the younger children or the charity, and new clothes are purchased. The celebration lasts for a total of 13 days with the first 5 days being most intensive. In preparation for the arrival of the New Year, which occurs at different times, progressing by 6 hours each year, special spread of fruits and sweets is displayed.

They are called "Seven S's" which count for the first word of seven items, which in Persian starts with an "S." They include sabzi (sprouting grains and wheat); sweet, vinegar (Serkeh); somagh, apple (Seeb); seer (garlic); shirini (sweet/candies); sharab (wine); and samanu (cereal). It also includes shamh (candle) and mirror for light and good luck and book, which can be a Book of Poetry by Hafez or a copy of The Holy Book.

The family members and friends are gathered around the spread of sweets and fruits, kiss each other at the time of the arrival of the New Year (similar to the arrival of the New Year in Western culture), kiss each other on both cheeks, and wish each other a happy and healthy and prosperous year. The family members and friends call on the older people in the first day of the New Year and wish them a happy Nowruz. They receive a coin from the older person as a blessing (Barkat). The coin supposedly has been kept in The Holy Book for a period of time to endow with divine blessings. The older people will visit the younger people in the subsequent days as a payback. They usually taste some wine and eat some fruit and some sweets. There is obviously a big overlap between older and younger people, because the younger people to one generation are the older people to the next generation.

By the 13th day of the New Year, the celebration is complete, and people get together for a picnic around running water and creeks and toss the sprouting greens in the wind, which is to take away any ills or bad odds from the family and wash it away. The 13th day obviously has some meaning.

Winter Solstice: Yalda Night

The second very important celebration is Yalda Night, which refers to winter solstice. It coincides with December 21st of the Gregorian calendar. It marks and celebrates the longest and the darkest night of the year, which is the winter solstice. The family and friends assemble to support each other and celebrate that the long and dark nights are behind them and they will become shorter with the daytime. They eat and drink their favorite foods. Two major items are the inclusion of pomegranate, which is representative of winter, and watermelon, which together with pomegranate is to contrast in the dark nights with red color. The fruits are stored in deep cellars for this particular occasion.

The participants read poetry, play music, participate in dancing, and particularly try to tell the future by reading the poems of the most popular Persian poet Hafez (Divan Hafez). The poetry of Hafez can be interpreted on many levels, which can coincide with the everyday happening, as well as the long-term killing of the future. The wine is tasted, and the fruits and sweets are presented [35, 36].

Fall Solstice: Mehregan

The beginning of fall coincides with Mehregan. Mehr is the Goddess from the pre-Zoroastrian time that has been incorporated as a holy and bounteous deity by Zoroastrians. Mehr is the moon and representative of friendship, love, and affection. It usually coincides with October 21st. Mehr or Mithra is responsible for the sanctity of covenants, oaths/contracts, and obligations. The protection of cattle in a positive way is entrusted to Mithra. She takes the sanctity of the contracts very seriously. She punishes people who break the contracts and acts very decisively. Mehr or Mithra has been incorporated by the Greek Mithra and in the Indian religion too. The Mithra in Greek religion is depicted by killing a bull as a sacrifice by Mithra, which will be alien to the Persian culture.

Summer Solstice: Tiregan

Tiregan is on July 3rd and is attributed to Tishtrya, the God of Sun. This coincides with the summer solstice and is celebrating by dancing, reciting poetry, and particularly splashing water on each other. The special food would include the spinach soup and a particular sweet dish called Sholezard, which is cooked with saffron for its bright yellow color and sweet rice and made in a pudding. Related to the Tiregan celebration is the Tir, which means the Arrow, and it was a deity, who was the messenger of God and was good in telling the future. He was also a guide for the soul of the dead. It has connected with the legendary Persian hero with the name of Arash Kamangir,

who was the strongest hero of the time and was particularly unmatched in his skills for shooting an arrow. He sacrificed himself in order to save people and the world from evil.

Zoroastrian Thoughts in Contemporary Literature

The competition between good and evil, light and dark, and evil and virtue is predicted throughout the writings of many famous writers. This represents the close affinity of Zoroastrian thinking with overall human thoughts 2700 years later or possibly 3700 years later. The book by Victor Hugo, Les Misérables [37, 38], a masterpiece, has depicted the difference between good and evil, enlightenment, and lack of enlightenment (remaining in the dark). Jean Valjean, the primary hero of the book, threatened by the impending deaths of his sister's child steals a loaf of bread. He served 19 years in a dungeon for punishment. After having served his penalty, he is being hunted by a policeman for violation of parole when he is seeking a job. He acts as a real villain when he robs a priest, and the priest "buys his soul" by lying to protect him and giving him the silver candlesticks from the church. He transforms into a highly righteous person, becomes the mayor of the town and owner of a factory, and provides jobs for many people.

Jean Valjean's moment of real trial comes when he has to choose between the expediency of keeping his mouth shut and letting a person who has been erroneously accused to be Jean Valjean. He would have saved the fruits of all his efforts and could rationalize it very well by the amount of good that he was doing for others. Instead, he chose to tell the truth and be haunted again by the policeman, Javel.

Later, when he could have eliminated Javel and ensured his own safety, he decided to save the life of Javel, who attempted to persecute him subsequently. He endangered his life again to save the young man who was in love with his "adopted daughter Cozette" and ensure them a glorious future, although his own life was cut short by this sacrifice.

The novel describes in the highly dramatic way the change from the light side to the dark side, which is forced on a person by the society to criminalize the behavior and promote darkness. It also shows the ability of the priest and the mother to recognize the light in him and make appropriate judgment and sacrifice in terms of salvaging his future.

Star Wars

In this very popular movie, the major teacher Ben Kenobi recognizes the internal spark in a young boy and trains him as a Jedi in order to fight for rightness and light. He sacrifices his own life to empower the boy, Luke, to overcome the representative of the force of darkness, namely Darth Vader. Initially, Luke is able to save the universe by destroying the Star Wars, which was the most potent destructive force. In a rematch, he is at the mercy of Darth Vader, but Darth Vader switches from the dark side to the side of light and saves Luke. It turns out that Darth Vader was on the light side himself and was the father of Luke, but has switched to the dark side. The movie and the book describe very sensitively the constant choices that one has to make between the dark and light sides and the wrong and light sides and the significance of a person's free will in the outcome.

Great Expectations: Charles Dickens

The book Great Expectations by Charles Dickens [39] has been one of the most popular and influential novels in English literary canons for generations of people since it was initially published, and it has many adaptations by different movies altering some of the outcomes.

This book describes two people who have been traumatized significantly in their personal lives, namely Ms. Havisham and Magwitch. Ms. Havisham was not able to resolve a less disastrous trauma, of being abandoned at the altar (by a villain), and chose a destructive/punitive way of ruining her own life as well as the life and the future of her adopted daughter.

Magwitch, who has suffered more disastrous double deaths of his wife and his daughter (which proved to be untrue), has maintained his goodness and sponsored the healthy development of Pip. Pip grew up to be a gentleman and eventually reconciled with the daughter of Magwitch in a partial or complete way, depending on the two different versions of the book. This book will be discussed in detail in the accompanying chapter because of the significance of trauma in promoting abusive and evil behavior in the future.

An Enormous Number of People Are Almost Zoroastrians

Most people living at the present time are not aware that their views on significant current life issues are identical with the emphases of Zoroastrian religion [30, 31, 33–35]:

1. To make thoughtfulness and reasoning the basis of your relationships.

    Make your comments and "word" to endorse and enhance the value of other people and productive of social problem-solving.
2. Make your thinking grounded on accurate observations, pragmatic evaluation of the perceptions in the context of environmental factors, and prevailing knowledge within a moral and ethical perspective.
3. Take actions to promote rightness and disempower falsehood, and avoid injury and destruction to people, animals, plants, and environment.
4. Honor animals that support you with their products such as milk, eggs, services, company, and plants for their fruits and other products [30, 31].
5. Maintain the purity of the water and avoid polluting it with the hazardous and waste materials [30, 31].
6. Maintain good quality of the air by refraining from polluting it with harmful and hazardous gases.
7. Produce light and fire from sources which are devoid of the smoke and impure sub-

stances and in harmony with the basic elements [30, 31].

8. Promote, maintain, and upgrade health and prevent, detect early, and treat diseases promptly to limit disability and death.

9. Protect the earth and its bounteous fruits, and do not pollute it with toxic and profane substances.

10. Make barren, dry lands and desserts green and blooming with water, lakes, plants, and forests.

11. Prolong life and prevent mortality in any forms: untreated disease, infant mortality, lack of prevention, violence, and war.

12. Endorse the equality of everyone's beliefs and rights, and do not accept the hegemony of any nation, race, or religious group over others.

13. We can be enriched by diversity rather than threatened by it.

14. The humans by nature are generous, joyful, and optimistic.

15. The lack of generosity, misery, pessimism, and hate are the products of stilted and distorted development by abuse, neglect, and violence and can be prevented and remedied.

16. Negative comments, demeaning others, are the products of greed and fearfulness. They are not inborn and fundamental human qualities. They should be prevented and remedied by cultivating sharing and collaboration to counter greed. Nurture courage against fearfulness. Fear results in untruthfulness and falsehood.

Epilogue

Zoroastrian religion emerged on the records in the second millennium BCE. The concept had been evolving over a period of 1000–1500 years before it entered the recorded history. According to the recorded history, Zoroaster, "The First Prophet," was born in 628 BCE and died in 551 BCE. After some initial strong resistance, he received the sponsorship of one of the kings, who was probably the father of the Darius the Great.

With his sponsorship, Zoroaster was able to present his ideas forcefully and deal with the resistance and opposition of the priestly group who were committed to protect their own interests, as well as the interest of their caste.

His idea was adopted quickly by two major emperors of the Persian Empire, namely Cyrus the Great and Darius the Great. They were at the process of extending beyond the regional domain and were well equipped to present a point of view, which was universal, had logical coherence, and most importantly was tolerant of the traditions of other religions. They respected the Gods and religions of other countries, particularly Babylonians and Hebrews, and entered a collaborative and respectful attitude toward other's beliefs. The history is very clear that Cyrus prevailed upon Babylonians to return the religious belongings and the images of the Gods of different nations to them. Most importantly, he charged his Satrap (governor) with rebuilding the Hebrew temple in Jerusalem, which was destroyed by Babylonians. The history is also clear that over a period of many years, Cyrus and his successor, Darius the Great, have charged three Satraps of Jerusalem to facilitate the building of the Hebrew temple and mediate between different Hebrew groups who were antagonistic toward each other's plans for temple.

Zoroastrian religion is not heavily burdened by metaphysical concepts as some other religions were burdened subsequently. Its teaching was built on conceptual organization that there is a ceaseless battle between right and wrong; light and darkness; truth and falsehood; and health versus illness and death. The purity of the basic elements, namely air, water, fire, and soil, was to be respected and protected against any impurity, decay, and destruction. It is particularly noticeable that the contemporary advance in the science represents the same ideas. Furthermore, the respect for other people's beliefs and refraining from demeaning other people's social and religious beliefs and dominating them by the power of the sword and government have proven to be a very fundamental belief. It is very noteworthy that the United Nations placed the cylinder of Cyrus the Great at the entrance to the United

Nations. There could be no better universal endorsement for his ideas.

The relationship between God, Zoroaster, and all the creatures, including human beings and animals, is voluntary and collaborative. There is no implication of a master and owner over the slave nor a paternalistic attitude toward lesser creatures. The collaboration and cooperation between humans and their best friends, namely the plants, horse, dog, and cow, are a good example of peaceful coexistence.

The number of Zoroastrians practicing has dwindled significantly since the three stages of Persian Empire, namely Achaemenians, Arsacid Dynasty, and the Sasanians. This mostly presents as a Zoroastrian diaspora, the migration of Young Zoroastrian to Western countries such as the United States, Canada, England, Australia, and New Zealand where their productive and virtuous lives can be more fruitful than living in countries with coercive practices against religious freedom.

Zoroastrians were subjected to the ruthless coercion by an invading force of Arab/Muslims who self-righteously put the follower of another well-regarded religion which was 2700 years older to the sword. Zoroastrians had to choose between getting killed, converting, paying high punitive taxes, or migration. The groups that escaped to India (and Pakistan), Tajikistan, and Turkmenistan were able to survive well in the new atmosphere. Following the division of India between India and Pakistan, the government of Pakistan proved to be much less tolerant and more coercive toward Zoroastrians, although the first mayor of Karachi, with nine million populations, was a well-respected Parsi. The level of discrimination has heightened significantly in recent years, leading to extensive immigration to the Western countries.

The latest wave of immigration of Zoroastrian diaspora has been to the United States (15,000 people), Canada (9847), England (5000–6000), Australia (2577), and New Zealand (1231). They have thrived in the new atmosphere.

The legitimacy of a religion is to help people to be better humans with higher ideals and get along well with each other. You can judge if the teaching of Zoroastrians passes this test.

References

1. Gerard R. The heirs to the forgotten religions. London: Penguin Books; 2013.
2. Ahura Mazda—Encyclopaedia Iranica. http://www.iranicaonline.org/articles/ahura-mazda. Retrieved 12 Jul 2019.
3. Ahriman. Encyclopaedia Iranica. http://www.iranicaonline.org/articles/ahriman. Retrieved 13 Jul 2019.
4. Zaehner RC. The dawn and twilight of Zoroastrianism. London: Phoenix Press; 1961. ISBN 978-1-84212-165-8.
5. Zoroastrianism. History.com, Editors, History. A&E Television Networks. https://www.history.com/topics/religion/zoroastrianism. 30 Jun 2023.
6. Alexander the Great ii. In Zoroastrianism—Encyclopaedia Iranica. https://iranicaonline.org/articles/
7. Alexander-the-Great-ii. Iranicaonline.org. Retrieved 30 Jan 2021.
8. Russell JR. Zoroastrianism in Armenia, Harvard Iranian series. Cambridge: Harvard University Press; 1987. IDBN 978-0-674-95850-9.
9. Zarathustra—Iranian prophet. https://www.britannica.com/biography/Zoroaster-Iranian-Prophet. Retrieved 9 Jun 2017.
10. Greece iii. Persian influence on Greek thought. Encyclopaedia Iranica. http://www.iranicaonline.org/articles/Greece-iii, Retrieved 14 Jul 2019.
11. Nigosian SA. Zoroastrian faith: tradition and modern research. McGill-Queen's Press; 1993. p. 95–97, 131. ISBN 9780773511330. https://books.google.com/books?id=p6c-TdNc69QC
12. Kohler K, Williams Jackson AV. Zoroastrianism, resemblances between Zoroastrianism and Judaism and causes of analogies uncertain. The Jewish encyclopaedia; 1906. https://www.jewishencyclopedia.com/articles/15283-zoroastrianism. Retrieved 3 Feb 2022.
13. Zaehner RE. The dawn and twilight of Zoroastrianism. New York: G. P. Putnam's DMS; 1961.
14. Boyce M. Zoroastrians: their religions believes and practices. London: Routledge; 2001. ISBN 978-0415239028.
15. Boyce M. The history of Zoroastrianism, vol. 1. Leiden: Brill; 1975. ISBN 978-9004-10474-7, (repr. 1996).
16. ASA (Asha "Truth"). Encyclopaedia Iranica. http://www.iranicaonline.org/articles/asa-means-truth-in-avestan. Retrieved 14 Jun 2017.
17. Druj. Encyclopaedia Iranica. http://www.iranicaonline.org/articles/drug. Retrieved 14 Jun 2017.
18. Hintze A. Monotheism the Zoroastrian way. J R Asiat Soc. 2013;24(2):225–49. https://www.researchgate.net/publication//271934655
19. Le Zend-Avesta, Ouvrage de Zoroastre, 3 vol. Paris, 1771, Berlin, 1858.
20. Kellens J. AVESTA i. Survey of the history and contents of the book. Encyclopaedia Iranica. http://

www.iranicaonline.org/articles/avesta-holy-book. Retrieved 13 Jul 2019.

21. Gathas. Encyclopaedia Iranica. http://www.iranicaonline.org/articles/gathas. Retrieved 13 Jul 2019.

22. Yasna. Encyclopaedia Iranica. http://www.iranicaonline.org/articles/yasna. Retrieved 13 Jul 2019.

23. Visperad. Encyclopaedia Iranica. http://www.iranicaonline.org/articles/visperad. Retrieved 13 Jul 2019.

24. Vendidad. Encyclopaedia Iranica. http://iranicaonline.org/articles/vendidad-parent. Retrieved 13 Jul 2019.

25. Khordeh Avesta. Encyclopaedia Iranica. http://www.iranicaonline.org/articles/khordeh-avesta. Retrieved 13 Jul 2019.

26. Zoroastrianism. Encyclopedia Britannica. Encyclopedia Britannica, Inc., 27 Mar 2023. www.britannica.com/topic/Zoroastrianism. Accessed 30 Jun 2023.

27. Irani KD. Domains of belief (Zoroastrianism). California Zoroastrian Center, YouTube.com; 1971.

28. Zoroastrianism, October 2022, Wikipedia.

29. Women ii. In the Avesta. Encyclopaedia Iranica. http://www.iranicaonline.org/articles/women-ii-avesta. Retrieved 13 Jul 2019.

30. Ataskada. Encyclopaedia Iranica. http://www.iranicaonline.org/articles/ataskada-new-persian-house-of-fire-mid. Retrieved 13 Jul 2019.

31. Zoroastrian rituals. Encyclopaedia Iranica. http://www.iranicaonline.org/articles/zoroastrian-rituals. Retrieved 13 Jul 2019.

32. Avesta: Zoroastrian scripture. Encyclopedia Britanica (n.d.) Google. Britanica Academics. Retrieved 29 Jun 2022. https://www.britannica.com/topic/Avesta-Zoroastrian-scripture

33. NIAC InSight, Washington insights for the Iranian-American community from the National Iranian American Council (16 Dec 2016). An old faith in the New World—Zoroastrianism in the United States. https://www.niacinsight.com/2016/12/16/an-old-faith-in-the-new-world-

34. Zoroastrianism-in-the-united-states. NIAC InSight. https://www.niacouncil.org/iranian-american-activism/an-old-faith-in-the-new-world-zoroastrianism-in-the-united-states/

35. What does Zoroastrianism teach us about ecology? Parliament of the World's Religions. https://parliamentofreligions.org/content/what-does-zoroastrianism-teach-us-about-ecology

36. Foltz R, Saadi-Nejad M. Is Zoroastrianism an ecological religion? J Study Relig Nat Cult. 2008;1(4) https://doi.org/10.1558/jsrnc.v1i4.413.

37. Hugo V. Les Miserable. New York: Modern Library; 1992.

38. Hugo V. Le Pacte/Rectangle Production. 2019 film.

39. Dickens C. Great expectations. Ware: Wordsworth Editions; 1992.

Zoroastrianism: Clinical and Literary Applications

G. Pirooz Sholevar

Introduction

The following principles of Zoroastrian religion have been described fully in the accompanying chapter in this volume and summarized here:

1. Asha: Life should be lived according to the principles of rightness, truthfulness, justice, and sustainability for humans, animals, plants, and the four principal elements.
2. The four principal elements are water, earth, air, and sun/fire. Their purity should be protected from pollution and profanity.
3. The humans and animals have the capacity for free and sound judgment to choose between joyous and wholesome living in contrast to decay, illness, and death.
4. The three principles of a virtuous life are to practice
   (a) Good thoughts
   (b) Good words
   (c) Good deeds
5. The three above processes are interdependent, and you cannot perform good deeds without good thoughts and good words.

6. There is a ceaseless struggle between righteousness, light, goodness, health on one hand and falsehood, deception, decay, disease, and death on the opposite.

Clinical Application of Zoroastrian Principles

1. The concept of good thoughts is very broad and embraces cognitive processes such as perception, reflection on the perceptions based on sound thinking and previous learning, affective and emotional processes which run parallel with cognitive processes and motivate it, and keen awareness that good thoughts are an instrument of health promotion and combine with environmental factors to ensure the welfare of all creatures and the four basic elements. The forces which underpin sound thoughts, wise selection, and protection of life have to struggle ceaselessly with forces of falsehood and evil (Ahriman/Angra Mainyu). That is where the struggle occurs and can only be managed satisfactorily by keen awareness of the power of the adversary.
2. Impulsivity, explosiveness, abuse, coercion, neglect, and abandonment are the territory of the evil/Ahriman who guards all the territories with strong dedication. Greed, self-interest, and fearfulness are the devil's three potent instruments.

G. P. Sholevar (✉)
Division of Child, Adolescent and Family Psychiatry, Jefferson Medical College, Thomas Jefferson University, Philadelphia, PA, USA

Nueva Vida Behavioral Health Center, Philadelphia, PA, USA

3. Zoroastrian religion is based on a collaborative partnership between the Wise Lord (Ahura Mazda) and all the creatures. It is significant that the relationship between the clinician and the patient is most productive within a collaborative frame entitled "Therapeutic Alliance" and "Working Alliance." Significant research indicates that the strong therapeutic alliance is producing the best treatment results [1].

The treatment occurs as an interaction between the clinician and the client/patient, within the framework of acceptable knowledge and values. The concept of Asha and its many tributaries can be used as the treatment frame, which would mutually examine the established goals. The goals are not written in stone and can be modified based on their feasibility and achievability rather than being a source of friction, hopelessness, and failure. They can be exchanged for more achievable goals. Once the goals are set, it will be translated into a general plan, which is further reduced to smaller segments. The clinical phenomenon will be jointly examined by the clinician and the patient to enhance progress and manage the temporary regressions within a workable framework. The forces of negation emerge as resistance and defensiveness against the progress and guide the person toward regression, backwardness, defeat, and distorted perceptions. The clinician will be well served by reminding oneself and the client that they are both on the same side, which is the side of righteousness, success, and maturity. Suffering and failure are their mutual enemy (engineered by Ahriman/Angra Mainyu).

A number of cases are presented to demonstrate Zoroastrian principles and clinical practice.

Case One: Courted by Devil on the Highway

William is a 23-year-old man from a highly principled and religious family. The family has a large number of children, and the grandchildren continue to emerge on the scene. The family is exceptionally committed to doing the right things. Against this background, an overwhelming major tragic death disrupted the family life. This trauma set in motion a number of subsequent family disasters with significant and long-lasting damage to family relationships, cohesion, and confidence. William had to drop out of college for not studying, drinking, and drug use. He returned to his town and tried to live on his own, which proved impossible due to high-risk unsupervised behavior. He moved back to the parents' house and could not wait to get out so he would have more freedom to use alcohol/drugs. (He receives SSRI and non-benzo anxiolytic.)

After a few months, he was able to secure a highly demanding job taking care of profoundly disabled people. His performance was outstanding. He embraced the unpleasant duties with a total dedication and soon was recognized by all the co-workers, the disabled patients, his family, and friends for his extraordinary committed dedication. Everyone noticed that he was doing "God's work." He recognized "the light of the Lord" in himself. The level of joy and ecstasy lasted for a few weeks. He then decided to meet with his friends out of town and have a weekend of celebration and enjoyment.

On his way to the trip, he stopped at the house of one of the friend's associates and picked up a large amount of drugs for the collective use over the weekend. While on the highway, he decided to use drugs while driving. Using drugs and driving, he did not recognize that his perception, evaluation, and judgment of possible consequences of his behavior were totally impaired. He was submerged in the wish to use more drugs while driving and would not even stop at the side of the road to do so. After a few hours, he ended up in a ditch next to the road and was too high to get rid of the evidence before the State Troopers arrived. He was arrested and taken to a nearby town, and parents came and bailed him out. He appeared in front of the magistrate judge the next day, and the court date was set with six charges against him, with the most important one being the UDI. Eventually, he was not sentenced to prison time and will continue his work and pay a heavy fine in addition to paying for college debts.

It was presented to him and his parents that he was initially lucky to end up on the side of goodness, working by serving others and aiding in their health. However, he changed sides and became the devil's disciple and agent while driving on the road under the influence of heavy drugs. He could have killed someone else or himself, or both, and he was clearly an agent of the devil and no longer an agent of God. The drop from the height of pride to the dungeons of shame, defeat, and failing everyone and all the principles was very noticeable.

He moved from the side of rightness/Lord to the side of destructiveness and the devil, from light to dark, very much like the movie Star Wars. The reference to the movie of Star Wars was used as a way of creating an impactful image and frame of reference. With the help of the court, the lawyer, and heavy fines, he has managed to move back to the side of rightness. He has a newly found recognition of temptation by devil which distorted his free will, perception, evaluation, and judgment, exposing himself, his family, and others to a new round of tragedy, which they can hardly endure. As his parents stated, if someone has died, it would have been the end of life for everyone in the family.

Case Two: Lie and Lifelessness

Richard is 38 years old and lives with his family. He is either in his room sleeping or doing nothing. He has not worked since he graduated college 15 years ago. He has been in intensive treatment with high doses of multiple medications and with several psychiatrists. He had inpatient and other intensive treatments. He smokes marijuana several times a day and goes to sleep right after smoking. He and some of his family members consider him a "pothead" ignoring his total confinement to the house in his room and very little work history.

In the second conjoint family session, he stated that either he or the psychiatrist is a "liar," in response to a very insignificant misunderstanding. The psychiatrist pointed out that Richard was preoccupied with a world full of "liars,"

which left him no room to succeed. He was afraid to go for a job interview because he thought that he would be denied a job because he appeared as a liar or he considered his potential employer to be a liar and he did not want to work with one. He then revealed his fantasy: If someone knocked at his door, a person was coming to strangle him and Richard and would try to strangle the intruder before he was strangled himself. There was no consideration of a friendly person walking in. He has lost all his friends and did not socialize with anybody including his brother whom he described in demeaning language.

Accepting the identity of a "pothead" denied that he "existed" as if he was already dead. He brushed his teeth once every 2 months and did not go out of his room and house as if he was confined to a tomb.

He had no motivation to seek or obtain a job or go out to walk his dog or spend a few minutes outdoors.

An interpretation was made that he acted as if he was already "dead" like to households of Egyptian Pharaohs who were entombed with their dead master. His life was very much like the life of the "underground man" described in the masterpiece book of Fyodor Dostoevsky [2].

The treatment plan included talking to and staying in the presence of his parents, going out of the house for very brief period of time, brushing his teeth and showering more frequently, changing cloths, reestablishing friendship or talking to 1 or 2 friends, and consideration of going for readily available jobs rather than the prestigious and difficult-to-obtain ones.

The provisions were made to protect the treatments against his ready cancellation of the sessions by agreeing on only three choices:

1. Attending in person, (2) virtually if he did not want to leave the house, and (3) being charged for the session. This arrangement eliminated his texting just before the sessions and canceling or asking for a call back and then overfocusing on lack of return of his text on time.
2. He tried to stay on the side of telling the truth and stay away from the lies and falsehood. The new guidelines are very much consistent

with Zoroastrian principles of staying on the side of righteousness, distancing from lies and falsehood, and adhering to the practice of maintaining the purity of body and its organs such as teeth and gums.

Case Three: Purification of Body

Ginger is a 13-year-old adolescent girl who has been in treatment for more than 2 years before being evaluated by the present child psychiatrist. She is very creative and has a number of unique ways of expressing her creativity particularly her perceptiveness about the qualities of other people. She is doing fairly well academically.

She has been diagnosed with obsessive-compulsive disorder (OCD). She has many obsessive symptoms, and some of them are disabling.

She has to clean her bottom repeatedly and for a very long time in the only family bathroom. She enters the bathroom after 8:30 PM and stays there for 2–3 or 4 hours cleaning herself. She goes through the whole roll of toilet paper every night.

Another obsessive symptom is that she cannot touch her foot, socks, or shoes because they are "dirty."

She is receiving 80 mg of Prozac, and her symptoms increase significantly if she misses her medication. The medication was augmented with Abilify which improved her symptoms, but the family could not afford the augmentation because of limited finances and lack of insurance coverage. She continues to see her psychotherapist of 2 years, but they have not been able to address any of the above symptoms.

Interventions

The recommendation was made to replace wiping herself clean in the bathroom with taking a shower and let the water purify her body and remove the impurities. She should make herself increasingly aware of the pleasure of the water on her body with pleasant fantasies such as being in a warm ocean in Caribbean. She would then remain wrapped in the bathroom towel and goes to bed if the towel is not too damp.

Three interventions were recommended for her shoes, socks, and feet. She will clean her shoes once a day and put the clean shoes in a special place to remain untouched. She would massage her feet and toes and soles for 5 or more minutes every night in the bathroom and take notice of how shapely and attractive her feet are. She then washes them in a combination of washing, massaging, and enjoying the sensations in her feet, hands, and the rest of her body. She will then put on a pair of totally clean socks and enjoy the pleasure of being very clean. She will change her socks into a pair of new clean socks when entering the bed while thinking of her clean feet, clean socks, and clean sheets.

Case Four: With the Help of the Best Friend

Jacky, a 12-year-old adolescent gymnast, sustained a head injury during a practice. She suffered with the symptoms of dizziness, headache, and loss of balance when dizzy and had to be confined in her house. She could not do her work on the computer because of lack of concentration and forgetting what she was working on. All her close friends were members of the gymnastic team, and she could not get together with them because she was not allowed to practice gymnastic activities for 3–6 months and maybe longer. Lack of school attendance made her feel excluded from the place where she belonged.

She was diagnosed with post-traumatic stress disorder (PTSD) and anxiety. Insomnia was a disturbing symptom with frequent sleep interruption and awakening.

The evaluation revealed that the family had a dog and she was moderately attached to him.

No medications were prescribed because it could have made her dizziness and headache worse.

The family was advised to enlist the assistance of the dog as the agent of togetherness, reduction of isolation, a pleasant and constant company, and comfort by hugging the dog as she has done with her stuffed animals.

The dog was invited to sleep in the bed with her, which remedied her initial insomnia and fragmented sleep, and she was able to sleep in the morning for longer period of time. The dog essentially lived in her room all the time. She took over feeding and walking the dog, and she did not suffer any dizziness or headache while doing those activities.

The mother was very welcoming of the recommendation. She revealed that she herself has had head injury as an adolescent and "my dog was my psychiatrist and she cured me."

The dog who was designated as "psychiatrist in residence" proved to be very helpful throughout the treatment and the next 4 months. We obtained a variance from the practice to allow the dog to participate in the sessions every 4 weeks. The dog proved very professional and on target in the sessions too. The patient was able to return to the school in 2 and 1/2 months. The course of the treatment was considered to be very accelerated by the use and constant and continuous presence of the dog as a company to the patient.

Case Five: Another Helping Friend with Another Teenager

Anne is a 13-year-old teenage girl who has been a competitive swimmer for almost 8 years. She injured her head accidentally against the pool wall and sustained a cerebral concussion. She went through multiple symptoms and isolation from peers and classmates. In her total isolation, she became extremely close to her dog, which helped her through a period of 3–4 months of recovery. She and her dog have remained exceptionally close for several years until she went to college. She repeatedly joked about taking the dog to the college as her best friend.

Case Six: Maltreatment of Best Friend

Roger is 37 years old and lives with his parents. He has been unemployed for several years after dropping out of college for lack of academic performance. He spends most of his time on the Internet and has a group of virtual "friends." He does not talk much about his difficulties with them. He has no contacts in real life except for his parents and the mother's friends. The father is very self-absorbed, and the mother is very self-centered.

Roger has the delusion that the devil(s) poke him on his behind. He then revealed that he was forcing the family dog into sexual act when he was 12 years old. The dog was frightened of him and would run away when he came around. He now feels "horrible" because he feels that he has "ruined the life of the dog." His own life has been compromised by lack of accomplishment and failures. His parents complained constantly that he was on the computer with his Internet friends and did not talk to them.

He was started on Seroquel, and the dose was increased. He complained of excessive sleepiness although he was taking the medication only at night. The medication was changed to Abilify and subsequently to Vraylar, and the dose of the last one was increased to 6 mg.

Roger's mental health improved quickly, and he obtained a job in a factory. He proved to be a good worker, and people were pleased with his performance. However, he felt that devil-like creatures were poking him on his behind, which would make him have an erection. He was terrified that people would see his erection. This proved to be a fear with no basis in reality. He was afraid to masturbate to decrease the sexual tension. (It was suspected that his masturbation fantasies were probably related to sexual acts with dogs.)

He continued progressing in treatment and had to be encouraged to spend time with his parents and talk to his Internet friends about his life activities rather than pretend socialization. His hygiene, taking showers, changing his clothes on a regular basis, and brushing teeth, required frequent interventions. These Zoroastrian principles of good thoughts, good talks, and good deeds were emphasized as clean cloths, body, and teeth.

Marital disengagements of the parents, mental status of the father (schizoid), and maternal behavioral instability were limiting factors. Roger emerged as the best force in negotiating family disagreements.

The closeness of the dogs in the family can provide a vehicle for being abused by others and obtaining gratification in a deviant fashion. The guilt feeling of Roger is a good indicator that he knew that the basic rights of the dog were being violated and the dog could not tell on him and reveal the secret. The parents were oblivious to the events around them.

Roger proved to be capable of empathy with the dog subsequently particularly when the resolution of his guilt feelings, mediated by his conscience, reduced his defensiveness.

Case Seven: When the Technology Reveals Abuse

Michael was a 12-year-old adolescent boy who lives with his mother, stepfather, and five siblings who are a combination of full siblings and half siblings. He was oppositional and defiant behaviorally but did not argue much with his parents. He was aggressive with his siblings. He was in outpatient treatment for oppositional and defiant behavior.

The house was wired and monitored by cameras so the parents know where the children were. They were surprised to find that Michael was sexually abusing the family dog. They then noticed that the dog was afraid of Michael and would run away when he came near him. Attempts at correction were unproductive, and the dog had to be given away with great hardship for the siblings.

The treatment of Michael was elevated to partial hospital level, which proved unproductive because he had no problem during the day and the problems continued in the evening. He was placed on major tranquilizers to increase self-control. His level of care was next elevated to residential program. The family could not continue to support for residential program due to physical distance.

Case Eight: "My Kingdom for a Horse"

The intense relationship between horses and teenage girls is well-recognized. However, people seldom pay attention that the lives of a man and his horse were intimately related throughout the history. Stealing a man's horse, particularly in the wilderness, was punishable by hanging, because taking a man's horse condemned the victim to unavoidable death. Shooting a rider's horse was equivalent to shooting him directly because the falling horse would pin down the rider and end his life quickly. The statement in Shakespeare play of Richard III offering his kingdom for a horse is a testimony to this partnership.

The close association of the horse and the rider is very eloquently and sensitively examined in the book and the movie of Horse Whisperer. Two teenage girls ride their horses in the middle of ice and snow, and they slide into a huge moving truck. One of the riders and her horse die immediately. The second rider loses a leg, and her horse is enormously injured. The mother declines the trainer's advice of putting the horse down, feeling that the horse belonged to his daughter, but unconsciously sensing that the loss of a leg, the horse, and her best friend would be too unbearable for the daughter to tolerate, and her vitality and fire of life would die out.

The mother located a "horse whisperer" to help the severely traumatized horse to resolve his overwhelming trauma. The horse whisperer accepts the task only if the daughter is a total and active participant in the treatment process as it unfolds. He is particularly moved by recognizing the agony in the eyes of the horse and observing the horse's many scars.

The book and the movie [3] sensitively reveal five parallel and interconnected lines of trauma:

1. The horse, whose extreme trauma exhibits by a turbulent mind and wild behavior.
2. The daughter, who has lost her best friend, her leg, and the pleasure of riding her horse with her friend; the attendant survivor's guilt and feeling unlovable due to the loss of her leg.
3. The trauma of the mother, who has lost her greatly beloved father as an adolescent, lack of transferring her love to her husband, and now the possibility of losing her daughter. A daughter without a soul and vitality.

4. The trauma of the horse whisperer, who has lost his beloved wife, who could not live on a ranch.
5. The trauma and pain of the father; lacking the love of his wife. The wife has become very self-absorbed following the death of her father.

The five people address their losses as the horse is recovering from his turbulent mind and gaining tranquility, allowing the girl to ride her again, reuniting ride and horse. It is reminiscent of the experience in cultures who have not seen a man riding a horse previously and thought of them as a single creature. When the horseman and the horse separated and reunited, they felt there was magic-in-action and were terror stricken.

The five-dimensional resolution of the trauma, propensity of the trauma to promote self-centeredness, and isolation relationally, socially, and in treatment were resolved in parallel with each other. "Working through" trauma required becoming more aware of the needs of other people. Empathy for people and other creatures around is a potent remedy for trauma resolution.

The horse maintains its central and exalted position endorsed by Zoroastrian religion. It reminds us of the long history: partnership between the two creatures.

Case Nine: Saved by a Black Stallion

Alex in the movie of Black Stallion [4] is about 11 years old. He is traveling with his father aboard a large ship, which catches fire which destroys the ship. There are moments of great closeness between the father and him prior to the fire. The father gives him a bronze replica of Alexander Great's horse: Bucephalus. He also meets a great black Arabian stallion who is being transported on the ship. Everyone in the ship dies, but Alex holds on the black stallion's ropes and is saved by him. Arriving at an isolated island, he later frees the stallion whose ropes are caught between rocks, before the horse exhausts himself. This stallion saves Alex

from a cobra snake. They bond in a great and intimate relationship before they are rescued and returned to England. Alex develops a father-son relationship with a trainer, and they both train the stallion to win the championship over two champion horses from the East and West of England.

Millions of children across the world have watched this charming classic movie, which imprints them with intimacy of a horse and a child; a boy and a man; the horse saving the life of a child against all the odds; and resolution of the trauma of the tragic loss of the father and being left totally alone. The shared initiative between a young boy and an old man results in a glorious optimism replacing the pessimism of the loss and the death of the father.

Case Ten: Farmer Hassan's Cow

This Persian movie has claimed awards in three major international film festivals [5]. It has remained popular as a classic for many years.

Farmer Hassan has the only milk cow in the village. The villagers line up in the evening to receive fresh milk of the cow. The farmer's social standing as a leader is very high in the village because of his unique position of providing milk for everyone. He loves his cow and treats her like his favorite child. He takes her outdoors to a pool of water next to the village, washes and massages her, and sings to her like a lover serenading his beloved woman. On one such outing, the cow is observed by three nomads, which is an ominous sign. The farmer is terror stricken and retreats into great panic.

The cow is stolen by the nomads, and the farmer is immobilized by his tremendous grief. He regresses and sits in the cow's stall and eats straws as if he is a cow. He cannot express his grief to the elders and the village or his wife. He has lost his status and identity as a cow owner and identifies with the cow and the mechanism of identification with the lost object [6]. The villagers cannot help him with his tragic loss and cannot grieve or solve the problem because they are also indirectly victimized.

The farmer dies as he is being transported to the city for psychiatric treatment.

The whole village is dependent on the milk of the cow and loses this source of nourishment.

This story is directly out of Zoroastrian sacred scripture when the cow petitions Ahura Mazda that his contributions and generosity to people are not recognized and he is treated cruelly by mankind. They take what she has to offer and then subject her to horrible ending, with the nomads stealing her and selling her to be slaughtered.

Note: There were 92.1 million milk cows in the United States in 2022, which constitutes 1 milk cow for every 400 people. They are nourishing us today as much as they did 2000 years BCE before the birth of Christ and at the inception of Zoroastrian religion 3800 years ago.

Case Eleven: The House Inhabited by Two Adversaries

In Zoroastrianism, in the first 3000 years after the creation of the world, Ahura Mazda and the forces of rightness and light (ASHA) occupied the sky and heavens. Angra Mainyu/Ahriman resided below, and they were separated by a huge void. They were aware of each other's existence, but they did not interact for 3000 years until Ahura Mazda decided to create the physical world. Ahriman then decided to create opposing creatures to destroy the creations of Ahura Mazda. The two forces struggle vigorously for victory over each other. At times, their powers are equally matched, and one cannot overcome the other.

The following case is an example of the forces of darkness and destruction coexisting with light and creation in a person, but neither force can prevail. One can gain the upper hand temporarily based on the environmental and contextual factors and reverse places periodically repeatedly.

Case example: Laura is a 17–1/2-year-old adolescent girl who was born to an emotionally ill mother of several children. After a very turbulent and unstable early childhood, she was hospitalized in a supervision and attention center.

This behavior was understood in a psychiatric hospital at the age of 5–1/2 years. This proved to be the beginning of many institutionalizations in the form of repeated hospitalizations and residential treatments.

She was fortunate to be adopted by a very loving, resourceful, and committed family who provided her with sensitive and appropriate parenting and would not be discouraged by many treatment setbacks.

One of her symptoms was to eat dangerous and nonfood items such as rocks, pieces of pencils, metal objects and screws, and more dangerously staples and batteries. Everyone noticed her need for constant reenactment of her early childhood when she was left ignored, and she would eat plaster from the walls and objects on the floor. The mother would intervene only when she has done something very dangerous, and at that point, she would give her intense attention by rushing her to the emergency room.

Simultaneously, the enormous investment of the adoptive parents and multiple treatment facilities have enriched her healthy ego and the capacity to communicate with others and get them interested in her until the next crisis left the clinical staff discouraged.

The two parts of her ego, namely the self-destructive part and the protective ego, resided together with her simultaneously and in the same mind. However, they were totally separated by a "void" or strong boundary and did not interact with each other. Therefore, the cycles of self-destruction and healthy development marched in parallel with each part equal in their strengths. In reality, the destructive part was more effective in destroying long periods of relational gains and skill development.

The coexistence of the two independent forces was demonstrated by her emphasis on "boundary," which could be understood and hypothesized to refer to the boundary between the two parts of her ego. The following example describes this phenomenon:

Laura was sitting in the large living room of the treatment facility with a heavy weighting blanket over her head. Her head was down, and her face was not visible. She had an appointment with the psychiatrist who entered the room but noticed that Laura was not accessible for the session. The psychiatrist made a mistake of asking Laura if she still wanted to keep the session (the psychiatrist has traveled to meet with Laura in her unit). She became very angry and made angry comments, and the psychiatrist left without any further statements.

The next day, the psychiatrist ran into Laura who stated that "you crossed (or violated) my boundary." This was understood to be referring to the boundary of bringing treatment light in when and where darkness and self-destruction ruled.

The self-destructive part of Laura was understood and hypothesized to be the leftover of her destructive experiences with her mother. The destructive relationship between her and her mother was preferable to the feeling of total abandonment, which she tried to remedy by eating the plasters from the walls and dirt from the floor and the ground. This has been described as "attachment to painful affects" [7–9], which is a defense against more painful affect of being total abandonment and left in a void feeling that her existence was denied or erased.

The therapeutic gains were not sufficiently powerful to enter or illuminate this dark corner of her mind, and the two parts had to live together and tolerate each other. One can hope that with good luck in her future life, the progressive part of her ego will be supported and strengthened by the selection of a healthy and powerful partner. Conversely, bad luck in her future relationships can undermine the healthy ego and strengthen the destructive and regressive forces. This is a partial explanation of why some abused people repeat the cycle of abuse (one-third) and two-thirds refrain from recreating their painful past.

Conclusion and Epilogue

The above cases demonstrate several major aspects of mental health treatment particularly psychotherapy within the context of the family and the community. It illustrates that Zoroastrian framework is very similar to the best psychotherapeutic practices.

In case 1, William becomes aware that the temporary satisfaction of his urge for pleasure should not have been an individual decision because of its significant and serious consequences for a range of people from total strangers to very close family members. He could have lost his own valuable life and the lives of other travelers on the road as well as led to emotional/ psychological death for his beloved family members who have already suffered unbearable and devastating trauma in their lives. Furthermore, he noticed the enormous power of his adversary (Ahriman) who could bring devastation to so many people. He then compared it with virtuous life of helping very disabled people and be "on the side of angels."

In case 6, Roger's empathy and guilt feeling has been persistently present for 25 years, and his guilt feelings were put in the "appropriate frame" when he developed empathy for his own long suffering for so many years.

In case 7, Michael has suppressed and denied his feeling of empathy for the dog at the time. However, the pain was felt strongly by the parents and siblings. In family-centered treatment, Michael developed more empathy for the dog and his siblings as well as his parents.

In cases 4 and 5, the dog as the man's best friend brought about relief, companionship, and comfort and love on 24-h-a-day basis for several weeks. Such time and emotional investment could not be offered by the parents or a clinician. Furthermore, a much closer relationship was established between the teenage girls and the dogs, which constantly reminded the family of the important role of the dogs and filled them with gratitude for what they have done.

Case 8 is an amazing demonstration that no one can take a horse out in hazardous conditions and expose them to death and serious injury without accepting responsibility for their part in the tragedy. Shooting a severely injured horse when other remedies are possible is unacceptable. After all, you would not shoot your teenage daughter for missing a leg.

The mother could only make this major decision because she has recognized the long-standing effect of the trauma after the death of her father. The daughter participated wholeheartedly in treatment because she could see the parallel similarity between her suffering and the horse. The Horse Whisperer has become more sensitized because of his own trauma.

In case 9, the Black Stallion saves the life of Alex, which is very commonly done by dogs in cases of house fire, and the dog can rescue the young children or the older people. The intensity of the relationship between the father and the boy led to the intense relationships between the boy and the horse and the trainer as a father substitute, and together they made legendary achievement.

In case 10, the farmer has a highly elevated position in the village served by the only milk cow. The cow is stolen by the greedy nomads. The farmer loses his status, his function, identity, and mostly his loving relationship with his cow, which resembled the relationship between a mother and an infant child. In his profound grief, he identifies with "the lost object" and identifies himself with the cow, which subsequently leads to his death [5].

The cases illustrate the holistic nature of the Zoroastrian religion and its use in treatment. A thoughtful paper by Dr. Trishala Chopra [10] endorses the principle common to Zoroastrianism and holistic medicine that the best treatment happens when compassionate care is offered within an ethical and loving relationship between people in a collaborative relationship with the patient where the goals, strategies, and process are equally constructed by two people rather than controlled by asymmetrical measures. The physical, relational, emotional, and spiritual selves are viewed in unity.

References

1. Sholevar P. Psychoanalytic family therapy. In: Sholevar GP, editor. Textbook of family and couples therapy. Washington, DC: APPI Press; 2005.
2. Sholevar P. Psychoanalytic case studies. Madison: International Universities Press; 1991.
3. Horse Whisperer, Touchstone Pictures, 1998.
4. Black Stallion, MGM, 1979.
5. The Cow, Iranian Ministry of Culture, 1968.
6. Freud A. Ego and the mechanism of defense. London: Routledge; 1966.
7. Sholevar P. Essay book review; affects. Int J Psychoanal. 1997;78:1239.
8. Jones JM. Affects as a process. Hillsdale/London: The Analytic Press; 1995. p. 268.
9. Morton K. Affect, object and character structure. Madison: International Universities Press; 1995. p. 266.
10. Chopra T. The intersection of Zoroastrianism and holistic health. Parsi Times, special issue, 18 Mar 2023;12(49), Zoroastrians.

Basic Principles and Clinical Considerations of Jainism

Abhishek Jain

Demographics

Jains are a relatively very small population worldwide. While exact numbers vary by source and survey methodology, an estimated 5–seven million of the world's population, or less than 0.1%, are identified as Jain [1, 2]. Most live in India, yet still only constitute about 0.4% of India's population. Per India's most recent census, with about 4.5 million in 2011, Jainism is India's sixth largest religion, after Hinduism, Islam, Christianity, Sikhism, and Buddhism, respectively [3, 4]. At least an additional 250,000 Jains live outside of India [5], with Jain communities in 35 or more countries [6]. In the USA and Canada, for example, the Federation of Jain Associations in North America (JAINA) is an umbrella organization of 72 Jain centers that represent 200,000 members [7]. However, identified Jain populations may also be an underestimate, such as by possibly being counted among Hindu populations [8]. Trying to capture precise data may also speak to the complexity and fluidity of how religious identity itself may be defined [9, 10].

Nonetheless, with its small size, individuals from other faiths may not be familiar with Jainism. In a 2019–2020 Pew Research Center survey of about 30,000 adults in India, 92% of Jains said that they know "a great deal" or "some" about Hinduism, yet only 18% of Hindus said that they know at least "some" about Jainism. Likewise, only 25–27% of Jains said that they know at least "some" about India's other four major religions. One explanation might be that Hinduism is the most prevalent and visible religion in India. Similarly, 66% of Jains "say they have a lot in common" with Hindus, yet only 19% of Hindus "say they have a lot in common" with Jains, and only 19–23% of Jains "say they have a lot in common" with the other four major religions in India [11].

Moreover, Jains generally have two main sects: the larger *Svetambara* and the smaller *Digambara*. Svetambara ("white-clad") monks and nuns wear white clothes and do not believe monastics are required to practice nudity. Digambara ("sky-clad") refers to principles and practices in which traditional male monks do not possess or wear clothes [2, 12, 13]. While the core principles and philosophies of the two sects (and even several subsects) are largely the same, some practices, texts, and interpretations vary. For the purposes of this chapter, Jainism is discussed broadly. However, it is helpful to be mindful that subsect and regional variations exist, which ultimately may or may not be relevant depending on individual practices and beliefs.

A. Jain (✉)
Psychiatry, Columbia University Vagelos College of Physicians and Surgeons, New York, NY, USA
e-mail: aj2798@cumc.columbia.edu

Brief History

Jainism's origins are complex. Contemporary practices and teachings can be traced to about 2800 years ago in India. However, the universe and its "truths" are said to have always existed and been revealed over time through the teachings of 24 *Tirthankaras* ("ford-builders"), akin to prophets. While the first *Tirthankaras* are thought to be more mythical figures, historical records exist of at least the last two, Lord Parshvanatha (c.eighth century BCE) and Lord Mahavira (c.599–527 BCE), although exact dates may be disputed. For context, Siddhartha Gautama, or the "Buddha" (c.563–483 BCE), is commonly thought to be a younger contemporary of Lord Mahavira and lived in India during similar times. Jainism and Buddhism are both also *Sramana* religions and share principles such as *Karma* and the aim of liberating from eternal cycles of reincarnation, or *Samsara*, through spiritual and ethical self-discipline [2, 14–16].

Through the centuries, Jains have experienced varying periods of being oppressed, tolerated, and supported. For example, the third Mughal Emperor Akbar the Great (reigning 1556–1605), who was of the Sunni Islam faith and interested in various religious faiths, was also impacted by Jain scholars, such as following vegetarian practices and banning animal slaughter during holy Jain events [17, 18]. During the era of British rule in India (1858–1947), Jains were again permitted to pursue their faith while no longer facing persecution; however, some practices—such as nudity by Digambara Jain monks—were banned until India's independence in 1947 [19, 20]. Around that time, Mahatma Gandhi was also famously influenced by Jain principle of nonviolence [21]. In 2014, the Government of India conferred Jains with an official minority status under the National Commission for Minorities Act, further safeguarding constitutional and other fundamental rights [22].

The first Jain to travel to the USA is recognized as Virchand Raghavji Gandhi, representative to the World's Parliament of Religions in Chicago in 1893 [23]. The first US Jain temple, now relocated to Los Angeles, was originally built in 1904 for the St. Louis World's Fair [24]. The first wave of Jain immigration to the USA began in the 1960s. The first Jain Center of America was informally organized in New York in 1965 and was officially registered in 1976 [25]. Since then, over 100 Jain centers and temples have opened throughout the USA and are similarly found throughout the world [26].

Basic Principles

Jainism is derived from the Sanskrit term "Jina." This can be translated as "spiritual conqueror" or enlightened human being who, through self-discipline, has transcended worldly existence and has been liberated from the numerous cycles of reincarnation, or *Samsara*, experienced by all souls [14]. In Jainism, all living beings have souls with the capacity to eventually reach the enlightened, liberated state of *Nirvana* or *Moksha*. In this sense, every soul has the inherent quality of "Godliness." Similarly, the Jain faith does not ascribe to the concept of a "creator God," rather that the universe and all its matter, souls, and laws have always existed [2, 14, 27, 28].

An important doctrine in Jainism is *Anekantavada* or that truth is very complex and has multiple aspects. Truth can be experienced but not fully expressed through language. This doctrine is often illustrated by the parable of the five blind men describing an elephant—in which each blind person can only describe the elephant as the part (e.g., trunk, ear, tail) that they can touch—with each only partially right and truth requiring multiple viewpoints [2, 29, 30].

One of the earliest authoritative texts in Jainism is the *Tattvarthasutra* ("All That Is"). Written sometime between second and fifth century CE, it contains 350 sutras (aphorisms) in 10 chapters. It presents the major Jain philosophies, such as the seven categories of truth regarding the soul, karma, and path to liberation from the repeating cycles of rebirth. The concept of *karma* is particularly unique in Jainism. Karma is believed to be "good" and "bad" physical particles that are universally present and attach to the soul based on the soul's actions. The idea of reaching enlightenment and transmigrating from *Samsara*—the continuous existence of reincarnations—involves detachment and liberating oneself from all ("good" and "bad") karmic bonds. This purification and liberation of the soul are achieved through three jewels: *Samyak Darshan* or right faith, *Samyak Gyan* or right knowledge, and *Samyak Charitra* or right conduct [31].

In Jainism, right conduct is based on five core ethical principles or five vows, which apply more strictly to Jain monastics (monks and nuns) and to a lesser degree to laypersons. The first vow, and one of the main pillars of Jainism, is *Ahimsa* or nonviolence towards all living beings, including plants, animals, and even bacteria and other microorganisms. This applies to actions, speech, and thoughts [2, 14, 15, 31]. Regarding this practice of nonviolence, Mahatma Gandhi stated, "No religion of the world has explained the principle of non-violence so deeply and systematically, with its applicability in life as in Jainism . . ." [21].

A second vow is *Satya* or "truth." This involves speaking the truth, not lying, and not speaking that which is not true. This also includes not encouraging others or approving an untruth spoken by others. Another vow is *Asteya* or "not stealing," including not taking anything that is not willingly given even if it is unattended or unclaimed. A fourth vow is *Brahmacharya* or "celibacy." For Jain monastics, this applies to abstinence from sex and sensual pleasures. For laypersons, this means chastity and faithfulness to one's partner. A fifth vow is *Aparigraha* or "non-possessiveness," which involves not craving, not being greedy, and not having attachment to material and emotional possessions [2, 14, 15, 31].

Symbols

The Jain emblem (Fig. 17.1) was adopted by the Jain community around 1974, commemorating the auspicious 2500th anniversary of Lord Mahavira obtaining *Nirvana*. It captures many of the key Jain philosophies and principles previously described. The shape's outline depicts the

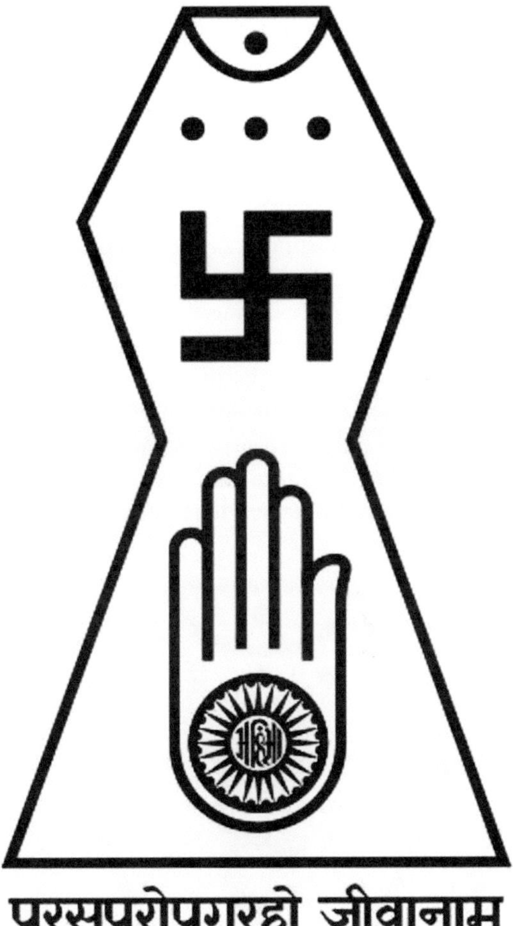

Fig. 17.1 The Jain emblem, with swastika. (Image obtained from https://www.jainheritagecentres.com/jainism/jain-symbols/universal-jain-symbol/)

universe in three sections—the lower portion is "hell," the middle portion is "the material world," and the upper portion is "heaven"—as described in ancient texts. At the top, the dot inside the crescent represents the liberated souls who occupy the apex of the universe in *Nirvana*. Below the crescent are three dots that symbolize the three jewels of Jainism described earlier: *Samyak Darshan* (right faith), *Samyak Gyan* (right knowledge), and *Samyak Charitra* (right conduct). The swastika, an ancient symbol from many religions before it was appropriated by the Nazi Party, in Jainism typically represents the cycles or reincarnation (*Samsara*) and four states of being into which the soul can be born before reaching

Nirvana: human, heavenly, hellish, and nonhuman (e.g., plants, animals, microorganisms). Due to sensitive associations with Nazism, the swastika is sometimes replaced with the Jain Om (Fig. 17.2), which represents the *Namokar Mantra*, the most significant Jain prayer (https://www.jaina.org/) [7, 32, 33]:

The hand is positioned as giving a blessing. In the palm is a circle, also representing *Samsara*, with 24 spokes representing the 24 Tirthankaras or teachers of Jainism. Within the circle, written in Devanagari script, is the central pillar of Jainism, *Ahimsa* or "nonviolence." At the bottom is the sacred phrase *Parasparopagraho Jivanam* from the Tattvarthasutra Jain text, which translates to "Souls render service to one another" or

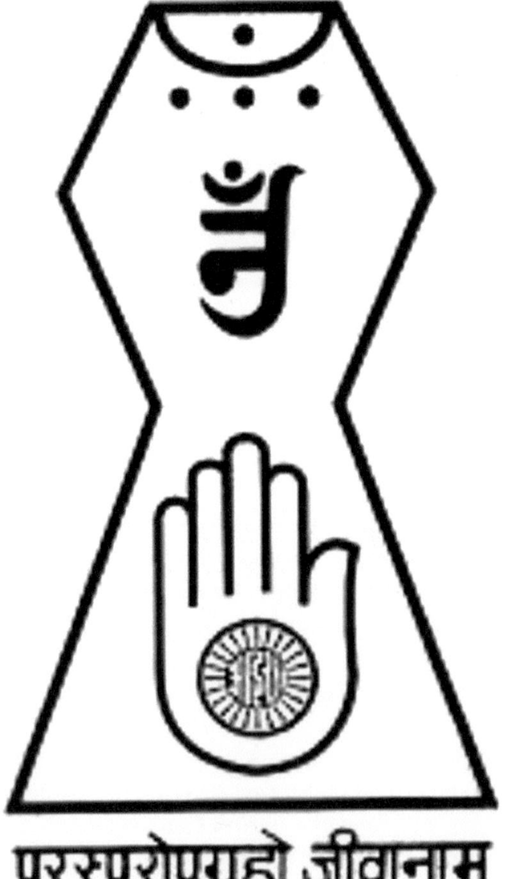

Fig. 17.2 The Jain emblem, with swastika replaced with Om. (Image obtained from https://pluralism.org/the-jain-symbol)

"All life is bound together by mutual support and interdependence" (https://www.jaina.org/) [7, 32, 33].

Practices

In the 2019–2020 Pew Research Survey in India, as with the other major religions, a large majority of Jains (89%) "Consider religion very important in their life" [11].

Vegetarianism is one of the most strictly adhered to practices in Jainism. This follows from the core ethical practice of *Ahimsa* or nonviolence towards all living beings. The Pew Research Survey found that 92% of Jains follow some degree of a vegetarian diet (e.g., not eating meat and fish) [11]. Traditional Jain diet also excludes eggs and dairy (i.e., veganism to avoid any harm when obtaining animal products) and often excludes products like honey and alcohol that involve large amounts of microorganisms (e.g., in the fermentation process). While plants are considered living organisms, the logic is that plants (e.g., fruits and vegetables) are lower sensed beings and do not experience the same sensation of pain and suffering as animals. However, even when eating plants, effort is made not to cause unnecessary harm to the plant (e.g., plucking fruit rather than harming the rest of the plant) [34]. In consideration of this, up to 67% of Jains also abstain from root vegetables (e.g., potatoes, onions, garlic) to avoid killing the entire plant [11].

Meditation is another practice in Jainism often incorporated into activities such as prayer and attending temple. It is also a concept in the vow of *samayika* or brief periods of concentration on religious activities (e.g., reading, praying, meditating). A common duration for this concentration is 48 min, though the exact reason varies, with one explanation that it is a reasonable duration to exercise full concentration and peacefulness. Another explanation is that it corresponds to 2 min for each of the 24 h of a day. While meditation in Jainism has further depth and meaning beyond the scope of this chapter, some goals are to practice detachment (i.e., stopping karmic attachments), focus inward on the soul, and reinforce core ethical principles [35, 36].

Some common practices in Jainism are generally sought to be incorporated in daily life, such as controlling one's desires; avoiding temptation and greed; not harming other living beings; and seeking forgiveness for any intentional or unintentional harm. Jains may practice further self-control and detachment, such as periods of fasting during certain festivals. Jain monastics (e.g., *Muni* or monk, *Upadhyaya* or teacher, *Acharya* or leader) have even stricter practices, like complete abstinence, limited diet, and detachment from worldly activities and possessions. When walking, cleaning their path with a soft brush (often made of fallen peacock feathers) to prevent stepping on insects is an example of another practice by Jain monks and nuns to avoid harming living beings. In the most common Jain prayer, the *Namokar Mantra*, respect is given to these monastic sages (e.g., Upadhyayas, Acharyas) and serves as a reminder of right conduct, eliminating sins, and the ultimate goal of reaching *Nirvana* [2, 13–15, 37].

Clinical Considerations

As with the clinical care of any patient, awareness and consideration of belief systems are important. An individual may not subscribe to all aspects of a particular faith, and similarly an individual's beliefs and behavior may not necessarily be attributed to a particular religious background. Nonetheless, when working with patients and families of a Jain background, clinicians can be mindful of common practices that may be relevant. These often flow from Jain tenets of nonviolence, truthfulness, not stealing, chastity, and non-materialism [15].

For instance, a vegetarian diet is very relevant when working with Jain patients. This may also extend to avoiding medications that have animal products (e.g., pill capsules with gelatin), though exceptions are often made depending on circumstances and individual beliefs (e.g., lifesaving medications) [38, 39]. Fasting in Jainism, especially during certain auspicious Jain holidays

(e.g., *Paryushan*, which typically occurs in August or September), may be relevant, but exceptions might similarly be made for health concerns. Healthcare providers can work with patients and their families to take these periods of fasting into account, such as with diabetes management [40]. Jains may also follow dietary practices like only eating during daylight (i.e., after sunrise and before sunset) [41]. Additional matters such as tube feedings may need further discussion with patients and/or their families [42]. Moreover, complex issues such as reproductive and end-of-life decisions likely require even more extensive and careful ethical consideration [2, 15].

Interestingly, many Jain concepts might already remind us of contemporary medical ethics and practices, such as *Ahimsa* (i.e., nonviolence and "first, do no harm") and *Anekantavada* (i.e., multi-sided truth and multidisciplinary collaboration). Brianne Donaldson of the Chao Center for Asian Studies at Rice University in Houston, Texas, also describes how, despite its emphasis on ethical action, consideration of living beings, and tradition of medicine, Jain ethics have been minimally present in broader medical bioethics discourse. While various reasons are considered for this absence, recently, there has been more attention to this interface, such as the "First Ever International Jain Bioethics Conference" in Claremont, California, in 2012. Donaldson specifically describes how Jain ethics of *Apramatta* or "carefulness" may contribute to modern bioethical discussions [2].

One example is the complex area of reproductive bioethics, such as in vitro fertilization and abortion. A 2017 survey of Jain medical professionals (e.g., medical residents, emergency surgeons, pharmacists), totaling 48 respondents, provided mixed opinions regarding when life begins and considerations of whether abortion could be justified and under what circumstances [2, 43]. Jain spiritual leaders have also described considerations of underlying motivations and ethical consequences when undertaking medical actions involving life or potential life. Such contemplations offer potential insight into Jainism's "tools of carefulness" (e.g., multiple viewpoints, considerations of all life forms, efforts to reduce harm) in these bioethical deliberations [2].

Another area that has drawn recent ethical and legal attention and is particularly relevant in psychiatry is a rare Jain practice called *Sallekhana* or *Santhara*—death through ritual starvation while facing the direction north. It translates to "thinning of the passions and the body" and is a conscious withdrawal from all human activities to detach from one's current life, purify the soul, and prepare for the next life. Whether it is considered the same as suicide has been debated for centuries. Even when accepted as distinct from suicide, Jain scholars only sanctioned it after scrutinizing the individual's motivations. Today, this is not a common practice, with an estimated 200 Jains in India fasting to death each year. In August 2015, the High Court of the Indian state of Rajasthan ruled that *Sallekhana* is illegal and equal to suicide (a crime in India); however, later that same month, the Supreme Court of India lifted the ban pending a full hearing in the future [15, 44].

While *Sallekhana* is an extreme and rare example, it highlights some complexities at the intersection of belief systems and medical ethics. It specifically brings forward how some core concepts in Jainism, such as detachment and transcending to a next life, may interact in the context of charged topics, such as declining and withdrawing care. At the same time, such deliberations are not unique to Jainism and are present in other faiths (e.g., refusing blood transfusions among Jehovah's Witnesses) [45, 46].

Overall, awareness of religious tenets can be helpful in patient care, though case-by-case nuances need to be considered. This is an area where psychiatrists may especially be involved, such as in considering how faith and belief systems may play a role in an individual's reasoning and medical decision-making. Considerations of underlying psychiatric or cognitive symptoms that may impair an individual's ability to provide informed consent or refusal are important, such as with complex cases in which religious beliefs and psychotic delusions need to be delineated [47–50].

Similarly, by better understanding a patient's Jain beliefs, as with other faiths, a clinician may be better able to engage that patient. This may also provide an opportunity to align with the patient's existing beliefs and practices (e.g., meditation, plant-based diets) that may also enhance healthcare and psychiatric outcomes. Discussion with patients, and when appropriate, families, ethical consultants, or even local faith-specific experts, can serve as important resources for clinicians to understand an individual's faith-based values and motivations [2, 47–50].

Conclusion

This chapter provides basic background on Jainism for mental health providers. While followed by a relatively small population worldwide, it is one of the oldest faiths with a significant historical and cultural context. Nonviolence and self-control are two of its central values, which translate to practices such as vegetarianism, fasting, and meditation. Other key principles are truth, detachment, introspection, and the goal of liberating from the cycle of reincarnation. As with any faith, the concept of religious identity may be complex and fluid. The role and the extent a patient's Jain beliefs may play in their healthcare and decisions often vary case by case, which can be especially important in psychiatry. Awareness of faiths and practices can help clinicians better engage with patients and potentially align towards shared positive healthcare goals. When appropriate, seeking additional input, such as from ethics consultants or even faith-specific scholars, can be helpful, especially when complex medical decisions are being considered.

References

1. Pew Research Center. The future of world religions: population growth projections, 2010–2050. Washington, DC: Pew Research Center; 2015.
2. Donaldson B. Bioethics and Jainism: from *ahimsā* to an applied ethics of carefulness. Religions. 2019;10(4):243. https://doi.org/10.3390/rel10040243.

3. Census of India. Religion data C-1 population by religious communities. 2011. https://censusindia.gov.in/nada/index.php/catalog/11361. Accessed 29 Jun 2024.

4. Pew Research Center. 21 Sept 2021. Religious composition of India. https://www.pewresearch.org/wpcontent/uploads/sites/20/2021/09/PF_09.21.21_Religious-Composition-of-India-FULL.pdf. Accessed 29 Jun 2024.

5. Pew Research Center. 2 Apr 2015. The future of world religions: population growth projections, 2010–2050. https://assets.pewresearch.org/wpcontent/uploads/sites/11/2015/03/PF_15.04.02_ProjectionsFullReport.pdf. Accessed 29 Jun 2024.

6. JAINA: Federation of Jain Associations of North America. Jain Diaspora. https://www.jaina.org/page/DiasporaHome. Accessed 29 Jun 2024.

7. JAINA: Federation of Jain Association. https://www.jaina.org/. Accessed 29 Jun 2024.

8. Babb LA. Understanding Jainism. Edinburgh: Dunedin; 2015.

9. Ammerman NT. Religious identities and religious institutions. In: Handbook of the sociology of religion. Cambridge: Cambridge University Press; 2003. p. 207–24.

10. Davidson LS, Ghosh D. Boundaries and crossings: religious fluidity in twenty-first century India. PORTAL J Multidiscip Int Stud. 2022;18(1–2) https://doi.org/10.5130/pjmis.v18i1-2.8245.

11. Pew Research Center. 29 Jun 2021. Religion in India: tolerance and segregation. https://www.pewresearch.org/wp-content/uploads/sites/20/2021/06/PF_06.29.21_India.full_.report.pdf. Accessed 29 Jun 2024.

12. Britannica, The Editors of Encyclopaedia. Shvetambara. Encyclopedia Britannica. 14 Sept 2012. https://www.britannica.com/topic/Shvetambara. Accessed 24 Sept 2023.

13. Britannica, The Editors of Encyclopaedia. Digambara. Encyclopedia Britannica. 20 Apr 2009. https://www.britannica.com/topic/Digambara. Accessed 24 Sept 2023.

14. Mark JJ. Jainism. World History Encyclopedia. 21 Sept 2020. https://www.worldhistory.org/jainism/. Accessed 29 Jun 2024.

15. Somasundaram O, Tejus Murthy AG, Raghavan DV. Jainism—its relevance to psychiatric practice; with special reference to the practice of *Sallekhana*. Indian J Psychiatry. 2016;58(4):471–4. https://doi.org/10.4103/0019-5545.196702. PMID: 28197009; PMCID: PMC5270277.

16. Dundas P. Jainism and Buddhism. In: Buswell RE, editor. Encyclopedia of Buddhism. New York: Macmillan Reference Lib; 2003.

17. Truschke A. III. A Mughal debate about Jain asceticism. In: Khafipour H, editor. The empires of the Near East and India: source studies of the Safavid, Ottoman, and Mughal literate communities. New York/Chichester: Columbia University Press; 2018. p. 107–24. https://doi.org/10.7312/khaf17436-011.

18. von Garbe R. Akbar, Emperor of India, Robinson LG (trans.). Chicago: The Open Court Publishing Company; 1909.

19. von Glasenapp H. Jainism: an Indian religion of salvation [Der Jainismus: Eine Indische Erlosungsreligion], Shridhar B. Shrotri (trans.). Delhi: Motilal Banarsidass (Reprinted: 1999); 1925. ISBN 81-208-1376-6.

20. Flugel P. Studies in Jaina history and culture: disputes and dialogues. New York: Routledge; 2006. https://library.oapen.org/bitstream/handle/20.500.12657/24126/1/1006005.pdf.

21. Dugar BR. Gandhi and Jainism. Indian J Polit Sci. 2013;74(2):319–22. JSTOR, http://www.jstor.org/stable/24701117. Accessed 24 Sept 2023.

22. Government of India. National Commission for Minorities. Last updated 18 Jul 2023. https://www.minorityaffairs.gov.in/show_content.php?lang=1&level=0&ls_id=216&lid=221. Accessed 24 Sept 2024.

23. The Pluralism Project, Harvard University. V.R. Gandhi at the world's parliament of religions. 2020. https://pluralism.org/files/pluralism/files/v.r._gandhi_at_the_worlds_parliament_of_religions.pdf. Accessed 29 Jun 2024.

24. Malaiya YK. The incredible journey of the 1904 St. Louis Jain temple. Jain Center of Central Ohio Pratishtha Sovenier; 2012. p. 81–4.

25. Jain Center of America—Ithaca Street, Queens temple. About us. https://www.nyjaincenter.org/About-Us. Accessed 24 Sept 2023.

26. The Pluralism Project, Harvard University. Buildings temples and networks. 2020. https://pluralism.org/files/pluralism/files/building_temples_and_networks.pdf. Accessed 29 Jun 2024.

27. The Pluralism Project, Harvard University. Jiva: the souls of all beings. 2020. https://pluralism.org/files/pluralism/files/jiva-the_souls_of_all_beings.pdf. Accessed 29 Jun 2024.

28. Sangave VA. Aspects of Jaina religion. 3rd ed. New Delhi: Bharatiya Jnanpith; 2001. ISBN 81-263-0626-2

29. The Pluralism Project, Harvard University. Anekantavada: the relativity of views. 2020. https://pluralism.org/files/pluralism/files/anekantavada-the_relativity_of_views.pdf. Accessed 29 Jun 2024.

30. Barbato M. Anekāntavāda and dialogic identity construction. Religions. 2019;10(12):642. https://doi.org/10.3390/rel10120642.

31. Tatia N. That which is—Tattvārtha Sūtra composed by Umāsvāti. San Francisco: Harper Collins Publishers; 1994.

32. The Pluralism Project, Harvard University. The Jain symbol. 2020. https://pluralism.org/files/pluralism/files/the_jain_symbol.pdf. Accessed 29 Jun 2024.

33. The Universal Jain Symbol. Jain Heritage Centres. https://jainworld.com/education/jain-education-material/jain-symbol/. Accessed 24 Sept 2023.

34. Shah A. Jain food struggles in America. Huffpost. 12 Jan 2017. https://www.huffpost.com/entry/jain-food-struggles-in-am_b_8961854. Accessed 24 Sept 2023.
35. Gada M. Jaina religion and psychiatry. Mens Sana Monogr. 2015;13(1):70.
36. JAINA: Federation of Jain Associations of North America. Samayika and Dhyana. https://www.jaina.org/page/SamayikaDhyana/Samayika-and-Dhyana.htm. Accessed 29 Jun 2024.
37. The Pluralism Project, Harvard University. Namaskara mantra: beginning with praise. 2020. https://pluralism.org/files/pluralism/files/namaskara_mantra-beginning_with_praise_0.pdf. Accessed 29 Jun 2024.
38. Prakash A, et al. Are your capsules vegetarian or nonvegetarian: an ethical and scientific justification. Indian J Pharmacol. 2017;49(5):401–4. https://doi.org/10.4103/ijp.IJP_409_17.
39. Khokhar WA, et al. When taking medication may be a sin: dietary requirements and food laws in psychotropic prescribing. BJPsych Adv. 2015;21(6):425–32. https://doi.org/10.1192/apt.bp.114.012534.
40. Saboo B, et al. Management of diabetes during fasting and feasting in India. J Assoc Physicians India. 2019;67(9):70–7.
41. Caring for the Jain Patient. Ashford and St. Peter's Hospitals, National Health Service (NHS) Foundation Trust. https://www.ashfordstpeters.info/images/other/PAS08.pdf. Accessed 24 Sept 2023.
42. Guidelines for Health Care Providers Interacting with Patients of the Jain Religion and Their Families. Metropolitan Chicago Healthcare Council. https://www.kyha.com/assets/docs/PreparednessDocs/cg-jain.pdf. Accessed 24 Sept 2023.
43. Donaldson B. Jain medical professionals' "reflexive ethical orientation": adaptive nonviolence, multiple sources of knowledge, and concern for five-sensed beings. Religions. 2022;13(11):1123. https://doi.org/10.3390/rel13111123.
44. McCarthy J. Fasting to the death: is it a religious rite or suicide? 2015. http://www.npr.org/sections/goatsandsoda/2015/09/02/436820789/fastingto-the-death-is-it-a-religious-rite-or-suicide.
45. Campbell A, Halpern D. Evaluating capacity in a suicidal Jehovah's witness refusing blood. Prim Care Companion CNS Disord. 2020;22(6):20l02595.
46. Barstow C, Shahan B, Roberts M. Evaluating medical decision-making capacity in practice. Am Fam Physician. 2018;98(1):40–6.
47. Sharma H, et al. End-of-life care: Indian perspective. Indian J Psychiatry. 2013;55(Suppl 2):S293–8. https://doi.org/10.4103/0019-5545.105554.
48. Geros-Willfond KN, et al. Religion and spirituality in surrogate decision making for hospitalized older adults. J Relig Health. 2016;55:765–77.
49. Rego F, et al. The influence of spirituality on decision-making in palliative care outpatients: a cross-sectional study. BMC Palliat Care. 2020;19(1):1–14.
50. Pierre JM. Faith or delusion? At the crossroads of religion and psychosis. J Psychiatr Pract. 2001;7(3):163–72.

The Theory and Practice of Chinese Confucian Mental Health Education

18

Kai Wang

Introduction

It may seem inappropriate to analyze Confucianism, which originated in ancient China, from a very modern perspective "mental health education". However, when we learn that Confucius, the founder of Confucianism, is widely considered to be the first private teacher in China [1], his advocacy of "Human becoming" is regarded as one of the most important educational ideas of Confucianism [2]. Under such circumstances, it is also clearly inappropriate to say that Confucianism has nothing to do with mental health education, which is centered on the human being. In fact, because mental health has long lacked a clear and universal definition [3], and with the development of cross-cultural psychology in recent years, psychologists have found it difficult to establish a mental health model that can be universally applied to all cultural communities, constructing a mental health model with local characteristics based on different cultures has become a new research trend. In this context, the construction of a mental health model based on Confucian culture has become an important topic in indigenous psychological research. These models can be divided into three categories: the first is the individual-centered mental health

model based on Confucian emotional theory; the second is the social-centered mental health model based on Confucian ethical theory; and the third is the state-centered mental health model based on Confucian political theory. Each of these models has its own limitations, and none of them can appropriately explain the Yin-Yang mental health model based on Confucian cosmology.

The Individual-Centered Mental Health Models and Their Limitations

The exploration of the psychological function of the individual is an ancient topic in Western philosophy. As early as ancient Greece, philosophers devoted themselves to illustrating the uniqueness of the human psyche through the soul. In modern times, influenced by the development of modern natural sciences, philosophers such as Hume began to distinguish the psyche as an mental entity as opposed to the physical entity based on an empiricist perspective and devoted themselves to exploring its structural features. In this context, when psychology diverged from philosophy as an independent science in the nineteenth century, it continued to follow the philosophers' path to study the structure of the individual psyche on the one hand, and devoted itself to constructing a more practical model of mental health from the perspective of empirical science on the other.

K. Wang (✉)
Institute of Traditional Chinese Culture, Ocean University of China, Qingdao, China
e-mail: wangkai5176@ouc.edu.cn

However, due to the complexity of human psychology, scientism can hardly replace humanism in the field of psychology. Therefore, two research directions have emerged in the construction of mental health models: one is to construct a negative mental health model from a scientific perspective; the other is to construct a positive mental health model from a humanistic perspective. Since Confucian culture is often seen as a representative of Eastern humanism in various philosophical and psychological works [4–6], when people began to study Confucian culture from the perspective of mental health, they tended to construct the Confucian models of mental health from the humanist theory of positive psychology. This led to the formation of an individual-centered mental health model based on Confucian emotional theory.

Since the end of the twentieth century, positive psychology research emerged, and influenced by this, happiness gradually became a separate research area in humanistic psychology research. In this context, many scholars began to analyze the Confucian concepts of mental health from the perspective of happiness, and formed two models of mental health with "Le"(happiness) as the core concept.

The first Le model is a physical and spiritual health model based on emotional balance and harmony. This model is constructed on the basis of an important Confucian work called *The Doctrine of the Mean*. As this work states:

Before the feelings of pleasure, anger, sorrow, and joy are aroused it is called equilibrium (chung, centrality, mean). When these feelings are aroused and each and all attain due measure and degree, it is called harmony. Equilibrium is the great foundation of the world, and harmony its universal path. When equilibrium and harmony are realized to the highest degree, heaven and earth will attain their proper order and all things will flourish [7].

This passage emphasizes that emotional balance and harmony are necessary to ensure the orderly development and prosperity of all things in heaven and earth. Therefore, in this model, how to maintain emotional balance and harmony becomes the key to happiness. For example,

Peng's theory of mind-body cultivation is a typical representative of this viewpoint, which can be summarized as a sagittal model.

In the sagittal model, both the unmanifest emotions and the harmonious state after the emotions have arisen are considered to be a psychological state that is in accordance with the law of nature and thus a psychological quality that a healthy person should possess. When emotions do not arise, all emotions are in a situation called equilibrium. In this case, the mind is calm, but as one is constantly exposed to the outside world and influenced by various life events, especially by the pursuit of political power, fame and status as emphasized by Confucianism, one's emotions such as joy, anger, sorrow and pleasure begin to arise and fluctuate from time to time and from event to event, making it difficult to be calm. At this time, the only way to bring the mind back to peace is to adjust the emotions and return them to a harmonious state according to the principle of the Mean. This method of adjustment is summarized by Guoxiang Peng in two ways: one is spiritual practice. This approach to practice is based on two of Mencius' concepts of spiritual practice: "maintain an unperturbed mind", "finding the lost mind". The former requires that the mind be able to concentrate on itself and not be moved by worldly matters, especially power, position, fame and fortune. The latter requires people who have been disturbed by the world to regain their original state of mind and to stimulate the moral energy of the mind, so that people can resist the disturbance of negative emotions [8]. The other is psychosomatic practice. This method emphasizes meditation and breath regulation. It is actually a method of physical and mental cultivation learned from Buddhism by Song and Ming philosophy, aiming to keep one's inner peace. Of course, Confucian scholars also made a point of emphasizing that this method of mind-body practice was to be done in daily life, rather than requiring a dedicated time and place for practice, as Buddhism does [9–11].

The second Le model is a model of moral emotion production that transcends external environmental stimuli. Since *The Doctrine of the Mean*, on which the first model construct is based, is widely regarded as a work revered by Confucian disciples after the Song Dynasty, many scholars believe that it does not represent the true spirit of primitive Confucianism. Therefore, they have constructed the second model based on a work called *The Analects*, which records the words and actions of Confucius, the founder of Confucianism. The most important statements in this book related to happiness are two passages that later became the " The Happiness of Confucius and Yan Hui":

Confucius said, "With coarse rice to eat, with water to drink, and with a bent arm for a pillow, there is still joy. Wealth and honor obtained through unrighteousness are but floating clouds to me" [12].

How good Yan Hui was, said the Master, living in a humble lane with only a handful of rice to eat and a gourdful of water to drink! Others could not bear such a wretched life, but Yan Hui was as happy as ever. How good Yan Hui was! [13].

These two passages show that, in the Confucian view, true happiness means that the mind is not influenced by external circumstances. Whether one is rich or poor, one is able to maintain inner peace and joy. Based on this concept, many new Confucian theories of mental health have been developed in the scholarship. These theories can be summarized as the stepped model of mental health.

This model reveals, first of all, that human beings do not exist independently, but survive and develop in the process of negotiating with their surroundings. Therefore, the ability to adjust one's behavior to maintain harmony with the surrounding environment is the key to achieving happiness and maintaining mental health. To reach this goal, people should make efforts in the following areas:

First, one should stimulate the love (benevolence) that is latent in the human spirit. Since people do not exist in isolation, focusing on others, not just on oneself, is a necessary prerequisite for people to create a happy life.

Secondly, one should learn the moral code and achieve certain achievements by the age of 30. This is the only way to stand firmly in the world.

Moral norms are codes of conduct for dealing with human relationships and can help individuals reconcile themselves with their surrounding interpersonal environment; secular achievements, on the other hand, reflect an individual's contribution to society and can help individuals reconcile themselves with their surrounding community environment.

Thirdly, when you are in your 40s or 50s, you should be able to not be bothered by external things and correctly grasp the nature and laws of nature, society and human beings themselves.

Fourth, after the age of 60, one should skillfully adjust one's inner self through introspection to a state that is consistent with moral norms and the laws of the world, so that all actions conform to the norms or laws, but one does not feel any discomfort in one's inner self by viewing these norms or laws as mandatory bondage.

Moreover, Confucianism emphasizes that only when all these requirements are fully implemented under the principle of sincerity can the individual truly achieve transcendence over his/her environment, be completely free from external stimuli, and reach a state of ultimate happiness.

Of course, in everyday life, ordinary people and intellectuals influenced by Confucianism have an easier and more direct way to maintain their mental health. For the people, using religious means to establish a connection with great Confucian figures or to obtain their spiritual help is a quick way to relieve psychological anxiety and maintain mental health. For example, in ancient China, many candidates would go to the Confucius temples to worship Confucius before their exams, and in Beijing, candidates would drink or grind the ink-stick with the water from the well inside the Confucius temple, which was said to make the candidates' thoughts flow and their writing flourish [14]. This tradition is also manifested in China today, where there are always various "tributes" in front of the statue of Confucius in some schools before final exams. This is a way for students to relieve their test anxiety. Sometimes, to get better results, students offer even more innovative tributes to please Confucius and ask for his blessing. For example, some students observed that the tributes in front of the statue of Confucius were a lot of fruits, milk tea and other foods, and they unexpectedly placed digestive medicine as tributes under the statue of Confucius [15].

In general, the individual-centered model describes in detail the Confucian concept of mental health in terms of well-being. However, as many scholars have pointed out, the individual is not the focus of Confucian theory. The individual in Confucianism is always the individual with social responsibilities, not the individual as a collection of social rights as stated in Western psychology based on individualism [16]. In light of this, the social-centered model has been constructed to describe the mental health standards of the social individual in Confucianism.

The Social-Centered Mental Health Model and Its Limitations

In Confucian theory, the individual always means not just the individual itself, but appears in some social role. It is for this reason that Confucianism's mental health means not only emotional harmony or psychological transcendence of the external environment, but also the ability to handle social relationships comfortably, especially the "human relations" that Confucianism regards as the fundamental basis of human beings. Based on this understanding, psychologists, represented by Yip, defined the Confucian understanding of mental health as a direction based on the classical Four Books of Confucianism, suggesting self-discipline and obedience to the social order in order to maintain one's inner balance and external harmony with others. The three levels of harmony and balance are shown in the triangular model. As the model shows, in order to maintain mental health, individuals need to achieve three levels of balance-namely, the individual, interpersonal, moral and ethical levels of balance [17].

In this model, it is clear that while mental health implies a balance of the three dimensions, for the individual it means more responsibilities in order to maintain good interpersonal and social relationships. This is very evident both in theory and in practice. In terms of practice, in today's Chinese national education, various emphases on family or social responsibility are used as one of the most prominent teaching elements. For example, many elementary schools in China use the *TwentyFour Examples of Filial Piety,* the well-known Chinese tale, portray a son's devotion to and sacrifices for his father or both parents, as well as a daughter's devotion to and sacrifices for her mother, motherinlaw, or father [18], as an important part of school education. This reflects the importance that Chinese education places on family responsibilities, which are an important part of Chinese social relations (see Table 18.1). Fei Xiaotong, a famous sociologist, even directly pointed out that Chinese social relations influenced by Confucian culture are interpersonal relationships based on family kinship relations with the existence of closeness and distance [19]. Therefore, in the context of Confucianism, the ability to maintain harmonious family relationships naturally becomes one of the important criteria for measuring an individual's psychological health.

This model also has a relatively easy means of practice. Ordinary Chinese people have had a strong concept of clan since ancient times, and they have used the maintenance of clan order to achieve harmony in family relations, which in turn promotes harmony in social relations. This concept is not limited to the maintenance of harmonious relationships between the living, but even between the living and the dead. For example, the Chinese often enshrine their dead ancestors in the living room of their homes, reinforcing the cohesion between family members (both living and dead). For ancient Chinese intellectuals, the ledgers of merit and demerit was another important means of maintaining individual and social harmony. These ledgers are merit-demerit calculation texts that use Confucian morality as one of its main foundations. It assigns separate points to an individual's moral and non-moral behavior. One of the most important criteria for determining whether an individual's behavior is moral or not is whether the individual can act in a way that is beneficial to others and to society. For example, a seventeenth-century book of merits and demerits stipulated that 100 merit points

Table 18.1 Content of family education in some Chinese elementary school

Number	Region	School	Teaching contents
1	North of China	Shenyang Shenhe District Culture Road Second Primary School	*New TwentyFour Examples of Filial Piety* Lectures[a]
2	North China	The Third Primary School of Zhongguancun, Haidian District, Beijing	Extracurricular practice: making rubbings of the "paintings of the *TwentyFour Examples of Filial Piety* "[b]
3	Eastern China	Taonan Road Primary School, Qingdao	Chrysanthemum Day Theme Activity: explaining and publicizing the *TwentyFour Examples of Filial Piety*[c]
4	Eastern China	Laogang Primary School, Shanghai	"Filial piety culture in the classroom" activities: (including group recitation of filial piety poems, calligraphy based on filial piety, origami flowers for parents, and gesture dance with music in memory of mother)[d]
5	South China	All primary schools in Guangzhou	*New TwentyFour Examples of Filial Piety* Painting Competition for Minors (Organizer: Guangzhou Municipal Committee of Spiritual Civilization Construction)[e]
6	South China	Fuxi school, Haikou	"Filial piety"birthday party[f]
7	Western China	Xincheng school, Pingliang	*TwentyFour Examples of Filial Piety* animation watching activity[g]
8	Central China	The Second Primary School of Huanghe Road and Fengwan School, Zhengzhou	Visiting the exhibition of brick sculptures of *TwentyFour Examples of Filial Piety*[h]

[a]https://mp.weixin.qq.com/s/ekw8vApwbivqNXIcmNYCoQ
[b]https://mp.weixin.qq.com/s/d7IaiKvhVb9aGwQ3f-gsbw
[c]https://mp.weixin.qq.com/s/FEq0SOCga03JrZoerEN8RQ
[d]https://mp.weixin.qq.com/s/DOivuWLSXHUBIFHucicrbw
[e]https://mp.weixin.qq.com/s/fZ6lgl-kG2vHZYs5AqTsWg
[f]https://mp.weixin.qq.com/s/bLuGnQGVoVIRsUgrcnaALg
[g]https://mp.weixin.qq.com/s/tkQ9IDsNPGDowtLuVFIz1w
[h]https://mp.weixin.qq.com/s/8mTB1tjC3oDTdwk7keKFHQ

should be given to a person who had saved another person's life, and 100 demerit points should be given to a person who was unwilling to give away his extra money to a person who was suffering in a time of war [20].

Although Confucianism attaches great importance to the family, maintaining good family relationships is not the ultimate goal of life that Confucian intellectuals seek. The famous Confucian classic *The Great Learning* begins with the statement that people should pay attention to "Self-Cultivation, Family Regulation, State Governance, Bringing Peace to All Under Heaven" [21]. Therefore, on a more fundamental level, achieving political success and contributing to the nation is the ultimate goal of Confucian education. With this in mind, some scholars have gone on to construct a state-centered model of mental health.

The State-Centered Mental Health Concepts and Their Limitations

Performing Great Deeds (mainly making contribution to countries), along with Set Moral Examples and Spread Noble Ideas, has long been recognized by Confucian elites throughout history as one of the three indelible virtues to be pursued throughout life. It is because Confucian followers are keen on acquiring political achievements that the ability to achieve political status and play a political role becomes a key factor influencing whether a person can become a healthy person (**in line with the Confucian Junzi [gentleman] personality**). It is because of this that in Chinese history we often see that only people like Dong Zhongshu, Zhu Xi, Wang Yangming and others who achieved great political success or had great political ambitions were seen as role models, while people like Li Bai, Du Fu, Xu Wei and others who were disillusioned in politics often only managed to stay famous in the world through artistic or literary achievements. Under the influence of this understanding, scholars have constructed a state-centered mental health concepts based on the personality of the Junzi.

On the whole, the Junzi plays an important moral influence and inspiration role in society and politics, and the Junzi's benevolence and love for the people with virtue is not only a moral obligation requirement, but also an active ideal pursuit and virtue realization. When a Junzi holds political power, he should pursue political virtues such as benevolence, righteousness, propriety and wisdom; when a Junzi lives in civil society, he is responsible for educating and teaching the people, regulating his behavior in accordance with Confucian rituals, using his words, virtues and demeanor to set an example for ordinary people and inspire the community. The Junzi's "virtue" as a moral example of intrinsic and universal, must cause the rulers and the general public to aspire to. The Junzi takes both personal and family moral norms as the meaning of his existence, the basis of his life and spiritual habitat, and the moral norms required in political practice, his own political activities as the way to achieve his values and ideals [22]. In this sense, becoming a Junzi is clearly an important means of achieving mental health. This is particularly important in the current Confucianism courses in Chinese universities, where one can easily find in the objectives or content of the courses about becoming a Junzi, assuming political responsibility, and contributing to the development of the country (see Table 18.2).

In ancient China, officials would also reinforce the pursuit of a Junzi personality among the

Table 18.2 Teaching objectives of Confucianism courses in some Chinese universities

Number	University	Course	Teaching objectives
1	Tianjin University of Technology	Confucian civilization and modern social management	Guiding college students to establish patriotism with the love of traditional Chinese culture as the core[a]
2	Hunan University	The Four Books and Life	To guide students to enhance their sense of cultural identity, to cultivate a sense of family and country, and to strengthen their sense of responsibility to inherit and promote excellent Chinese traditional culture[b]
3	China University of Political Science and Law	Introduction to the Four Books	Students are taught the latest research on Chinese culture, on the basis of which they can develop a discursive, rational and political approach[c]
4	Taizhou University	The ideal of life in *Analects*	The purpose of the course is to tell the Chinese story and carry forward the Chinese spirit[d]
5	Guizhou University	Introduction to the Wang Yangming's Philosophy	With the practical and responsible spirit of Wang Yangming's "Zhi Liang Zhi", the students will gain a deeper understanding of the state of the world, the state of the Party, the state of the people, and the state of the nation, so that they…… will be determined to join the great current of the times and contribute to the great rejuvenation of the Chinese nation[e]
6	Ocean University of China	Introduction to the *Analects*	Through the teaching of the Confucian idea of "Junzi", which is the core of the Analects of Confucius, students will be helped and guided to cultivate the character of "Junzi" through cooperative learning and research studies, taking into account the characteristics of the mindset of college students in the new era[f]

[a]https://mp.weixin.qq.com/s/uuqsU1W_1x1T0XQU9CAkWA
[b]https://mp.weixin.qq.com/s/FbV7COeHvAUbYTxotuNVKA
[c]https://mp.weixin.qq.com/s/3Y9QU_IvZn5VDDxUBwBAtA
[d]https://mp.weixin.qq.com/s/IYGQQTi8fBB_lZUdLzRf0Q
[e]https://mp.weixin.qq.com/s/a2vbNkPpQH5XTNH8ZVGa2g
[f]https://mp.weixin.qq.com/s/XG2RlTVLfwbC__aIP6yyYQ

elites through various religious ceremonies. Confucius himself, the founder of Confucianism, attached great importance to rituals and once put forward the principle of participating in rituals: "When sacrifice is offered to someone, act as though someone is just in front of you. When sacrifice is offered to a god, act as though the god is present." This actually requires that those who participate in the rituals participate in the rituals wholeheartedly, and through such participation at the spiritual level, the participants tend to have a sense of morality enhanced, which is, of course, one of the reasons why Confucianism attaches great importance to the reality of the sacrificial rituals [23].

This model accurately describes Confucianism's theoretical tendency to prescribe the state of human health in terms of political ends. But in general, Confucian theory did not begin by focusing on the state; what really constitutes the source of Confucian theory is a work that is widely considered to embody the Chinese cosmology: the *Zhou Yi* (*The Book of Changes*). This book describes the origin, development process and laws of nature and society in terms of Yin and Yang. Therefore, in order to present a complete Confucian theory of mental health, we should not start with the state alone, but should consider the overall Confucian view of nature, the individual, society, and the state in a comprehensive manner.

The Yin-Yang Model of Mental Health and the Education of Confucianism

It is an indisputable fact that Confucius regarded the *Zhou Yi* as an extremely important work. In this regard, it is necessary to construct a model of Confucian mental health theory and educational practice in conjunction with the thought of *Zhou Yi*. The so-called "*Zhou Yi*" is an ancient Chinese philosophical work. Its content depicts the fundamental understanding of the Chinese people about the universe and life, and has been passed down for thousands of years and is still highly respected today. The concept of Taiji and the the-

ory of Yin and Yang in the *Zhou Yi* is at its core. Among them, Taiji is considered the most fundamental element of the universe, while Yin and Yang represent the static and dynamic states of Taiji respectively. Everything that arises from the changes between the static and dynamic states of Taiji constitutes the essence of the world [24]. It is by observing the laws of heaven and earth that Confucianism constructs the norms of human behavior, following the example of nature. As all things in heaven and earth are created by the movement of Yin and Yang, human mental health should also be discussed in the context of the movement of Yin and Yang.

It is by observing the laws of heaven and earth that Confucianism constructs the norms of human behavior, following the example of nature. According to the observation of Confucianism, in nature, heaven represents Yang and earth represents Yin, and heaven and earth are in harmony, and Yin and Yang harmonize to produce all things **(enable all living things to perpetuate themselves)**. Human society depends on heaven and earth for its existence and must also follow its laws. In human society, the active and aggressive spirit represents Yang and the tolerant and altruistic spirit represents Yin, and only when everyone actively contributes to others can the world become a better place and the country become stable **(enable others to lead better lives)**. From this, it logically follows that the ideal Confucian state of personal health should be one in which Yin and Yang are harmonized and active service to others is the state of mind. In the process of serving others, people can shift their attention from themselves to others, thus avoiding the psychological pain of wanting more than they can fill because of excessive focus on themselves, especially excessive pursuit of their own desires [25].

With this in mind, Confucian mental health education should begin with nature education rather than directly subjecting students to some moral code such as helping others.

Starting from the overall Confucian theory, the first step of mental health education should be to let students get close to nature and understand the laws of natural growth of all things. The second step is to start from emotions, using music education, etiquette education and other means to stimulate students' inner feelings of respecting and thinking of others. The third step is family education, through the family as a basic social unit, let students initially establish the dedication to thinking of family members, and finally realize the good family atmosphere of father's kindness, son's filial piety, brother's friendship and brother's respect, so that people can acquire the ability to maintain harmonious interpersonal relationship. The fourth step is social education, in which students learn about moral norms, emulate the behavior of moral models, and contribute to social development and national progress.

Conclusions

The definition of mental health has been very vague since the beginning of the use of mental health terminology in Europe in the mid-nineteenth century. In this context, it becomes more difficult to summarize a pre-modern Confucian culture's mental health criteria. Previous studies of Confucian mental health education have been divided into three categories: individual mental health education with the goal of balancing individual emotions, social mental health education with the goal of harmonizing family and social relationships, and national mental health education with the goal of assuming social responsibility. These three types of mental health education are all based on one aspect of Confucianism theory to construct corresponding mental health models and standards, and thus all have the limitation of lacking wholeness and cannot correctly explain the Confucian Yin-Yang mental health model established based on cosmology in the context of traditional Chinese culture. Due to this limitation, this study proposes a Confucian model of mental health education centered on the Yin-Yang movement using Confucianism's multi-faceted discourse on nature, the individual, society, and the state. The model states that the basic Confucian view on mental health education is to follow the spirit of nature in fertilizing all things, transforming

the concern for the individual self into service and contribution to others, thus promoting the unity of man with nature or society and creating a good environment for his own survival, and thus achieving the goal of mental health. This model, presented for the first time, establishes a mental health standard that is more in line with actual Chinese thinking and provides cultural resources and pedagogical suggestions for the study of modern Chinese mental health teaching.

References

1. Yu-lan F. A short history of Chinese philosophy. New York: The Free Press; 1966. p. 39.
2. Ames RT. Human becomings: theorizing persons for Confucian role ethics. State University of New York Press; 2020, ebook.
3. Galderisi S, Heinz A, Kastrup M, Beezhold J, Sartorius N. Toward a new definition of mental health. World Psychiatry. 2015;14(2):231–3.
4. Lan F. Ezra Pound and confucianism: remaking humanism in the face of modernity. University of Toronto Press; 2005. p. 183–98.
5. Liu JH. What confucian philosophy means for Chinese and Asian psychology today: Indigenous roots for a psychology of social change. J Pac Rim Psychol. 2014;8(2):35–42.
6. Weiming T. The ecological turn in new confucian humanism: implications for China and the world. Daedalus. 2001;130(4):243–64.
7. Chan W-T. A source book in Chinese philosophy. Princeton University Press; 1963. p. 98.
8. Guoxiang P. "Realizing the Xin" and "cultivating the Qi". Acad Monthly. 2018;50(04):5–20.
9. Guoxiang P. Confucian tradition: crossing religion and humanism. Beijing: Peking University Press; 2007. p. 246–8.
10. Taylor RL. The cultivation of sagehood as a religious goal in neo-confucianism: a study of selected writings of Kao P'an-Lung (1562–1626). Columbia University; 1974.
11. Taylor RL. The confucian tradition of contemplation: Okada Takehiko and the tradition of quiet-sitting. Philos East West. 1990;40(3):413–5.
12. Chan W-T. A source book in Chinese philosophy. Princeton University Press; 1963. p. 32.
13. Yuanchong X. LUNYU YIHUA. BEIJING: Peking University Press; 2017, e-book, Retrieved November 7, 2023, from https://weread.qq.com/web/reader/0c43 2b6071dc8ee80c4779f?
14. Beijing Municipal Committee of the Chinese People's Political Consultative Conferenee. Beijing stories. Beijing: Beijing publishing house; 2020. p. 181.

15. Wang K. Exam student gives Confucius statue a stomach-boosting tablet. 2020. Retrieved November 7, 2023, from https://mp.weixin.qq.com/s/j44KrrjB445_TUPWsUzdzw

16. Yip KS. A Chinese cultural critique of the global qualifying standards for social work education. Soc Work Educ. 2004;23(5):597–612. https://doi.org/10.1080/0261547042000252316.

17. Yip K-S. Traditional confucian concepts of mental health: its implications to social work practice with Chinese communities. Asia Pac J Soc Work Dev. 2003;13(2):65–89. https://doi.org/10.1080/21650993.2003.9755929.

18. Hsu FLK. Confucianism in comparative context. In: Slote WH, De Vos GA, editors. Confucianism and the family. New York: State University of New York Press; 1998. p. 58.

19. Fei X, Hamilton GG, Zheng W. From the soil: the foundations of Chinese society. Oakland: University of California Press; 1992. p. 60–70.

20. Brokaw CJ. The ledgers of merit and demerit: social change and moral order in late imperial China. Princeton University Press; 1991. p. 61–109.

21. Legge J. Confucian analects: the great learning, and the doctrine of the mean. New York: Courier Corporation; 1971.

22. Yu J. The change of the concept of "the gentleman" and confucius' "politics of the noble" in the era of "six classics". J Cent South Univ (Soc Sci). 2022;28(1):13–20.

23. Zijie P. A confucian view of interactive interaction in sacrificial rituals. News Res. 2022;02:77–83.

24. Baynes CF, Wilhelm H. The I Ching or book of changes, vol. 31. Princeton University Press; 2011.

25. Field SL. The Duke of Zhou Changes: A Study and Annotated Translation of the Zhouyi. 周易: Harrassowitz Verlag; 2015.

Part III

Cultural Humility Perspectives on the Eastern Traditions from Western Psychiatry

A Christian Perspective on Eastern Religions and Mental Health

19

Deborah Y. Park and John R. Peteet

Introduction

Christian and Eastern religions have interacted for centuries. Here we briefly review historical and cultural aspects of this relationship, explore theological commonalities and differences, review paths to greater compatibility, and discuss some clinical implications.

History and Culture

According to tradition, the apostle Thomas founded one of the oldest existing Christian communities in Kerala, India. During and after the colonial era, missionaries received mixed reception with particularly violent conflict in Japan. However, despite Communist repression of religion, Christians have continued to worship as a vital minority in many southeast Asian countries. Eastern cultural adaptation of Christianity resulted as seen in Fig. 19.1. This art piece utilizes an Indian painting style, originating in the Deccan region of Central India, to illustrate the birth of Jesus Christ. Another art piece titled *An Angel Summons the Shepherds* (1940s, China) depicts the shepherds being called by angels to Jesus's birth using Chinese techniques on silk scrolls (Fig. 19.2). In 2018, the Chinese government declared that there are over 44 million Christians in China, which is likely an underestimate due to the large number of unregistered or underground churches.

Eastern religions spread into the West first through immigration and later through Westerners who followed Indian gurus, and learned meditation. During the twentieth century, the Japanese Buddhist monk D.T. Suzuki taught in a number of universities, interpreting and popularizing Zen Buddhism in the West. Subsequently, Thich Naht Hahn pioneered mindfulness, along with clinicians Jack Kornfield, Sharon Salzberg, and Joseph Goldstein who founded the Insight Meditation Society (IMS) in 1975.

In the 1960s, the prominent theologian Paul Tillich called for a dialogue between Buddhism and Christianity, around the time that the trappiest monk Thomas Merton went further to say "I want to become as good a Buddhist as I can," describing the impact on him of Buddhist insights into paradox, freedom, compassion, contemplation, and mysticism.

At the same time, some Christians find the now widespread acceptance of yoga and meditation as ostensibly secular practices within clinical and educational settings problematic. For exam-

D. Y. Park (⊠) · J. R. Peteet
Department of Psychiatry, Brigham and Women's Hospital, Boston, MA, USA
e-mail: dypark@bwh.harvard.edu;
jpeteet@bwh.harvard.edu

H. S. Moffic et al. (eds.), *Eastern Religions, Spirituality, and Psychiatry*,
https://doi.org/10.1007/978-3-031-56744-5_19

Fig. 19.1 Adoration of
the Christ Child

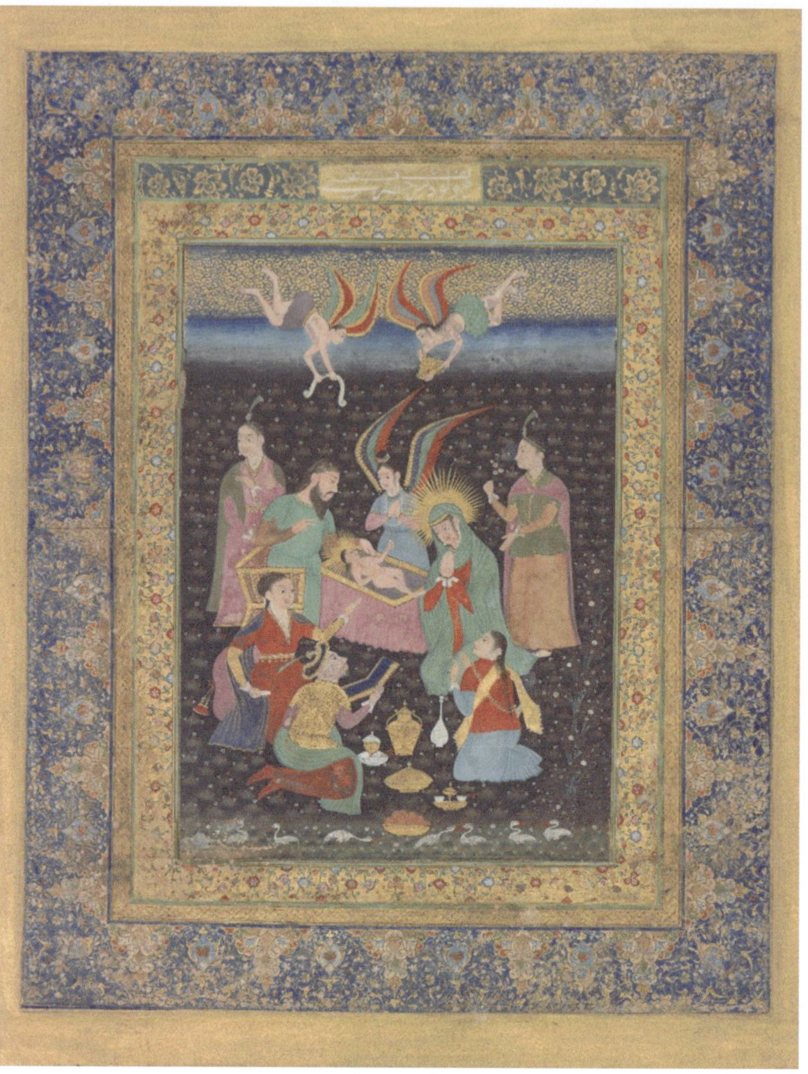

ple, Candace Brown in *Debating Yoga and Mindfulness in Public Schools: Reforming Secular Education or Reestablishing Religion?* [1] argues that inherent in training in these modalities are metaphysical assumptions which are often unacknowledged. Questions she raises include whether suffering is the central human dilemma, whether the answer to suffering comes in the form of self-cultivated enlightenment (renunciation of desire) or a realignment of desires and a restored relationship with God and others, and what implications a non-dualistic world view has for moral motivation and action.

Respect for Contributions and Common Ground

Respect for the values, beliefs, and worldviews of other religions contributes to a cohesive and diverse community. Christians can go further to appreciate a number of contributions of Eastern religions and their common ground. Consider some of these noted below, as well as some differences between Eastern and Christian perspectives.

Hinduism is heterogeneous by nature, but core Hindu beliefs include the interconnectedness of

Fig. 19.2 An angel summons the shepherds

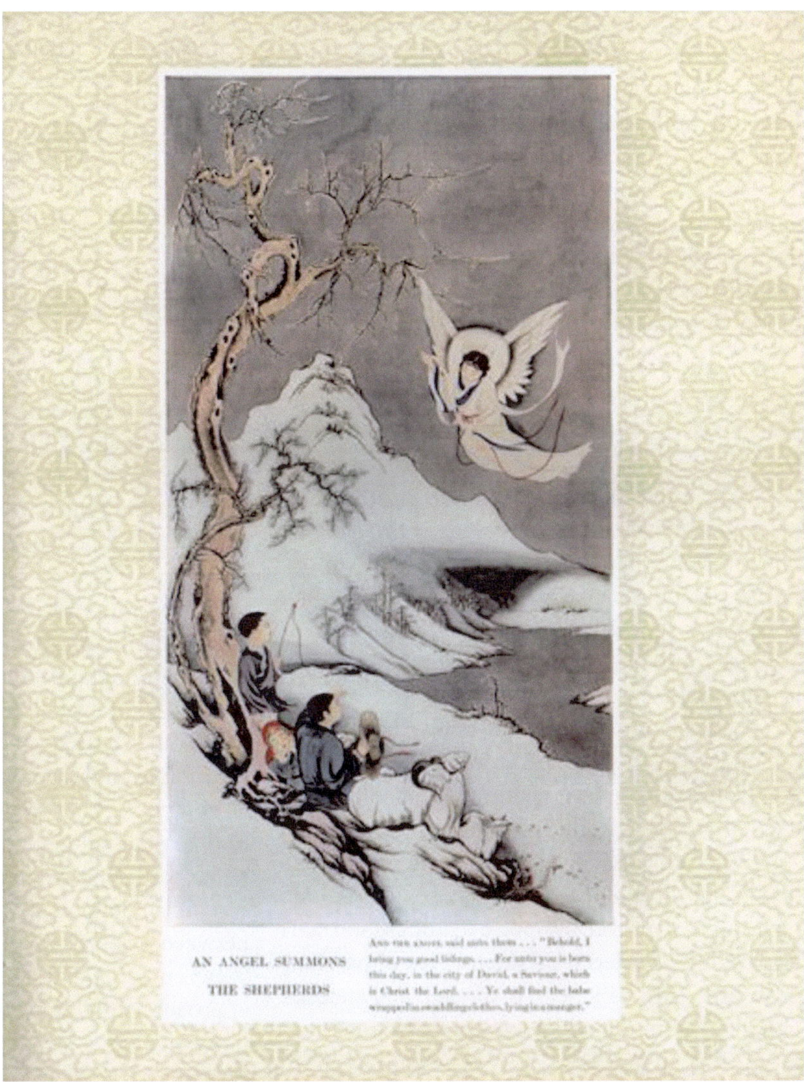

the universe and that no one religion holds a monopoly on the truth. This belief promotes a non-judgmental perspective toward other religious beliefs and can facilitate safe dialogue between religious communities. Hinduism additionally encourages people to care for other beings, to minimize harm, and to do so selflessly, without any expectation of reward, as demonstrated in Bhagavad Gita 2:47 [2]:

> You have a right to perform your prescribed duties, but you are not entitled to the fruits of your actions. Never consider yourself to be the cause of the results of your activities, nor be attached to inaction.

These Hindu values of compassion, love, and selflessness are ones espoused by Christians, who believe that encountering God's unconditional love compels people to love others selflessly as seen in Philippians 2: 3–8 [3]:

> Do nothing out of selfish ambition or vain conceit. Rather, in humility value others above yourselves, not looking to your own interests but each of you to the interests of the others. In your relationships with one another, have the same mindset as Christ Jesus: Who, being in very nature God, did not consider equality with God something to be used to his own advantage; rather, he made himself nothing by taking the very nature of a servant, being made in human likeness.

Two of the four virtues taught by the Buddha are loving-kindness and compassion. Christians similarly are called to follow Jesus by prioritizing the needs of others and to love others as much as themselves (Matthew 7:12).

Another central virtue emphasized by Buddha is equanimity, understood as an unattached and open-minded mentality that ultimately results in unshakeable calmness and the avoidance of suffering, as detailed in the *Dhammapada* [4]:

> Even as a solid rock
> Does not move on account of the wind,
> So are the wise not shaken
> In the face of blame and praise

Buddhist mindfulness and meditation practices cultivated to achieve equanimity recognize the impermanence and interdependence of all things. By abandoning's one's expectations regarding how things should be, one can achieve a state of *nirvana* consisting of a state of complete stillness and contentment.

Clarity about the nature of reality fostered by mindfulness is not limited to any religious tradition. Christianity has historically incorporated meditative practices that promote equanimity and self-transcendence. For example, desert monastics in the third and fourth centuries committed themselves to prayer, scripture readings, and self-deprivation in order to rid themselves of passions or desires [5]—practices of prayer and meditation upon scripture which continue in contemporary Christian practice. However, while the need for renunciation resembles the Buddhist notion of letting go of desires, a key difference is that Christian detachment from earthly desire is intended to enhance one's desire for God. Saint Augustine famous passage reads, "… yet would man praise Thee; he, but a particle of Thy creation. Thou awakest us to delight in Thy praise; for Thou madest us for Thyself, and our heart is restless, until it repose in Thee" [6].

Many North Americans, including Christians, are drawn to Buddhism's strong emphasis on inner experience. Rather than believing in realities that are unseen, followers are asked to experience its truths for themselves and accept what resonates with them. For instance, the Kalama Sutta [7] states:

> Now, Kalamas, don't go by reports, by legends, by traditions, by scripture, by logical conjecture, by inference, by analogies, by agreement through pondering views, by probability, or by the thought, "This contemplative is our teacher." When you know for yourselves that, "These qualities are skillful; these qualities are blameless; these qualities are praised by the wise; these qualities, when adopted & carried out, lead to welfare & to happiness" — then you should enter & remain in them.

While Christians are similarly encouraged to "test the spirits, to see if they are from God" (1 John 4:1), they also are reminded that they "walk by faith, not by sight" (2 Cor 5:7). By contrast, many Buddhists view the pursuit of God or higher powers as a manifestation of craving, and thus an obstacle in the path to emptiness/selflessness (salvation, or *nirvana*). The freedom offered by Buddhists to achieve salvation through one's own efforts (meditation and the development of the mind) can be appealing to those reluctant to accept accountability to an omnipotent deity.

Another core teaching in Buddhism concerns the middle path, which lies between two extremes as something that exists and does not exist. The middle path neither supports nor rejects the existence of the permanent self. Rather, the middle way is explained through the interdependency between oneself with everything else and even between being and non-being. This non-dualistic approach highlights the interdependency of all things existing in the world as seen in the *Majjhima Nikaya* [8]:

> When this exists, that comes to be
> With the arising of this, that arises;
> When this does not exist, that does not come to be;
> With the cessation of this, that ceases

Buddhist teaching emphasizes that all things in the world depend on each other and that nothing exists by itself. Similarly, Christianity does not see people as isolated beings but rather as parts of a larger whole, as seen in the biblical description of Christians as one body:

> For just as the body is one and has many members, and all the members of the body, though many, are one body, so it is with Christ. For in one Spirit we were all baptized into one body… there may be no division in the body, but that the members may have the same care for one another. If one member

suffers, all suffer together; if one member is honored, all rejoice together. (1 Cor 12: 12–13, 12:25–26)

At the beginning of creation, God created man and women to be mutually dependent. Genesis additionally records that God created mankind in his own image. Therefore, all humans are related to each other and ultimately reflect God's image. Everything in the world was made by and for God:

For by him all things were created, in heaven and on earth, visible and invisible, whether thrones or dominions or rulers or authorities—all things were created through him and for him. (Col 1:16)

Thus, the relational emphasis in Christianity resonates with the interconnectedness in Buddhism.

Tensions and Reservations

Three prominent sources of disagreement between Christians and followers of Eastern traditions involve the meaning of suffering, the class system of Hindu castes, and the nature of yoga.

Consider the differences between Christian and Eastern perspectives on the origin of and answer to suffering. In Hinduism, suffering is the result of *karma* that has been accumulated in one's prior and current life. The cause of suffering is ignorance (or *avidya*), with no doctrine of sin as found in Christian tradition. Therefore, rather than turning to God for a solution to suffering, one must seek to cease the accumulation of *karma* in their succession of lives. Liberation from suffering comes by realizing our true reality as *atman* in Hinduism (similarly *anatta* in Buddhism) [9]. In Christianity, while ignorance can play a role (Jesus referred often to spiritual blindness and asked forgiveness for those who did not know what they were doing), suffering is understood to be the result of original sin and the subsequent brokenness of creation, ultimately addressed by Jesus' suffering for humankind. Suffering due to mental and other illnesses is not attributed to past transgressions or stigmatized as a punishment.

As he passed by, he saw a man blind from birth. And his disciples asked him, "Rabbi, who sinned, this man or his parents, that he was born blind?" Jesus answered, "It was not that this man sinned, or his parents, but that the works of God might be displayed in him." (John 9:1–3)

Buddhists find the cause of suffering in the Four Noble Truths [8]:

And what is the origin of suffering? It is craving, which brings renewal of being, is accompanied by delight and lust, and delights in this and that; that is, craving for sensual pleasures, craving for being, and craving for non-being. This is called the origin of suffering.
And what is the cessation of suffering? It is the remainderless fading away and ceasing, the giving up, relinquishing, letting go, and rejecting of that same craving. This is called the cessation of suffering.

Here again we see that suffering results from cravings, attachments, or emotional investments in things, and the answer is self-cultivated enlightenment, with the renunciation of all desires as the way to set things right. Rather than seeing salvation in detachment, Christians instead invite individuals into a relationship with a God who understands and has taken on their suffering in Jesus and who helps them respond to the suffering of others. Rather than aiming for the elimination of desire as in Buddhism, Christians aim to increase desire for God.

The caste system in several Hindu communities offers another area of disagreement with Christian values. *Manusmriti*, widely acknowledged as one of the key texts in Hinduism, asserts that the caste system is the basis of order and regularity of society. The caste system divides Hindus into four main castes: Brahmins, Kshatriyas, Vaishyas, and Shudras. Believed to have originated from Brahma (Hindu god of creation), Brahmins were teachers and intellectuals (Brahma's head), Kshatriyas were the warriors and rulers (Brahma's arms), Vaisyas were the traders and landowners (Brahma's thighs), and Shudras were the bottom class who did unskilled tasks (Brahma's feet) [10]. Those outside of the Hindu caste system were the Dalits or the untouchables. This caste system (while not in all

Hindu texts) is woven into the social fabric of many Hindu societies. In some orthodox Hindu practices, the Upanishadic path of knowledge was only accessible to the males of the upper three caste groups. It is believed that placement in lower castes was bad *karma* in past lives while higher castes were earned with virtuous behavior. As Brian Smith writes, "the belief in karma and the cycle of rebirth whereby one's social position in this life is ethically determined by moral actions in past lives" [10]. While lower castes are not excluded from salvation, the caste system led to social injustice with the lower castes facing discrimination and oppression. The consequences of the caste systems conflict with Christian ideals of equality and justice for the poor. Christianity asserts that all people are made in the image of God (Gen 1:27) on equal footing and saved by grace rather than by virtuous behavior. One's social standing in life is not reflective of faith or righteousness. Wealth is rather seen as an obstacle for attaining faith: "It is easier for a camel to go through the eye of a needle than for a rich person to enter the kingdom of God" (Mark 10:25). It should be noted that Hinduism contains a diversity of views within its belief system; the religious canons of some Hindu communities do not support the caste system and its values.

As noted above, some Christians are skeptical of yoga due to its religious roots in Hinduism (yoga is also practiced in Buddhism and Jainism). Their concern is that yoga is an act or prayer or worship toward other gods and thus a form of idolatry, based on the biblical prohibition: "You must not worship the Lord your God in their way" (Deut 12:4). Critics note that the Sun Salutations were developed as prayer to the solar deity, Surya, and that many postures are modeled after animals associated with divine beings. By adopting these postures, it is argued that the body becomes more receptive to other spiritual beings. Albert Mohler, president of Southern Baptist Theological Seminary, contends that "the physical is the spiritual in yoga, and the exercises and disciplines of yoga are meant to connect with the divine" [1].

Paths to Compatibility

Both Christians and followers of Eastern faiths urge responding to human suffering with compassion, regardless of one's responsibility for their own suffering. In practice, of course, health care systems in all cultures and inspired by all traditions reflect the inequities of the cultures of which they are a part.

Some Christians have modified yoga to align with Christian values. During their postures, practitioners pray to Jesus or embrace *prāṇāyāma* (breathing techniques for regulating impersonal "vital energy") as breathing in the Holy Spirit [1]. At Wheaton College, Christian modified yoga is taught as a spiritual supplement to Christian disciplines, or "bodily-kinetic prayer," recognizing its Hindu roots but emphasizing that the Hindu gods do not "make it onto my mat" [11]. These efforts to consolidate Christian faith with yoga offer a potential path to compatibility.

While some Christians also have reservations regarding mindfulness practice due to its Buddhist roots, mindfulness like yoga can be adapted to fit a Christian worldview. Divesting these practices of their Buddhist and New Age associations and reframing them in Christian terms [[as ways to "take every thought captive and make it obedient to Christ" (2 Cor 10:5]).] can enhance their acceptability to Christians. When Ford and Garzon [12] compared the experience of a 3-week Christian accommodative mindfulness (CAM) program to a 3-week conventional mindfulness program in a sample of university students and campus staff, they found significantly positive outcomes in the cohort receiving CAM compared to the conventional mindfulness program. Notably, biblical encouragements to meditate (in Hebrew, to ponder, speak, or mutter) led the Desert Fathers to memorize, recite, and sing the scripture [13] —searching for peace in a deeper relationship to God— a contemplative tradition which has recently received more appreciation in the West.

> His delight is in the law of the Lord, and on his law he **meditates** day and night (Ps 1:2; emphasis added)

This Book of the Law shall not depart from your mouth, but you shall **meditate** on it day and night (Josh 1:8; emphasis added)

Let the words of my mouth and the **meditation** of my heart be acceptable in your sight, O Lord, my rock and my redeemer. (Ps 19:14; emphasis added)

Offering meditation (e.g., Buddhist mindfulness or contemplative prayer) based on an individual's own tradition is a constructive way to minimize tension between faiths over differing practices.

Clinical Implications

The commonalities and differences between Christianity and Eastern religions have several implications for patient care. Comparing the theologies which ground their values can help clinicians from different faith traditions to realize that they may have differing preferred virtues which shape the direction of the treatment they provide [14]. For Christians, these might be love and grace; for Buddhists, equanimity and compassion; and for Hindus, appreciation of *Dharma* and *Karma*. Examples of Christian virtues being introduced into Chinese culture can be found in posters distributed in the 1920s and 1930s; many such as "Wheat and Weeds" aimed at moral instruction (Fig. 19.3).

Understanding a tradition's specific challenges and available resources can help clinicians tailor their recommendations. For example, patients burdened by judgmental expectations might benefit from approaches that teach compassion. Those whose religious practice seems arid because it is cognitive may benefit from practices emphasizing lived experience. And those struggling with ruminative anxiety may benefit from learning meditation.

More religious individuals may more easily accept approaches which are rooted in or integrated with the teachings of their own tradition Examples for Buddhists include Mindfulness Based Stress Reduction (MBSR) and dialectical behavior therapy (DBT), for Christians spiritually integrated (Christian) CBT [15], and for Hindus psychotherapy that incorporates the Bhagavad Gita [16]. At the same time, some have expressed concern about the potential risks for narcissistic personalities to engage in Buddhist practice [17] and for overly scrupulous individuals to engage in Catholic rituals [18].

The helpfulness of a given spiritual resource ultimately depends on the patient's relationship to their faith. Is it deeply formative of their identity, superficial, ambivalent, or even hostile? If it is changing, in what way, and why?

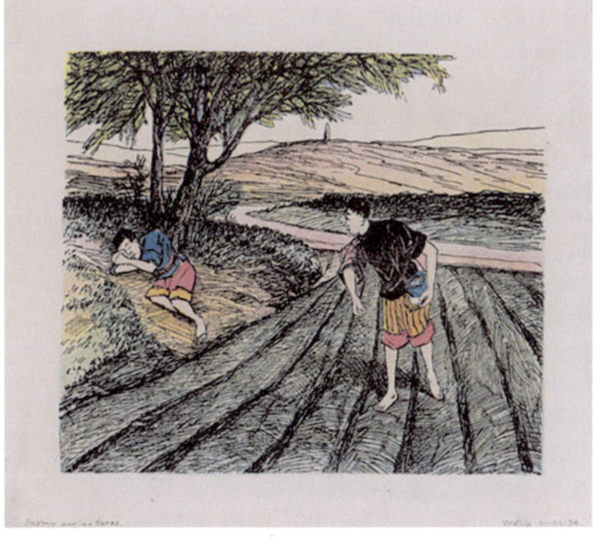

Fig. 19.3 Wheat and weeds

A patient in her 70 s with complex PTSD, estranged from her family, presented feeling hopeless, and that she could no longer believe in "a God who could leave me so damaged". She had graduated late in life from a Christian seminary, but after despairing of God felt drawn to Buddhism, and spent time in a meditation center. While there, she found some relief of anxiety, but was not able to feel embraced by others. She eventually discovered a small church where she felt loved, was able to voice her objections to conservative positions of the pastor when she had them, and to re-engage in a relationship with God.

This patient's therapist was able to help her not by encouraging a particular faith or resource at any given time, but by acknowledging that her spirituality was an important part of her life and healing, helping her explore options and understanding her responses to each of them—in this case, an experience of transformation through love.

A fictional example of an Asian Christian moving toward Buddhism in a crisis is the character Winnie in Lan Samantha Chang's novel *The Family Chou,* [19] who although a longsuffering Christian leaves her husband after learning the extent of his abusiveness, to join a local Buddhist monastery. She finds safety and community there but also continues to participate in Christian traditions, such as the local Chinese Christmas party, at which the Bible is read.

When religious differences contribute to family rifts, clinicians may need to understand the intertwined spiritual and emotional issues involved. These may include the virtues championed by each tradition, resources they contain for finding common ground and reconciliation, spiritual and emotional struggles that may need attention, dynamics of the biological family and the family of faith, and the values and countertransference of the clinician.

Consider a final example of the value of combining Eastern and Christian resources in the service of recovery. Marsha Linehan, the developer of DBT, has described how, as a Catholic who was repeatedly hospitalized for suicidality and self-harm, she was unable to value herself until she suddenly experienced being loved by God [20]. She found this realization to be transformative, but later also incorporated Buddhist ways of cultivating mindfulness and compassion into DBT in order to help others heal.

In conclusion, both Christians and followers of Eastern religions have much to gain from understanding and appreciating what each uniquely and together can contribute to human flourishing.

References

1. Brown C. Debating yoga and mindfulness in public schools: reforming secular education or Reestablishing religion? Chapel Hill: University of North Carolina Press; 2019.
2. Mitchell S, editor and translator. Bhagavad Gita: a new translation. New York: Three Rivers Press; 1988.
3. Bible. English standard version. Wheaton: Crossway Bibles; 2001.
4. Carter JR, Palihawadana M. The Dhammapada: the sayings of the Buddha. New York: Oxford University Press; 2008.
5. Mckay F. Equanimity: the somatization of a moral sentiment from the eighteenth to late twentieth century. J Hist Behav Sci. 2019 Oct;55(4):281–98.
6. Augustine S. The confessions of S. Augustine: revised from a former translation by EB Pusey: with illustrations from S. Augustine himself. London: J.G. and F. Rivington; 1838.
7. Thanissaro B. Kalama Sutta: To the Kalamas. Access to Insight (BCBS Edition). https://www.accessto-insight.org/tipitaka/an/an03/an03.065.than.html. Published 1994. Accessed 9 Apr 2023.
8. Nanamoli B, Bodhi B, editors and translators. The middle length discourses of the Buddha: a new translation of the Majjhima Nikaya. Somerville: Wisdom Publications; 1995.
9. Thatamanil JJ. The immanent divine: god, creation, and the human predicament. Philadelphia: Fortress Press; 2006.
10. Smith BK. Classifying the universe: the ancient Indian Varṇa system and the origins of caste. London: Oxford University Press; 1994.
11. Tennant A. Yes to Yoga. Christianity Today. https://www.christianitytoday.com/ct/2005/mayweb-only/42.0b.html. Published May 19, 2005. Accessed 12 Feb 2023.
12. Ford K, Garzon F. Research note: a randomized investigation of evangelical Christian accommodative mindfulness. Spirit Clin Prac. 2017;4(2):92.
13. Wortley J. How the desert fathers "meditated". Greek Roman Byzantine Stud. 2006;46(3):315–28.
14. Peteet JR. What is the place of clinicians' religious or spiritual commitments in psychotherapy? A virtues based perspective. J Relig Health. 2014;53:1190–8.

15. Pearce MJ, Koenig HG, Robins CJ, Nelson B, Shaw SF, Cohen HJ, King MB. Religiously integrated cognitive behavioral therapy: a new method of treatment for major depression in patients with chronic medical illness. Psychotherapy (Chic). 2015;52(1):56–66.
16. Pandurangi AK, Shenoy S, Keshavan MS. Psychotherapy in the Bhagavad Gita, the Hindu scriptural text. Am J Psychiatry. 2014;171:827–8.
17. Jennings P. East of ego: the intersection of narcissistic personality and Buddhist practice. J Relig Health. 2007;46:3–18.
18. Buchholz JL, Abramowitz JS, Riemann BC, et al. Scrupulosity, religious affiliation and symptom presentation in obsessive compulsive disorder. Behav Cogn Psychother. 2019;47(4):478–92. https://doi.org/10.1017/S1352465818000711.
19. Chang LS. The family Chou. New York: W.W. Norton; 2022.
20. Linehan M. The power of rescuing others. New York Times, June 23, 2011. https://www.nytimes.com/video/health/100000000877082/the-power-of-rescuing-others.html. Accessed 13 Apr 2023.

A Muslim Psychiatrist's Perspective on the Eastern Traditions

Omar Reda and Imam Mamadou Toure

Background

My first direct encounter with someone from the Sikh faith was during a recent visit to Canada. He happened to be my taxi driver.

I was going to start a friendly conversation, hoping to learn something new about him, but my fellow passenger, who happened to also be Muslim, told me that whatever it takes we cannot fall asleep because he had a negative experience with a Sikh who told him and his hijabi wife that killing them was something that was encouraged in his religious beliefs.

I was conflicted, as I did not view the young man driving us as a threat. He was quite polite and courteous. I have to admit that there was an awkward energy in the car though. I wish I had not heard that story from my taxi partner, because fearing someone can provoke strong emotions, and can even feed into prejudice and hate.

Soon after my return from that trip, I came across the book *See No Stranger: A Memoir and Manifesto of Revolutionary Love* by Valarie Kaur, and what a beautiful gift to the soul it was [1]. The book is a powerful source of hope and inspiration as the author invites all of us to make the intentional decision to embrace love even when we are targeted by hate.

I have always been intrigued by diversity and the "Asian culture," and I am deeply grateful for the opportunity to write this chapter about my brothers and sisters who adopt "Eastern" religious, faith, and spiritual ways of life.

I need to make a disclaimer that I am not an expert on Eastern religions by any means. My hope in writing this chapter is to look for common ground through examining the similarities, major differences, and historical relations between Islam and three of the Eastern religions, namely Buddhism, Hinduism, and Sikhism.

Islam literally means submission, that is to totally submit oneself to the will of God, and to be willing to accept the Divine destiny and wisdom even if it is not what one is expecting or hoping for. Islam also means peace. These definitions will come in handy later in the chapter as we reflect on how Muslims view their religion as a comprehensive way of life and how they are called to treat followers of other religions with dignity, justice, and compassion [2].

Researching the topic, I have been enriched and enlightened through the exposure to many religious rituals, faith beliefs, and spiritual practices of Eastern religions. For that, I am deeply humbled and forever grateful.

O. Reda (✉)
Healing Trauma Institute, Fort Collins, CO, USA

I. M. Toure
Portland, OR, USA

Introduction

Rabbi Abraham Joshua Heschel said: "If religion is a heirloom, rather than a living fountain, if religion speaks with the power of authority, rather than with the voice of compassion, its message becomes meaningless [3]." And in their essences, this is the meeting place of all religious systems [4].

The word "religion" comes from the Latin word "RELIGARE" consisting of the prefix RE (which means doing something again, a second time, for example: re-connect, return), and the word "LIGARE" which means to tie, to bind (this is where the word ligament comes from).

So in essence the role of religion is to re-connect, to re-bind:

(a) The human being to the Divine
(b) The human being to the human being (by focusing on what unites and heals, as opposed to what separates and harms)

Every religious system has three components:

(a) Theology: Consists of the body of belief systems of the said religion system, addressing questions such as the nature of the Divine, the concept of afterlife, etc…
(b) Rituals: Ways of worship, of encountering the Divine in a personal and intimate relationship.
(c) Ethics: The moral dimensions of faith, and how the "believer" encounters the world.

Although there are many differences among religions in the areas of theology and rituals, it is the ethical dimension that unites them and this unifying principle has the greatest impact on the day-to-day functioning of society. What is most important with regard to your neighbor? Whom he worships? (Theology). How he worships? (Rituals). And is he one from whom you and your family are safe? (Ethics).

Similarities

1. One thing that Islam has in common with Eastern religions is the emphasis on morality, ethical conduct, and engaging in acts of grace and kindness. Living a virtuous life means that the best way to worship the Creator is to serve the creation, tending to the needs of the voiceless and the forgotten through acts of kindness and community service.
2. The concept of an ultimate reality or high power. Although different religions have different understandings of who or what God is, they all offer a path to connect with the Divine, through engaging rituals like prayer and meditation.
3. Emphasis on self-improvement. All four religions advocate for excellence through refining one's soul and character. It is through working on oneself that one can attain spiritual enlightenment and "liberation."
4. Respect for life. All of these traditions prioritize collective well-being and respect for all forms of life, through encouraging their followers to extend compassion and mercy to all living beings.
5. Importance of community. All four religions emphasize the importance of family, community, and shared values. They advocate for social service, charity, and altruism as means of creating a harmonious and healthy society.

Differences

In terms of differences, Islam is monotheistic, and its central scripture is the Quran, a sacred text believed to be God (Allah)'s exact words revealed to prophet Muhammad (peace be upon him) through the angel Gabriel. Buddhism's central teachings come from the Buddha's insights into human suffering and liberation. Hinduism has a range of deities and texts, although it generally regards the Vedas as its sacred scripture. Sikhism emerged from the syncretic blending of other diverse faith traditions, and its central text is the Guru Granth Sahib.

Despite these differences, the four religions share a commitment to promote peace, show compassion, and offer respect for all beings, and despite challenges, they continue to shape the spiritual lives and values of hundreds of millions of people around the world.

Historical Relations

The reality is that tension does exist between Islam and Eastern religions, and that can be explained by a variety of complex factors, including:

1. Historical conflicts. Islam and Eastern religions have a history of conflict dating back to early Islamic conquests in the Indian subcontinent. That has led to a persistent cultural and religious divide between these communities that continues to exist until today.
2. Differences in worldview. Islam and Eastern religions have different values and belief systems which sometimes have led to tension. For example, Islam places great emphasis on monotheism, while Eastern religions might consider many deities and the belief in reincarnation.
3. Political and social issues. Contemporary political and social conflicts often fuel tensions between Islam and Eastern religions. For example, the ongoing conflict between India and Pakistan has a strong religious aspect, with India being predominantly Hindu and Pakistan being predominantly Muslim.
4. Geopolitical factors. The tension between Islam and Eastern religions is often driven by geopolitical factors such as territorial disputes, demographic competitions, and economic interests. Take, for example, the current situation in Kashmir, and that of the Rohingya Muslims in Burma and the Uyghur Muslims in China.

Violence

There have been numerous incidents of violence between Muslims, Buddhists, Hindus, and Sikhs throughout history. Some of the key incidents are as follows:

1. India-Pakistan Partition. In 1947, the region was partitioned into India and Pakistan, which led to communal riots between Muslims and Hindus, resulting in the death of thousands of people from both sides.
2. Temples and mosques demolition. Multiple incidents of targeting places of worship led to riots between Hindus and Muslims resulting in the death of hundreds of people.
3. Rohingya Crisis. The Rohingya, a Muslim minority in Myanmar, had faced persecution and violence at the hands of the Buddhist majority army forces for decades. Thousands have been killed, and hundreds of thousands have fled Burma to neighboring countries, especially Bangladesh.
4. The current struggle of Uyghur Muslims in China. Millions of Muslims are reported to have being forced into "re-education camps" by the Chinese government.

These incidents highlight the deep-rooted religious tensions that exist in that part of the world and the need for peaceful coexistence between different communities. There is no secret that some of the tension and hostility had followed religious communities to their new homes in North America, Europe, and Australia.

Proposed Solutions

1. Respect for, and celebrating, differences. Each religion should have an open and accepting, not just tolerant, attitude toward "others," and understand that there will be always differences in beliefs, practices, and traditions which should be a reason for all of us to cele-

brate and build bridges, rather than alienate and erect walls. There should be respect for these differences without attempting to impose one's own beliefs on others. Islam, for example, makes it very clear that there is no compulsion in the religion.

2. Dialogue. Interfaith dialogue between leaders and members of different religions can be an effective way to promote understanding and peaceful coexistence. Discussions can be held on shared beliefs, moral values, and cultural practices, and on finding ways to address common social justice issues and challenges.

3. Education. Educating individuals about different religions, when coupled with genuine curiosity and interest, can promote mutual respect and understanding. Schools, places of worship, and community centers can provide opportunities to learn about different religions and cultures through books, documentaries, and guest speakers. I do believe that education is a powerful tool to heal the wounds of ignorance, but strengthening human connections through shared humanity can also bring much needed communal healing.

4. Shared values. Many religions share similar values such as compassion, kindness, and social justice. Promoting these shared values and working together toward common goals can create a sense of unity and cooperation among different religious groups.

5. Healthy communication. In order to work toward peaceful coexistence and respect for different beliefs and practices, it is important to avoid confrontation, prejudice, and discrimination toward each other as that can lead to religious tensions and eventually conflict, hostility, and violence. Active listening, curiosity, empathy, and being genuinely interested in someone else's story can serve as powerful connection tools.

Mental Health

I remember a young patient I met during one of my consultation-liaison assignments. She was diagnosed with an advanced case of eating disorder, was quite ill, and also "difficult to engage" due to "selective mustism." Her parents were devout Sikhs, and through honoring their dedication to their daughter and respecting and celebrating their strong beliefs in a high power and through engaging their spiritual healing rituals and traditions, we were able to make a decent progress toward improving her overall prognosis and quality of life.

I had the pleasure of bearing witness to a Hindu community leader who was regularly consulting with an imam on how to heal his own daughter who was struggling with some sort of psychosis. Despite their diverse belief systems, they united in prayer and sharing a moment of intimate and sacred tenderness in the midst of severe suffering.

As a psychiatrist, I wanted to see what do Eastern religions say about mental health, illness, and wellness. I intend to use what I learned to better connect with clients and coworkers from these faith traditions.

1. In Islam, mental health is considered an important aspect of overall well-being. Quranic and prophetic teachings emphasize the importance of maintaining a sound and balanced state of body and mind. Islamic teachings encourage seeking remedies for mental illness through medical and spiritual means, including seeking professional help, engaging in prayer and meditation, practicing self-care, and participating in healthy social interactions. Healing in Islam is comprehensive, taking the needs of the body, mind, heart, and soul into consideration.

2. Buddhism places a great emphasis on mental health and the need to develop a clear and peaceful mind. Buddhist teachings highlight the importance of maintaining mental and emotional balance, practicing mindfulness, and engaging in spiritual practices such as meditation to cultivate inner peace and self-awareness. Buddhism also teaches that mental illness can be overcome through the practice of insight and wisdom.

3. In Hinduism, mental illness is believed to be caused by an imbalance in the three doshas of

the body (Vata, Pitta, and Kapha). Hindu teachings emphasize the importance of maintaining physical and mental wellness through Ayurvedic practices, including yoga and meditation and also the importance of spiritual healing and seeking guidance from spiritual leaders.

4. In Sikhism, mental health is considered an important aspect of the overall health and well-being. Sikh teachings emphasize the importance of a balanced and disciplined lifestyle, including a healthy diet, regular exercise, and meditation and also the importance of seeking professional help and engaging in healthy social interactions to overcome mental suffering. Sikhism encourages meditation and prayer to promote mental and emotional balance.

Conclusion

Golden rule in these four religious [5] systems:

Islam: None of you is a believer until he loves for all mankind, what he loves for himself (saying of prophet Muhammad peace be upon him)

Buddhism: Whatever is disagreeable to yourself, do not do unto others (Udna-Varga 5.18-6th century BC)

Hinduism: This is the sum of duty: do naught unto others what you would not have them do unto you

Sikhism: I am a stranger to no one, and no one is a stranger to me

As I mentioned at the beginning of the chapter, I am by no means an expert on Eastern religions. I am a student of knowledge and still have too much to learn. I am however keenly committed to do so. It is only through educating oneself, working on unconscious bias and blind spots, and reaching out to "the other" that we finally can open channels of communication, build bridges of trust, and not only coexist and survive, but collaborate and thrive.

References

1. Kaur V. See no stranger: a memoir and manifesto of revolutionary love. New York: One World; 2021. Reprint edition.
2. Asad M, author, translator. The message of the Qur'an. The Book Foundation; 2008.
3. Heschel A. The wisdom of Herschel. New York: Farrar Straus Giroux; 1975.
4. Kripal J, editor. Comparing religions. Hoboken: Wiley-Blackwell; 2014.
5. Neusner J, Hilton B, editors. The golden rule: the ethics of reciprocity in world religions. London: Continuum; 2009.

A Jewish Psychiatrist's Perspective on the Eastern Religions, Spirituality, and Mental Health

H. Steven Moffic

It's a very ancient saying.
But a true and honest thought
That if you become a teacher
By your pupils you'll be taught

As a teacher I've been learning -
You'll forgive me if I boast -
And I've now become an expert
On the subject I like most

Getting to know you!

—Getting to Know You from the musical The King and I

"The King and I" is a very popular musical from 1951 that explores cross cultural relationships. A female British schoolteacher is hired by the King of Siam, now called Thailand, to teach the country's children, as she says and sings in this song. The relationship between the teacher and the King is fraught with conflict, trust, mistrust, and hidden love. The ending has the teacher comforting the King as he is dying and grudgingly westernizing some of his policies. If this sounds somewhat cliched, out-of-date, and even inappropriate, remember that it originated over 70 years ago.

Though the musical is a plea for tolerance, occasionally some critics convey that there is a cute sort of condescension toward the exotic "east" by playwrights from the "West." The Thailand we visited about a decade ago was, of course, much different and westernized, with downtown traffic in Bangkok worse than major cities in the United States.

The musical was based on the 1944 novel by Margaret Landon [1], which in turn was based on the memoirs of a Christian governess and King in the early 1860s. Mongkut, who was King of Siam in 1861, founded a new order of Buddhism and lived half his life as a Buddhist monk.

My wife loved and participated in musical theater, so I saw this play many years back and, with some embarrassment can say that it was my main source of information about the "Eastern" faiths for some time. Perhaps such limited and even erroneous insight is common. Even so, many years later, the relational challenges in the play seemed to presage those that I later experienced in teaching cultural and spiritual aspects of psychiatry to residents in training as well as in establishing a clinician patient alliance with patients of much different backgrounds than myself.

Personal Exposure to Eastern Religions and Spirituality

Once upon a time, after a few years of living in a changing area, I grew up in an all Jewish twelve block area of Chicago. My family joined a

H. S. Moffic (✉)
Private Pro Bono Community Psychiatrist, Milwaukee, WI, USA

Conservative Synagogue, that being the denomination between the more liberal Reform movement and the more historical and traditional Orthodox denominations. However, it is important to know that, by now, it is recognized that Judaism can be described as a community of people, or a spiritual perspective, in addition to or instead of a religion that was characterized by an ethical covenant with a monotheistic God. Humanistic Judaism is an example of secular Judaism. As an adolescent, it meant so little to me that I was kicked out of Sunday school for a time for my behavior. I did manage to get a Bar Mitzvah, though I don't recall my speech at all.

While in high school, I read Freud's Interpretation of Dreams and also became familiar with his secular Jewish identification. When I got married in 1968, my wife was from a Reform background and that is what we followed. Its liberal nature suited me much better and after some years, our synagogue even had a seminar on psychotherapy and religion, for which I spoke.

Much later, about a decade ago, the Rabbi of my new synagogue gave me a new Jewish name, neither of us recalling what mine had previously been. He gave me the name Hillel, which couldn't have been more moving to me, given the contributions of Hillel the Elder centuries ago, including this saying:

If I am not for myself, who will be?
If I am only for myself, what am I?
If not now, when?

My exposure to people of other faiths and cultures was minimal, at least until high school, where I met students of the Christian faith. But students of Eastern faiths? I don't think so. I don't think I even knew that word or what it meant, or even what its controversial predecessor "Orientals" was back then. But as part of late adolescent discussion with friends about life and its meanings, I did have a brief fascination with Alan Watts, who was coming out of the West, and his writings about Zen Buddhism, especially his classic 1957 introductory book The Way of Zen [2]. The primary goal of Buddhist and Zen enlightenment seemed to be the reduction of suffering and the freedom to enjoy life as it is. Perhaps I didn't understand the depths of the book or hadn't yet suffered enough.

In the 1960s, I also read about the Jewish psychologist Richard Alpert who, along with Timothy Leary at Harvard, experimented with psychedelics, something I never did. After being dismissed from Harvard, to continue his psychedelic revelations, he traveled to the east for more spiritual enlightenment and methods to relieve suffering, being disappointed with the Judaism of his childhood. In the Himalayas, he met Bhagavan Das, the yogi who gave him a new name of Ram Dass, meaning "Servant of God." He added knowledge of Zen Buddhism, Hindu mysticism, Christ consciousness, various forms of yoga, and other traditions and became a teacher and guru himself, writing a best seller book of his ideas [3]. Later, in the 1980s, he came back to Jewish mysticism and connected that both to his new spirituality and to the Judaism of his youth. Many other Jews had the same experience of rediscovering their Jewish identity in travels to Buddhist India [4]. My own reconnection to Judaism occurred later and in a different way.

Currently, my childhood neighborhood and its stores are mainly composed of people of the Eastern faiths. They are mostly Hindus, often coming from India, along with some Muslims coming from India and Pakistan. Along with some from Russian immigrants, going down Devon Avenue seems a little like visiting a foreign country.

A few years back, my lifelong best friend visited Chicago and we decided to stop in our old neighborhood to see his old house. I had passed mine off and on once we moved to Milwaukee over 30 years ago, but never went inside. In an article, he wrote for a series I curated for Psychiatric Times on Earth & Psychiatry, he wrote about it [5].

Barry nostalgically described how he—and sometimes I with him—played in his background Eden that he called "The Woods." One day sometime later, his father gently gave him the fearful news:

They are going to cut down your trees, Barry. I am so sorry.

It happened. As the Joni Mitchell song went, they paved paradise with a parking lot.

His father had a plan, though. He found a spot behind their house to plant another, a small one at the edge of the woods. Barry planted it and it grew to have a canopy of leaves where we could look up at the stars.

Some 60 years later, we actually returned, bravely ringing the front doorbell to get permission to go into the backyard. Had the tree survived? The owners turned out to be from India, with the Hindu artifacts I had come to know in the rooms we passed through.

What we saw in coming out into the backyard was all tree, the sturdy oak that had been planted there. We sat under it for a while.

The elder woman of the house came forward to speak giggling as if a bit embarrassed:

> You know, that tree is sacred to our family. Our young boy sits under it all the time. He insists that it is his tree.

By this time, I had become a climate activist and even visited India about 10 years prior. While there I learned more about the Hindu religion and its depictions in artworks. I also learned of the cycles of life and our guide said that the Hindu thought was that we were in an age of destruction in the eternal cycles of creation and destruction. Was she right, I wondered, and still do: can't we do anything about it?

Barry and I always talked about the serendipity in our lives that two unconnected things happened around the same time and seemed to have great meaning. At the same time, I recently googled up his article on Google, I saw another article titled "Our Trees of Life" by Lalitha Sridhar, about the uprooted trees in Chennai, India from Cyclone Vardah in 2016. Of course, I had to read it. Those who lived there suddenly realized how much the trees had meant. Someone concluded:

> Saving trees and planting more is, naturally, the best way to replace regret with recompense.

Recompense? Recompense can mean to make compensation for something lost. In a way, I am trying to do that with this chapter and my best friend, as our cycle of creation recently ended with his unexpected death.

Barry and Buddhism

One of the reasons that I was interested in editing this volume was because of the one area where Barry and I seemed to have had a difference. That was Buddhism or, really Buddhism and Judaism. I was hoping that not only would Barry illustrate this book with his original images, as he had done in our prior three volumes on religions and psychiatry, but that he would write a chapter on his own Eastern spiritual journey.

His sudden death ended that, but continued our discussion, at least on my side. Usually living far away from each other, we still had discussed our potential deaths off and on, and more in recent years. However, I didn't know what he preferred as far as burial. It turned out that he was to be cremated. That isn't a typical Jewish custom, which prefers the sacred body to be buried in a coffin, but it is a common Buddhist practice. Buddha himself was cremated. The Buddhist belief is that death leads to rebirth, in reincarnation when a person's spirit seeds a new body and life. In Judaism, there is less certainty about after death, but some sense one's soul will continue and perhaps join others.

Even if his after death was more Buddhist, there was no doubt that Barry always felt Jewish, even if he didn't regularly participate in organized Jewish activities. He wrote a chapter in our edited book *Anti-Semitism and Psychiatry* [6]. There was quite a bit of focus in its content and images on his Anti-Semitism fears. Interestingly enough, Buddhism wasn't mentioned. I can't recall if that was my editorial decision or his to leave that out.

What I remember of his journey is that when he lived with his wife for a few years in Colorado Springs many years ago, he attended the Naropa Institute in Boulder and felt a spiritual connection. We often discussed his teacher and he eventually took "refuge" in Buddhism, which didn't mean he gave up Judaism. This combination of being Jewish and Buddhist, though it almost always came with Jews also becoming Buddhist rather than the other way around, came to have many designations: JuBu, Jewbu, Jewboo, Buddhist Jew, or even Jewish Buddhist, depending on which was the adjective and which the noun. In later years, his teacher ran into some cultish trouble and Barry's interest seemed to wane, at least in our discussions.

Professionally, he was trained as a psychiatric social worker and specialized in setting up artistic creative communities for troubled children. Of course, his patients, like mine, seemed to have suffering as a major component of their psychiatric problems. And it was in suffering that we had the most difference of opinion.

Barry presented his interpretation that Buddhism knew that suffering was a necessary occurrence in life and acceptance of that was best. In Western literature, perhaps that was illustrated most strikingly in the well-known play by Samuel Beckett, Waiting for Godot. Yes, the two tramps are waiting, but as they wait they undergo hunger, homelessness, and unrelenting pain. They are locked into a world of seemingly arbitrary suffering, for which no explanation is provided. However, since Beckett was always reluctant to explain his intentions, it leaves the interpretation of whether the suffering should be accepted up to the listener.

I, from my Jewish perspective, felt that our people had suffered much too much over thousands of years, including in comparison to other cultural and religious groups, and that the suffering was caused by the Anti-Semitism of others and not an absolute necessity to happen. How could we accept as a necessary part of life the suffering of the Holocaust as the most recent example, for instance?

The Story of Job

Perhaps, I thought, we could come to a consensus in this book project as we crept closer to our own inevitable deaths. Without that opportunity, as it turned out, was there any way for me to resolve our differences, at least in my mind? Eventually, as our proposal was accepted not long after Barry died, I thought maybe so.

First the story of Job, one of the oldest books in the Jewish bible, comes to mind. Actually, it only comes to mind because my son Evan

became a Rabbi and that led to my interest in learning more about Judaism, its history, and its connection to psychiatry. Job suffered horrible losses even though it seemed like he lived a basically righteous life. He loses family, wealth, and health for no apparent reason. At first, Job seems to accept the tragedies in a Buddhist sort of way:

> The Lord gives and the Lord takes away. Blessed is the name of the Lord. (Job 1:21)

Then, in the following more poetic section of the story, he rails against the suffering and challenges God to explain why:

> God has wronged me. He has besieged me. I cry out, but get no response. I shout out, but can get no justice. (Job 19:6–7).

His friends argue that he must have done something to bring on the tragedies. God then resolves the story. He conveys that Job's suffering was unfair and his protests appropriate, but that the cosmic reasons may not be understandable by mankind. Then the book ends with Job's family, health, and wealth restored by God. As such, the book doesn't clarify why bad things happen to good people, but encourages the reader to try to trust God's wisdom and hidden reasons. So, it seems to me the story of Job both maintains the necessity of bearing suffering, but also protesting against it, with the hope that God will intervene eventually for reasons we may not know.

In our time, Rabbi Kushner has become well-known for his books that try to consider "why bad things happened to a good person" [7]. He concludes that God is moral, but nature is not, and that we can find God in our resilience and ability to find meaning in life regardless of circumstances. That seems to affirm the place of compassion and caring in the role of clinical psychiatry to relieve suffering, does it not?

In a way, Rabbi Kushner's conclusions are not unlike that which the Jewish psychiatrist Viktor Frankl drew from being a concentration camp survivor in World War II [8]. He discovered that finding meaning even in such a traumatic situation was valuable. It led after the war to a school of psychotherapy called logotherapy.

The Stories of Mark Epstein, MD

But is there a fellow contemporary psychiatrist who might teach me a lesson from my professional standpoint? Is there available a conceit of a substitute psychiatrist that I could use for some resolution following Barry? I might have been primed for that as a psychiatrist brother-in-law of my wife had become interested in Buddhist meditation practice many years back and felt that it helped him psychologically, though I had no interest myself. Now, as I thought about Buddhism as one of the foci for Eastern traditions, I came to learn more about the popular author on Buddhism and psychiatry, the psychiatrist Mark Epstein.

You may know that the last name Epstein is usually a Jewish one, but that can also be misleading at times. The limited comments I could find about his early religious background suggested that his father was of the Orthodox Jewish faith [9]. Dr. Epstein himself clearly had come to Buddhism not as a child, but as a developing adult.

Without successfully contacting Dr. Epstein, I began to examine his published psychiatric and spiritual background as best I could. First came an article in the Chicago Tribune in 1998 [10]. He apparently became interested in Buddhism as an undergraduate at Harvard, feeling it was both psychological and spiritual, but not about a God. His age at the time predated the age when Barry became interested in Buddhism.

Then, when he was 21, Epstein studied meditation at the Naropa Institute in Boulder, Colorado. Check! Barry, some years older, did the same.

Epstein went back to Harvard for medical school and trained to become a psychiatrist, whereas Barry became a psychiatric social worker.

Early in his psychiatric career, Dr. Epstein was interested in Freudian theory, but felt that it fell short in changing behavior, as Freud himself came to conclude. He found that training in meditation allowed freedom from habits and therefore an increased ability to change behavior. A

fusion seemed to exist in Insight Meditation (Vipassana), a kind of universalized and sanitized Buddhism in America.

Over 40 years later, after many other books, in his last book, Zen and Therapy [11], in a certain kind of introspection, Dr. Epstein wondered how his Buddhist perspective made a difference in therapy sessions, perhaps by providing an alternative perspective beyond traditional psychoanalysis.

Actually, he also realized that a Freudian therapist seemed Buddhist in the attention given, as in "give impartial attention to everything you observe" or an "analytic attitude" of "evenly suspended attention."

That is how I was trained, too, about 50 years back.

Dr. Epstein's current conclusion is that the therapeutic relationship can become a kind of spiritual friendship. He says:

> Therapy is not something that psychiatry does with a patient, nor is it solely a place to complain about the indignities that one has suffered; it is a space in which a person can listen to their own voice.

In one of the clinical vignettes, Dr. Epstein wanted his patient to be willing to suffer in the sense of being able to hold her uncomfortable feelings. The Buddha's first noble truth is that there is always something uncomfortable for any of us, and that there cannot be any full escape from that. That acceptance is not unlike Freudian psychodynamic understanding that the suffering can be processed helpfully, but never go away completely, as in the saying of the psychiatrist Frieda Fromm-Reichman to a patient: "I never promised you a rose garden" [12].

Now the traditional Judaic belief in regard to suffering is that there is a faith in God's ultimate goodness and that a messianic age is to come. The Buddhist response is to mentally detach from the suffering, meditation being one of the means to doing so. Judaism, too, has meditative practices, though they are much less well known. I've never used any meditation practice, Jewish or Eastern, but it seems that my listening to jazz music serves some similar calming and centering purpose for me. Jazz meditation?

Where does this portrait of Dr. Epstein leave Barry and me in terms of suffering then? Closer than I thought. Certainly I am suffering as I grieve his dying. I am not in a hurry to detach myself from that, but expect that to happen over time in the grieving process. Then, I will be left with whatever introjected memories and experiences I will like to recall.

My Professional Career in Cultural Psychiatry

I'm quite sure I will learn more about the Eastern traditions as this book develops and I review the other chapters. Though my prior exposure was limited, there was other learning and curiosity along the way beside my personal relationship with Barry. This other exposure came more through my professional career than personal relationships.

There is a Jewish value called Tikkun Olam. It essentially means to try to heal the world. As I was thinking about what I wanted to focus on in my psychiatric career, Tikkun Olam was a guiding focus.

Back in 1970, and still to an extent, it was clear that certain cultural groups were underserved in psychiatry. These were cultural or ethnic groups such as Black Americans, Hispanic Americans, Native Americans, and perhaps Asian Americans. Jewish Americans were not among them; in fact, we used psychiatric treatment extensively. Perhaps that reflected the fact that Jews were over-represented in the founding of modern psychiatry, starting with Freud. Before modern psychiatry, Rabbis often counseled congregants about their personal lives. With the Mexican Americans common in Houston, it could be curanderos as folk healers.

As a consequence of my interest in minority groups, early in my career at Baylor College of Medicine I was asked to put together the new seminar series for residents on Community & Social Psychiatry. Clearly, cultural aspects of psychiatry had to be part of that. How did different cultural groups view psychiatry, from psychotherapy to the use of medication? What about some specific "Eastern" therapeutic techniques that were becoming more popular in America, especially various forms of meditation?

Eventually, that beginning led to a Black psychiatry resident and I teaming up to lead a seminar series specifically focused on the cultural aspects of psychiatry. There we started with describing our own cultural identities and how that might be relevant to psychiatry. Fortunately, there was an increasing variety of residents with diverse cultural backgrounds, sort of a reflection of the growing international diversity of Houston. That led to the first national model of psychiatric education on cultural psychiatry [13].

Off and on, our religious backgrounds were discussed. Over time, the questions arose whether that was being ignored more than it should be, whether religion was part of culture, or whether religion should have its own series. Freud had put a damper on studying religion, deeming it an opium for the masses or a neurotic obsession, but religion could positively provide community and meaning to one's life.

Nevertheless, Christianity, Judaism, and Islam continued to be part of these cultural explorations. When some residents came who had grown up in Asian countries and mentioned their Hindu, Buddhist, and other Eastern traditions, those also got explored. Nationally, as Freudian influence died down and biological aspects increased, in psychiatry more psychiatrists became interested in religion and spirituality.

The same principle of exploring and knowing oneself culturally and religiously could be applied with humility to understanding patients of different faith backgrounds. However, it is crucial to use general knowledge about Eastern religions and faith as a potentially relevant backdrop to the care of an individual patient. Clinicians, let alone the general public, take a risk by assuming that someone is of a given religion given appearance, name, or background. Moreover, as my colleague and chapter writer Vincenzo Di Nicola reminded me, don't assume if you know their religion or ethnicity that you really know anything about them. Each patient is an individual and requires personal exploration of whatever faith is held.

The professional organization that seemed to fit these interests seemed to be the Society for the

Study of Psychiatry and Culture, but it turned out to have its own bias at the time. It was mainly devoted to research of cultures outside of the United States, and religion was relatively ignored. Leadership was mainly Western and white. However, many years later the foci have broadened and there is much leadership by Asian Canadians and Americans.

Given my national work with cultural aspects of psychiatry, I often became the Jewish representative in interfaith projects and presentations. That included annual meetings of the Americana Psychiatric Association seminars of interfaith panels on forgiveness, death and dying, and discrimination within psychiatry.

Eventually, after a similar interfaith panel on Islamophobia, that led me to being asked by an acquisitions editor at Springer in 2017 to be a lead editor for a volume on Islamophobia and Psychiatry. Immediately, that evoked the question of whether it takes one to know one in a cultural or religious sense. This question had long been explored in cultural psychiatry. Potential problems could come both from a culturally similar or different ethnic and religious background of patient and clinician. Differences could lead to ignorance about values, where similarity could cause misleading mutual assumptions.

By this time, there were many more psychiatrists of various cultural and religious backgrounds. Therefore, it was no surprise when a prominent Muslim psychiatrist said that I had no right to lead such a project, and that it had to come from a Muslim because this was about their belief system and personal lived experiences. I actually didn't disagree and asked if that psychiatrist or other Muslim psychiatrists wanted to take over, but none did, and we decided to try to work together and learn from each other. That worked.

Some of the same challenge came up as this project emerged with the question of whether a Western imperialistic attitude might be pervading some of the plans. I certainly did not feel knowledgeable enough about Eastern religions or spirituality. I never even meditated, one of their major contributions to American life and mental wellbeing. But I was curious, respectful, and hopefully humble enough to again offer up the lead editorship up. Once again, a compromise developed to make this as much of an interfaith project as possible, but also to rely on psychiatrists from each given Eastern tradition to take responsibility for accuracy of information and inclusivity.

What I had learned in our second volume on Anti-Semitism and Psychiatry was also crucial to my interest in this project. As in a chapter on the relationship of Hinduism and Judaism was being written, the authors claimed that there had never been any Anti-Semitism in Hindu India. Some other psychiatrists doubted this could be true, so I joined these as a co-author to examine that myself. I couldn't find out any historical information to dispute their claims. Though the number of Jews in India historically were relatively small, it was not insignificant, and Anti-Semitism indeed did not seem to exist. Currently, there is a very small number of Jews remaining in India since the state of Israel emerged.

Other colleagues wondered about the other Asian countries like China and Japan. Historically, they had even fewer Jews living there, but the information was not as clear. Anti-Semitism could exist even if Jews were not present, given whatever information was available, accurate or not.

And so, we and I are left with this idea of East and West and their separate histories of religious and spiritual developments. East and West are just cultural and psychological reflections, because there really is no east or west geographically in an earth that is round and rotating. We in the United States could just as easily be designated as being east from India, could we not?

What is indisputable historically, though, is that religious and spiritual developments developed mainly separately in the east and west thousands of years ago, but with global travel, immigration, and communication, much has become intertwined. It seems that the flow from Judaism to Christianity to Islam involved much competition, perhaps in an Oedipal sense writ large, as Hinduism, Buddhism, and others could have experienced in the east. However, that could leave the east and west religious and spiritual traditions to be more complementary than competitive, leaving me wondering with whether we have a unique opportunity to understand what we have common from a faith perspective, but also what we can learn from our differences. This consideration is not to ignore those who are atheist or agnostic, or come from more isolated native spiritual beliefs, as once again there are similarities and differences. Perhaps, too, this aspect of globalization is leading to less involvement in formal religious practices and more individuality and spirituality.

Other Sources of Eastern Knowledge

Intermittent exposure to other faith traditions followed through teaching cultural psychiatry, colleagues, editing, writing, art, and travel.

I viewed Eastern religious and spiritual art on trips to other countries as well as museums in the United States. The Rubin Museum in New York is a favorite and recently had an exhibit on healing practices, with an accompanying publication. The magazine will continue to be available after the exhibit ends and includes such personal practical applications as a sound practice, plant ritual, writing prompt, and receipt to potentially try [14].

Travel, whether for personal or professional reasons, provides real-life exposure to other lands and ways of living. That was true in visiting China when the World's Fair Expo was being held in Shanghai in 2010. The potential power of religion was indicated by its official banning in China. While there, the East and West seemed to connect in an unexpected visual way. Confucian thinking was still popular and so was Colonel Sanders chicken from the United States. Take a look at a picture of the Colonel and Confucius and see how similar they looked. Despite the relative banning of religion, we quietly heard some about Taoism, too, a Chinese philosophy or religion, depending on your definition, but which we were told advocates the way for living in harmony with humility and piety.

Travel to India also helped me to learn about Hinduism. It strikes me so far that although Hinduism has a top deity or life force, Brahman, all of the Eastern faiths are much less centralized and open to wide interpretations. Hinduism has countless small g personal gods and goddesses. In India, we heard some about Sikhism, a relatively new major monotheistic religion and philosophy, with the goal to become one with God by reverence, hard work, service, and sharing. It originated in the Punjab region of India, with many converts from Hinduism and Islam. It became better known in the United States from a mass murder in my hometown of Milwaukee. Also in India, I was fascinated by the reverence for all life that seemed to be the essence of Jainism.

Much closer, in our prior home of Houston, the husband of a neighbor was a Zoroastrian from India. He reported that his belief was within the framework of a monotheistic ontology, promising an ultimate triumph of good over evil.

Moreover, with the development of various meditative techniques, these traditions have contributed much to mental well-being in a different way than Judaism. In particular, I have been buoyed that Hinduism has not displayed Anti-Semitism, meaning that this is not inevitable. Even so, some of these traditions have been involved in deadly conflicts, including between Hindus and Muslims in India, as well as Buddhists and Muslims in Myanmar.

Conclusions

Over time, there was no wavering from my family and ancestral Jewish background, although a bit like Ram Dass experienced, the intensity of my commitment and involvement varied. I've thought the most important aspects were the more liberal Judaism commitment to social justice, the ability to overcome great trauma over time, and the ethical monotheism.

Perhaps due to the diaspora of the Jewish people over so much of the world, with its current large representation in the United States, Judaism is thought to be a Western religion. But it really is a Middle Eastern religion. Its home has always been in Israel, whether in mind or reality. That is true of all the so-called Western religions, coming out of the same area in the Middle East, all being monotheistic in addition. Unfortunately, or consequently, there has been much conflict among these religions.

Certainly, too, there remains a challenge and controversy as to who should speak for the "West," generally speaking Euro-Americans, and "East," generally referring to Asians, both having presence in the "North" and "South," too. These are conceptual, not geographic, concepts. Perhaps it was inappropriate to assume what I was learning from my friend Barry, as well as the substitute conceit of psychiatrist Mark Epstein, was adequate, given that they are both from the "West." Then, there is the "South," Africa and South America, let alone all the indigenous spiritual belief systems around the world.

My exposure and knowledge of the so-called Eastern religions and spirituality have been slow and more sporadic. My lifelong best friend embraced Buddhism to complement his Judaism, so that enabled me to learn about it through our relationship, as specific and limited as that was. That personal relationship was supplemented by reading about other Jews who had immersed themselves in Eastern religions and spirituality, most especially certain sects of Buddhism, like the psychiatrist Mark Epstein, the poet Rodger Kamenetz, and the psychologist who became Ram Dass. Though data is limited, by the turn of the new millennium at least 5% of American Jewry had seemingly embraced Buddhism, and that about 15% of American Buddhists were Jewish. While I was surprised and pleased to not find Anti-Semitism in Hinduism, it can be found in Buddhist teachings.

With a globally connected world, it seems that countries, leaders, and belief systems need both a solid base, but also humility, curiosity, and the embrace of aspects of other traditions. Combined with atheists and doubters, all faith traditions in their own ways can potentially supplement one another in order to produce a more unified and safe world for the future.

If any generality holds true for reducing prejudice, it is what is conveyed in the song "Getting to Know You." Getting to know someone who is different generally reduces prejudice not only toward that person, but everyone in that cultural group. However, it can't be just a one way street in any direction in getting to know the other, nor an a priori expectation of change in one direction, especially likely for the one in power.

Assumptions about cultural and religious beliefs need checking out, including for this reflection. Though general knowledge can help, understanding has to be a quest with every individual patient or stranger. Faith, or its lack thereof, matters, and a religious and spiritual history is indicated for any patient. Paradoxically, suffering needs to be both accepted and rejected, which is where clinical psychiatry comes into place. Religion, spirituality, and psychiatry in all their manifestations can be connected and contribute wisdom and well-being.

The gift of knowing the Eastern other is built into the idea and process of this book, as well as in psychiatry in general, but is only available if you look for it with a curious mind.

References

1. Landon M. Anna and the king of Siam. Harper Perennial; London. New York, NY. 1999.
2. Watts A. The way of Zen. Vintage; Watts. Visalia, CA. 1999.
3. Dass R. Be here now. Harmony; Dass. Easton, PA. 1978.
4. Kamenetz R. The Jew in the lotus. HarperOne; Kamenetz. San Francisco, CA. 1994.
5. Marcus B. Our trees of life. Psychiatric Times, posted April 16, 2021.
6. Marcus B. An artistic view of anti-Semitism. In: Moffic HS, et al., editors. Anti-Semitism and psychiatry: recognition, prevention, and interventions. Springer; 2020.
7. Kushner H. The book of job: when bad things happened to a good person. Schocken; Kushner. New York, NY. 2012.
8. Frankl V. Man's search for meaning. Beacon's Press; 2006.
9. Kisel B, Kisel M. A Jubu-ish journey toward transcendence. The Dayton Jewish Observer, posted October 24, 2019.
10. Lauerman C. 'Buddhist psychiatrist' brings spirituality and psychotherapy into closer harmony. Chicago Tribune, August 6, 1998.
11. Epstein M. The Zen of therapy. Penguin Press; Epstein. Penguin Press, London, United Kingdom. 2022.
12. Greenberg J. I never promised you a rose garden. Penguin Classics; Greenberg. Penguin Classics, London, United Kingdom. 2022.
13. Moffic HS, Kendrick EA, Lomax JW, Reid K. Education in cultural psychiatry in the United States. Transcult Psychiatr Res Rev. 1987;24(3):167–87.
14. Rubin Museum. Spiral: "healing practices". Rubin Museum, Spring; 2022.

How Did a Nice Jewish Girl Like You Get So Interested in Asia?

Sharon Packer

Introduction

The origins of my intrigue with Asia can be summed up in three words: Chicago Art Institute. Then one thing led to another. But before I elaborate on this link, let me tell you a bit about my own background.

I was born, reared, and educated in Chicago (until starting psychiatry residency in New York and subsequently permanently relocating to New York). In Chicago, I attended the Chicago Jewish Academy and later studied at the Women's Division of Hebrew Theological College (aka Skokie Yeshiva). I earned certification in Orthodox Jewish Education—via the Jerusalem Exam, under the auspices of Hebrew University. I did not have the slightest interest in teaching Hebrew—I planned to be a physician/psychiatrist from a young age—but I was always interested in Judaism and especially in Jewish history, so preparing for this exam was not unpleasant. Plus, it was the highest religious degree available to women in that pre-feminist era.

When I grew up on the North Side of Chicago, near Devon Avenue, and near to Skokie, Chicago was said to be the second most segregated city in the world, second only to Johannesburg, in South Africa. What an ignominious association!

According to rumor, two Chinese families who owned local restaurants lived in what was otherwise an all-Jewish neighborhood that supported only two sit-down kosher restaurants, also on Devon Avenue. The restaurant culture that we enjoy today, especially in New York, had not yet blossomed in the Midwest, and budgets for eating outside the home were much more modest. Even if kosher restaurants were in short supply, there was no dearth of synagogues in this specific section of Chicago, for a different synagogue sprung up on each city block. Plus, several kosher butchers were nearby, as well as a Sabbath-observing kosher bakery, which, unfortunately, employed me on Sunday mornings when I was in high school. My shift started at the ungodly hour of 5 AM, but it prepared me for the standard 5 AM start time of surgery rotations in medical school.

Decades later, when I returned to Chicago to attend our 25th medical school reunion, a former medical school classmate drove us around to our "old haunts." He editorialized throughout the trip, as if he were a seasoned tour guide rather than an experienced M.D. I learned that Devon Avenue's once-omnipresent kosher butchers had been replaced by South Indian vegetarian eateries. The older Jewish population had migrated away, mostly to warmer climes, while persons of South Asian ancestry took their place. Many newer arrivals had come to Chicago for medical residencies. While still in med school, two resi-

S. Packer (✉)
Icahn School of Medicine at Mount Sinai,
New York, NY, USA

dents were kind enough to escort my classmate Joel and me to an early iteration of those Indian restaurants. They patiently explained each dish on the menu and added enough extra intriguing info about India that both Joel and I eventually (separately) made several trips to India and visited every Indian state.

I cringed when I saw those restaurants and realized how much airfare and jet lag I could have saved myself, had this cuisine been available while I still lived in Chicago but after I acquired an unremitting affection for spicy Indian food (rather than the Chinese food that Jews are said to enjoy). Yet I surely never regretted visiting India so many times interim.

From Chicago's Art Institute to Its Little India (and Actual India in Asia)

So how did we go from the Chicago Art Institute to Chicago's version of Little India, with its expanding selection of South Indian vegetarian restaurants? Let me explain.

The Chicago Art Institute boasted the world's second largest collection of Chinese art, surpassed only by the museum in Taiwan. That is not bad for the "second city," as it was known, even though Chicago did not acquire its old time nickname for that reason alone. But there is more to explain why Chinese art appealed to me so strongly.

For someone from as Jewish a background as mine, a "neutral" East Asian aesthetic was a welcome respite from the Christian iconography depicted in so many of Europe's greatest masterpieces. Eventually, Christian themes fell out of favor in Western art, but until then, so much art revolved around imagery that was either forbidden to Jews or that evoked painful recollections of religious persecutions, forced conversions or mass murders, some of them orchestrated by the Church or condoned by Church officials. Greco-Roman "pagan" art was a different matter, one which deserves discussion in an art history forum, rather than in a study of Asian spirituality. Suffice it to say that Greco-Roman or even Egyptian art

never moved me the same way as Asian art, although the mummy cases intrigued me as a child, in much the same way that the dinosaurs on display at the Field Museum "spoke" to me and most other children.

Thankfully, Asian art was free of troubling historical associations and could be enjoyed by someone like me, guiltlessly. Although some Chinese art revolves around religious icons such as the Buddha, the Bodhisattvas, Prince Shakyamuni, or any of the other 200-plus deities of Buddhism, the stylized geometrical designs of early Asian metalwork or stoneware were far removed from Western religion. Botanical imagery from later dynasties was similarly free from sad associations evoked by European art, as were the Tang dynasty porcelain horses, or any of the many funerary figures excavated from burial grounds, only to be displayed at the museum. And even if images of Buddhas appeared in such art, those images were thankfully not tainted by association with persecution. I should add, these museum visits took place long before Americans and Europeans became self-conscious about trespassing on sacred sites or exporting their totems—which we called "art and artifact"— before requesting appropriate permission.

When a college professor insisted that we study Chinese philosophy as well as art history, to better understand the significance of the imagery from this very ancient culture, I could not have agreed more. I also came from a very ancient culture that informs my daily life and so I recognized that even seemingly secular surface ornamentation can carry more connotations than meet the eye. So, I dutifully studied the basics of Confucianism, Taoism, and the many manifestations of Buddhism that evolved in varying countries. I memorized differences between Hinayana; Mahayana; Vajrayana; and Zen and learned where each variant evolved.

Tibetan art, with its kaleidoscopic mandala imagery, and towering demonic figures, was still a step-child of Chinese civilization, and did not appear in this collection. It deserved a separate study and appeared in different collections located as far away as Switzerland, Staten Island, and even Newark, New Jersey. Still, Tibetan art appealed to me on a very different level, enough to merit a trek to India's northernmost "Little Tibet" or Ladakh, at a time when the Chinese government forbade tourism in Tibet itself, which it had annexed.

Some decades later, after 9/11, many young Chinese-Americans sought psychiatric treatment with me, in my downtown New York City office. Most hoped to relieve the distress they experienced from witnessing the fall of the Twin Towers, which were visible from their families Chinatown apartments. Some had sat outside on their balconies, or simply peered through windows, watching trapped workers jump from burning buildings while they themselves were breathing in ash that floated through the atmosphere. They could not push those images out of their minds, no matter how hard they tried. The flashbacks were often so intense that they decided to try psychiatric care, even though their culture disdained psychiatry and felt that it was reserved only for persons with serious mental illness, which in turn was stigmatized.

Hoping to connect with these patients, I attempted to display my knowledge of those nuances of Buddhism that I had studied early on. And so, I asked each new patient about the specific school of Buddhism that they practiced—yet no one could answer. Virtually all seemed amused that I would be concerned about such details. Initially, I was surprised, because in Judaism, we argue incessantly about nuances of observance and belief, and draw sharp distinctions between different "brands" of Judaism. Yet there seemed to be no parallel among my patients of Asian ancestry. They were more impressed to learn that I had studied Chinese art in college, and some said that they sought treatment with me because they saw that I spoke Hebrew, which, to them, meant that I also appreciated ancient traditions, and would be more inclined to respect their ancient heritage than a psychiatrist who was more secular or more "All-American."

Apart from that, it seemed that "ancestor worship"—rather than formal religious affiliation and temple worship—was more common among my patients than "official" or organized religion. For many, home-based incense-burning shrines,

bedecked with photos of the departed, sufficed. For them, the elaborate temples depicted in travel brochures about Asia were irrelevant, although I myself enjoyed wandering around New York's Chinatown, peering into dusty windows populated with statues of Buddhas, where burning incense and billowing smoke made the scene seem even more exotic to me. For Jews like me, incense was reserved for a single short ritual on Saturday night, performed as the Sabbath ended, although frankincense and myrrh were standard in the long-gone Jerusalem Temple described in the Hebrew Bible.

Let me return to my initial references to Chinese art, which were mentioned at the start of this essay. I had additional reasons for choosing to study Chinese art (along with other Asian traditions much later). For one thing, I was intent on getting a reasonable humanities education before embarking on the strictly scientific studies I expected to encounter in medical school. Equally importantly, the museum's art collection contrasted with the so-called art scattered across the walls of my mother's apartment, where cheap plastic "Shalom" signs substituted for actual (and otherwise unaffordable) art. Each Shalom sign was indistinguishable from the next, and each was decorated with large fake gold letters, in Hebrew, of course. Words were painted on striated plastic meant to simulate higher quality wooden plaques, as seen in synagogues. Framed prints of Chagall paintings hung side by side with those Shalom signs.

Looking back, I did not expect to explore Asia, and my interest in Asia—its art, its people, its religions, its cultures—did not arrive through the usual routes. Unlike some co-religionists, I never embraced an Asian religion, never practiced meditation, and never entertained trading Judaism for Hare Krishna or other Eastern religions that proselytized heavily in the 1960s. The closest I came to "observing" Asian spiritual traditions was via yoga, but as a medical treatment rather than a spiritual journey. Dr. Harold Benson's adaptation of Tibetan and transcendental meditation, as described in his best-selling book about *The Relaxation* Response [1], was also appealing, for pharmacology-free stress reduction, and not because I aped Asian approaches to so-called higher consciousness. If someone had told me back then that I would eventually visit India seven times, I would have laughed, not because there was anything objectionable about India, but because the airfare seemed so exorbitant for someone of my modest circumstances.

Using a Specialized Jewish Education to Understand Asia

So, where does that leave us? (Or me?)

On the surface, my particularistic and specialized Jewish education seemed limited and clearly ethnocentric. Everything in my early universe revolved around Judaism or Jewish history, as if this was the earth encircled by the sun, as seen in the pre-Copernican imagination. Yet things are not always what they seem, for Jewish history is almost always contextualized. Even when they occupied their own land, before the earlier Babylonian Exile and before the final destruction of the rebuilt Jerusalem temple in 70 C.E., my Jewish ancestors (or the Twelve Tribes or the Hebrews) lived in the proximity of other peoples and other cultures. Canaanites, Egyptians, and Philistines are described in detail in the Hebrew Bible, known as the Tanach. The Amorites and the Hittites and others also appear in the sacred Hebrew canon. The Persians, the Greeks, be they Saracens or Hellenes, have prominent places in our history, even if not always positive places. And who could ever forget the Egyptians of the Passover story?

Early Hebrew history was typically contrasted with local cultures, and sometimes the newly settled wandering tribes coopted religious rites—as well as agricultural practices—from their immediate neighbors. Sometimes other nations attempted to cannibalize (or assimilate or outlaw) the Hebrews' culture and sometimes they succeeded. Sometimes the Hebrews sought out those forbidden foreign deities on their own accord, despite admonitions against them. These constant comparisons in the official Hebrew canon made me to wonder about religious rites and beliefs of

other people who lived elsewhere, not necessarily in the vicinity of the Twelve Tribes.

The Hebrew prophets of old repeatedly chastised the Children of Israel for attempting to emulate "other nations," and for abandoning the one and only Yahweh, the invisible deity who guided them through the desert, on their way to the Promised Land. Specifically, the prophets admonished the Israelite nation for "lusting" after deities worshipped by the locals. They wrote about pagan goddesses such as Asherah or Ashtoreth, and made repeated allusions to the Babylonian Baal, the so-called rider on the storm who was lionized by The Doors' moody music. In short, the incident surrounding the Golden Calf, which was smelted from women's jewelry when Moses was away on Mount Sinai, and awaiting delivery of the Ten Commandments, was not a one-off event. Whether or not this intrigue with bovine animal effigies anticipated the Hindus' sanctification of the cow or simply inspired latter day expressions about "sacred cows" is a question for linguistics as well as history scholars.

At the time, these recurring accusations about "lusting" after pagan deities perplexed me. (The Hebrew word refers to "lusting," in all translations.) Were they alluding to the proverbial pagan orgies? Those were details that the rabbis who taught our Bible (Tanach) classes did not share, and which we students did not dare ask about. My own answer: maybe yes, maybe no, but my later life visits to India's incense-laden Hindu temples, bedecked with fragrant marigold petals, and painted in a prism of colors, reminded me of those Biblical allusions to sensuousness of idols. But more about that later.

Many years would pass before I entered a Hindu temple, initially to see the artwork and architecture (or what I called "artwork," but which believers identified as deities). I was initially deterred by my own religious proscription against visiting religious sites of other religions, but I rationalized that this visit functioned more as research than religion. I relished the pageantry seen in those temples and contrasted those celebrations with less flamboyant Jewish religious rites. Temple festivals held on the night of the full moon especially intrigued me, because they reminded me of the Biblical harvest festivals that were always scheduled during full moons, when bright moonlight made pilgrimages to the Jerusalem's Holy Temple possible.

Some years later, still in pursuit of middle-of-the-night moonlight celebrations, we made our way to Malaysia, where some Tamils from South India established a large emigrant community, and observed an annual festival called "Thaipusam." Celebrants danced themselves into a trance, while heavy melons and smaller fruits hung from hooks attached to their skin. The concept of trance dancing was not unique—I knew of Chasidic Jewish sects that sought to achieve ecstatic trances via circle dances, and I had read whole books about *Music and Trance* [2] in varied cultures, and I had previously witnessed Sufi trance dancing in Turkey. Yet the concept of such self-mutilation initially seemed strange to me, until I compared those Hindu rites to the Jewish practice of "laying tefillin," when men wrap sanctified leather straps around their arms during morning prayer, sometimes so tightly that the skin beneath turns blue and the surrounding flesh bulges besides the leather.

Yet almost everything else in Hindu temples and rituals was as different as imaginable. In Judaism, graven images are officially forbidden (although Rabbi Burton Visotzky cites curious examples of deviation from those standards in his book about *Aphrodite and the Rabbis: How the Jews Adapted Roman Culture to Create Judaism as We Know It* [3]). In contrast, images are intrinsic to most approaches to Hinduism. Moreover, Judaism demands allegiance to one G-d only, whose true name is never spoken, but is transliterated as "Yahweh," whereas Hinduism acknowledges a pantheon of deities, with some more important than others. Some subsects revolve around specific deities, such as Rama, or Krishna, or Shiva, or Vishnu or Hanuman, the Monkey deity, and so on, and some families worship one deity in particular.

The closest I could come to understanding other parallels between Hinduism and Western religion (including my own) came by way of Wendy Doniger's book on *Hindu Myths* (2014)

[4]. Among many other things, she details the Ganesh-Shiva-Parvati story, enough to make me draw comparisons (and contrasts) to the Oedipus myth, which is a more familiar "family romance" that has played so important role in the origins of Freud's psychoanalytic theories. By her own admission (during our short personal discussion at one of her readings at New York's Asia Society), Doniger is more partial to Jungian ideas than to Freudianism, even though the father–mother–son triad of that Hindu story begs for Freudian interpretation. Unlike Oedipus, who loses his vision because he autonucleates to expiate the sin of inadvertently sleeping with his own mother, Ganesh acquires the head of an elephant after his incensed father decapitates his human head. Ganesh also became one of Hinduism's most popular deities, if not the most popular.

An Indologist who has authored 40 books on the subject, and a professor at the University of Chicago Divinity School, Doniger subsequently came under attack for her 2011 book on *The Hindus: An Alternative History*, not because this publication lacked the impeccable scholarship that underlies her earlier works, but because some people, especially conservative Hindus in India, believed (erroneously, according to Doniger) that her 2011 volume is "anti-Hindu" [5, 6] Her publisher was sued and put under pressure—well before our current American concerns with academic freedom and book banning peaked. Mainstream media as well as the internet followed the lawsuit closely, and the publisher— Penguin—eventually withdrew sales of the book to comply with a legal settlement. The courtroom arguments surrounding these accusations, republished on both social media and in the official press, highlight the potential perils of dissecting the religious beliefs of others, even if no offense is intended.

To this day, I doubt that I could ever fully understand Hindu spirituality, even though I could memorize terms from the Vedas or Upanishads or various sutras, and even though I learned to identify many Hindu deities on sight. The concept of being at one with the universe— that noetic experience described by philosopher/

psychologist William James or by Freud's friend, the Nobel Prize-winning novelist Romain Rolland—was foreign to me, no matter how well I mastered the terminology. I could wonder all I want if James' nitrous oxide-induced perceptions paralleled the results of "true" Hindu meditation, or if his descriptions detailed in *The Varieties of Religious Experience* (1902) were nothing more than perceptions popularized by the 1960s drug culture, perceptions that desecrate true Hindu belief systems. I accepted that I would never know the answer. For me, Hindu ragas performed at the World Music Institute were lovely, relaxing music, with pleasing acoustics, but for practicing Hindus, such melodies carried spiritual connotations that extended beyond aesthetics and that were beyond my grasp.

Curiously, Buddhism was birthed in Northern India some 2500 years ago, but never gained a strong foothold in its country of origin, although Buddhism in general interacted with local Hindu belief systems. Instead, Buddhism traveled to China, where it enjoys the largest number of followers. The version of Buddhism that took hold in Japan and Korea—Zen, which means "meditation"—stresses nature and simplicity and the pursuit of enlightenment via intuition and meditation. For several reasons, Zen has had special appeal in the West and has played a prominent role in specialized approaches to psychiatry and psychoanalysis, as we will see below.

Erich Fromm's Trek from Orthodox Judaism, Chasidic Mysticism, and Zen Mindfulness

My intellectual—as opposed to experiential—approach to Asian religions led me to the writings of Erich Fromm, a lay analyst and social psychologist who was among the first to introduce Buddhism to American psychoanalytic audiences. Fromm collaborated with Shunryu Suzuki, a Zen master, and with Richard de Martino, to write his book on *Zen Buddhism and Psychoanalysis* (1960) [7]. That book evolved from a psychoanalytic seminar on the subject, held three years earlier. As for Suzuki, he became

a pioneer in his own right: his teachings reached devotees outside of his native Japan when he opened the first Zen monastery outside of Asia. The San Francisco Zen center, founded by Suzuki, remains one of the most influential Zen centers in the United States.

Curiously, Fromm acquired his early knowledge of Buddhist practice by reading books about Buddhism and from studying the Buddhist canon or Pali while at university in Europe, rather than from consulting practicing Buddhists or observing their rites or attempting those rites himself [8]. Much later in life, he met a Buddhist monk, Nyanaponika Thera, who, like Fromm, had been born Jewish in Germany. His new friend narrowly escaped the Nazis before emigrating to Sri Lanka, where he was ordained as a Buddhist monk. Fromm adopted his friend's version of Buddhist meditation, having become skeptical of Zen's promise of instant enlightenment or "satori," which bypassed the need for character change and thereby cheapened the concept of "mindfulness," as per Fromm.

Initially, Fromm's publication piqued my interest, not because of Zen per se, but because his background was so strongly rooted in Jewish tradition—or I should say, rooted in varied Jewish traditions. I could not help but wonder how he made these disparate journeys.

Fromm's later life infatuation with Zen was shared by Beat poets who preceded him, and whom he obliquely disparaged in his text. For instance, Allan Ginsberg, author of "A Buddhist Kaddish," syncretized Judaism and Buddhism, at least temporarily, and his fellow Beat writers Jack Kerouac and Neal Cassidy added a Catholic tinge to their Buddhist belief system. The Beats' literary influence from the 1950s stands to this day, and their life stories continue to intrigue younger readers as well as those who are closer in age to the "Beat Generation" [9].

Fromm's collaborative book would be one of many volumes on Zen and psychoanalysis to surface over the decades. He foresaw potential pitfalls in promoting Zen as a "feel good" therapeutic practice—or religion—without demanding the personal growth that he deemed necessary, and some say that he predicted today's explosion of [meaningless] "mindfulness." Fromm's stature vis-a-vis Zen Buddhism has since been overshadowed by later writers who tackled similar subject matter, such as psychiatrist Mark Epstein, author of the best-selling *Thoughts without a Thinker* [10] in 1995, *The Zen of Therapy* in 2022 [11] and other related works.

Erich Fromm's personal history is intriguing, albeit less sensational. Long before I encountered his collaborative book about *Zen Buddhism and Psychoanalysis* (1960), Fromm's surname surfaced in Hannah Green's cult memoir cum novel—*I Never Promised You a Rose Garden* [12]. The semi-autobiographical novel, which later became both a movie and a play as well as required reading in many college classes,—revolved around Fromm's one-time supervising analyst, and future wife, Frieda Fromm-Reichmann. Fromm and Frieda Fromm-Reichmann divorced after a short marriage—and he married two more times—but she retained Fromm's name. Besides gaining celebrity through Joanne Greenberg's thinly disguised account of her hospital stay at Chestnut Lodge, Fromm-Reichmann was well-known in psychiatric circles for her since-debunked but once popular concept of the "schizophrenogenic mother" whose behavior (rather than genetic endowment) allegedly produced schizophrenia in her progeny.

Not long after reading *Rose Garden,* I meandered into a university bookstore, and spotted Fromm's book about the Hebrew psalms sitting on the shelf. As the title implies, *You Shall be as Gods: A Radical Interpretation of the Old Testament and its Tradition* (1966) [13], links his later Marxist and humanist views to his earlier, intensely religious Jewish background. He condemns the totalitarianism of this religion—just as he indicts totalitarianism wherever it appears—but he praises its occasional forays into mysticism. His endorsement of mysticism is consistent with his approach to Zen, which he articulated a few years earlier. This preference for personal religious experience may also link to his one-on-one studies with a mystically inclined Chasidic rabbi, conducted after he broke with the organized religion of his earlier years. He identified

this rabbi as being the greatest influence on his life, as per an article in an Israeli newspaper, Haaretz [14].

Fromm's journey from Jewish scholar to (non-medical) lay psychoanalyst to refugee from the Reich to social psychologist to established academician to Zen devotee followed a convoluted path. Fromm was born into an Orthodox Jewish family in Frankfort-am-Main, a descendent of a long line of rabbis. Long before embarking on psychoanalytic studies and joining the staff of Chestnut Lodge, he earned a Ph.D. in sociology. His dissertation concerned sociological investigations of three very different and distinctive Jewish communities—the Karaites, the Hasidim, and Reform Jewry—each of which evolved in different time periods and each of which had completely different approaches to Jewish practice and Jewish law.

Even though his topic was particularistic, in that it focused on Judaism, his research nevertheless testified to his interest in the sociological influences on religious schisms. He later came to link any totalitarian system—be it religious, governmental, or political—to fascism. His apparent appreciation of the wide variations in Jewish ideology also paved the way for his study of Zen's approach to consciousness, as did his individual studies with his mystically-inclined Chasidic rebbe.

Working in conjunction with Freida Reichmann at "The Lodge," the two offered what was jocularly and informally known as "Torah therapy" or "Torapeutics." On a more formal level, they conducted their program at the Therapeuticum, which was an experimental, residential, psychoanalytic institution that combined therapy with Orthodox Jewish observance. Fromm and Fromm-Reichmann's forays into this unique approach did not persist, for each embraced socialism and abandoned strict adherence to Jewish tradition. Erich Fromm introduced Freida to his evolving socialist and humanist ideals, just as she familiarized him with psychoanalytic concepts and treatment approaches when she functioned as his supervisor at The Lodge. Although it had been a bastion of psychoanalysis in its heyday, Chestnut Lodge has since shuttered its doors for reasons that are beyond the scope of this essay [15]

Fromm's forked path from Judaism and then to "official" psychoanalytic ideology and finally to Zen's approach to "mindfulness" and individual enlightenment is worth exploring. The parallels between the traditional Jewish valorization of the collective history of the "Children of Israel" and psychoanalysis' emphasis on childhood history are clearcut: each is rooted in the past. Fromm's later studies with his Chasidic rebbe are more relevant to his belated enthusiasm for Zen. It is worth explaining the distinctions between the Chasidim and "traditional" Talmud-based orthodox Jews (who were also called "mitnagdim," to signify their opposition to Chasidism), for there was—and still is—a wide chasm between the "mitnagdim" who reared and formally educated Fromm, and early Chasidism, which emerged in mid-eighteenth century Eastern Europe. With its mystical mindset, its emphasis on an individual's communing with nature, outside, in forests or fields (rather than inside, in a synagogue), and its preference for personal experience over collective prayer services, Chasidism stood in opposition to the more mainstream "mitnagdi" approach to Judaism. With their text-based and ritual-bound practices, and their unwavering devotion to the written words of the Talmud, which is still called the "Oral Law," even though it was canonized many, many centuries earlier, the "mitnagdim" who opposed Chasidism could not have been more different from their Chasidic opponents— or from the Zen masters whom Fromm exalted. On the other hand, crossovers between the Chasidic mindset described above and the Zen mindset are apparent.

The contrast between those historical approaches of traditional (mitnagdi) Judaism— and Freudian-influenced psychoanalysis—and Zen's emphasis on the moment and on immediate experience is profound and could explain Fromm's detour from standard psychoanalytic approaches to mental distress (as well as traditional Judaism), in pursuit of alternative approaches offered by Zen Buddhism. (We could speculate why he pursued Zen meditation, as

opposed to the mysticism of Chasidism, which eventually evolved into a rigid hierarchical system, with "totalitarian" "rebbes" situated at the helm of each Chasidic sect—but such speculation is beyond our scope here.) Nevertheless, I should point out that Fromm was not a complete renegade vis-a-vis psychoanalysis, even if he was not a complete conformist either, for he was one of the founders of the William Alanson White Institute, a breakaway psychoanalytic school in New York City.

Fromm's peregrinations as a social psychologist were equally convoluted. At one point, he turned his attention to the psychology of fascism. His tome on *Escape from Freedom* (1941) attempted to explain why the authoritarian personality epitomized by Hitler appealed to otherwise rational people and especially to a German culture that was previously renowned for its contributions to literature, music, philosophy, and science. Although Fromm's study emphasizes his reactions to the Nazi regime, it was World War I, rather than World War II, which impacted his point of view most strongly. He had been born in 1900, and so he experienced adolescence while World War I—The Great War—was in progress [14].

By returning to embers of The Great War, rather than highlighting World War II, which was still raging when he wrote this volume, and which would prove to be far more devastating than ever expected, Fromm attempted to address a world that wanted to know how Hitler and other fascists exacted such an unwavering hold on advanced nations. In 1941, when his book on fascism hit the press, the Nazi death camps had just started. Predictions about the impending Holocaust that would claim the lives of six million Jews were still lacking.

In hindsight, we can understand why such questions would vex Fromm on a very personal level—he himself escaped the Reich, and would have faced death, had Nazi restrictions on practicing psychoanalysis (which was dismissed by the Nazis as the "Jewish science") not motivated him to emigrate when Hitler first took power and well before the mass murders began. More data about the Shoah and its subsequent influence on

American psychiatry are available in my chapter published in the first book in this series [16].

Despite this dramatic history and his authorship of 20 books in total, Fromm gained the most fame from a best-selling book about *The Art of Loving* (1956). This book went into print a few years before his book on Zen. For many of his admirers, his studies of social and political psychology remain the most important of his many accomplishments.

Marsha Linehan's Route to the Discovery of DBT: From Personal Agony, to Catholic Ecstacy, to Zen Meditation

With all respect for Fromm's profound contributions to social, political, and even religious psychology, when we look for the link between psychiatry, psychology, psychoanalysis, and Zen, we find the most impressive, most pervasive, and most enduring influence coming from Marsha Linehan, Ph.D. Linehan, a troubled soul during her teens, used Zen as a foundation for creating DBT (dialectical behavioral therapy) after standard therapeutic techniques (and even ECT) failed to relieve her internal pain and acting out. DBT therapy is currently a mainstay in the treatment of people with otherwise difficult-to-treat borderline personalities, with their mood instability, impulsivity, and baseline suicidal ideation.

Linehan's personal history is as striking as her professional accomplishments—she endured repeated and lengthy psychiatric hospitalizations as an otherwise "incurable" adolescent with a presumptive (but since disputed) diagnosis of schizophrenia. Then something changed. Some years after leaving the hospital, she had an ecstatic experience while praying in a chapel in her religion of birth (Catholicism). As the New York Times tells it, "[she] was kneeling in [the chapel], looking up at the cross, and the whole place became gold. . . and [she] said, 'I love myself.'" Finally feeling loved by G-d. she "felt transformed" [17]. She accepted herself as she was, embracing the principles of what we currently call "radical acceptance." She stopped cutting and burning herself for the next year, weathering the storms of her raging emotions and forestalling her impulses to self-harm, but still not completely free from psychic distress that had haunted her for so long.

Undaunted by her supposedly "intractable" psychiatric condition, she subsequently "found" Zen, perfected her techniques of "mindfulness" over time, and reevaluated her symptoms and her diagnosis. She pursued advanced education in psychology, earning a doctorate degree. She tested her theories experimentally and published her results, thereby paving the way to treat previously "untreatable" patients and cementing her legacy in psychology. Many consider her to be one of the most influential psychologists of her era. She also became a Zen teacher, and a practitioner, in addition to maintaining her more mainstream academic posts.

Conclusion

When starting this study on Asian spirituality and psychiatry, I planned to zero in on Fromm and his travels from Orthodox Judaism to Zen meditation, to show how "unorthodox" routes can exert indelible—albeit unexpected—influences on society, on psychiatry, and on spirituality. And then I digressed and pursued a broader and more personalized path, while retaining Fromm as the backbone of this essay, and using him as an example of outsiders who injected Asian spirituality into American psychiatry, psychology, and psychoanalysis.

Although some disagree with the appropriateness of such "outsider influences" on reinterpreting (or misinterpreting) the sacred traditions of another's society (as exemplified by the debates surrounding Doniger's scholarship), the fact of the matter is that syncretism has been more the norm than the exception since the start of history. History is remade again and again by the creative misinterpretation of events and ideas from other times and other peoples.

Regardless, my experiences highlight how one's own background provides the lens through which we perceive other cultures, other religions, and other spiritual systems. It is entirely possible that this lens is clouded, to the point of being so opaque that it lets us look inward only, while deceiving ourselves that we can indeed see what lies outside. Yet it is also possible that such a lens leads to a greater focus and a clearer vision of whatever lies ahead.

References

1. Benson H. The relaxation response. New York: William Morrow & Company; 1975.
2. Rouget G. Music and trance: a theory of the relations between music and possession. Chicago: University of Chicago Press; 1985.
3. Visotzky B. Aphrodite and the rabbis: how the Jews adapted Roman culture to create Judaism as we know it. New York: St. Martin's Press; 2016.
4. Wendy Doniger, Hindu Myths: A Sourcebook Translated from the Sanskrit. New York: Penguin Classics, 2004.
5. Podcast | 'My Book Was Pro Hindu. Those Who Had Attacked Me Hadn't Read It': Wendy Doniger. https://thewire.in/books/wendy-doniger-podcast-hindu-book. Accessed 01 May 2023.
6. Gottipati S. Indian publisher withdraws book on Hindus after court case. https://www.reuters.com/article/us-india-hindus/indian-publisher-withdraws-book-on-hindus-after-court-case-idUSBREA1A1D220140211
7. Fromm E, Suzuki S, de Martino R. Zen Buddhism and psychoanalysis. Condor Books; 1960.
8. Helderman I. Heeding Erich Fromm's Warning, in Tricycle.org, Winter 2020. https://tricycle.org/magazine/erich-fromm/. Accessed online.
9. Strausbaugh J. The village: 400 years of Beats and bohemians, radicals and rogues. New York: Ecco/Harper Collins; 2013.
10. Epstein M. Thoughts without a thinker. New York: Basic Books; 1995.
11. Epstein M. The Zen of therapy: uncovering a hidden kindness in life. New York: Penguin Random House; 2022.
12. Green H [Greenberg J]. I never promised you a rose garden. New York: Holt, Reinhart, & Winston; 1964.
13. Fromm E. You shall be as Gods: a radical interpretation of the old testament and its tradition. New York: Henry Holt; 1966.
14. This Day in Jewish History | 1900: A Psychoanalyst Who Couldn't Understand War Is Born. Haaretz, March 23, 2015. https://www.haaretz.com/jewish/2015-03-23/ty-article/.premium/1900-analyst-who-couldnt-understand-war/0000017f-dc57-d856-a37f-fdd7aced0000
15. Packer S. A belated obituary: Raphael J. Osheroff, M.D., Psychiatric Times, June 28, 2013.
16. Packer S. How anti-Semitism and the Shoah helped shape twentieth-century psychoanalysis. In: Moffic S, Peteet J, Hankir A, Seeman M, editors. Antisemitism and psychiatry. Cham: Springer; 2020.
17. Carey B. Expert on mental illness reveals her own fight. The New York Times (nytimes.com), June 23, 2011.

Integrating Judaic and Buddhist Insights into Psychotherapy and Counseling

Ronald W. Pies

Introduction

As a child raised in a mostly secular Jewish home, I had very little exposure to the religious traditions of the East. Only much later in life, having made a study of Buddhism, did I learn that Jews have been prominent American Buddhist leaders from the early days of Buddhism's appearance in the United States, as a recent book by sociologist Emily Sigalow points out. In *American JewBu*, Sigalow traces the complicated nexus between these two ancient spiritual and cultural traditions [1].

When considered from a purely theological perspective, the affinity for Buddhism among many American Jews—or Jews anywhere else—may seem rather surprising. After all, traditional, Orthodox Judaism is a covenantal faith in which an omniscient and omnipotent deity, the Creator of the Universe, demands strict adherence to the laws and regulations of the *Torah*—narrowly defined as the first five books of the Hebrew Bible.

In marked contrast, Buddhism—at least in its earliest forms—posited no such Creator God and entailed no such covenant. Nor was Buddhism grounded in a single "holy book" that was widely accepted as the revealed word of God. Indeed, Siddhartha Gautama—who came to be known as the Buddha or "awakened one"—is sometimes described as an "atheist"—though "non-theist" or "agnostic" might be a more apt description [2].

The issue is complicated, as Zen priest and psychologist Seth Zuihō Segall makes clear:

> You often see the claim made that Buddhism is a non-theistic religion. As is often the case, however, things are never quite so simple. There are ways in which the claim is true, ways in which it's untrue, and even ways in which it's just quasi-true…The claim of Non-theism is true in the sense that there is no God in Buddhism who is a Creator, Judge, or Deity-in-Charge…There's no Divine Intercessor putting one's merits and demerits onto a permanent record card that follows one around over countless lifetimes. [3]

On the other hand, Segall notes that

> The claim of Non-theism is not completely true because the Buddhist *suttas* and *sutras* make reference to all sorts of supernatural beings who inhabit the universe… The Buddha, himself, is often described as "a teacher of gods and men. [3]

These theological and metaphysical issues are intriguing, but are beyond the scope of this chapter. The complex issue of "God in Buddhism" is discussed in detail in the chapter by Prof. Harold G. Koenig, M.D., including research on the belief in God among Buddhists worldwide. In any case, perhaps it is worth hypothesizing that the non-theistic nature of Buddhism is what allows it to

R. W. Pies (✉)
SUNY Upstate Medical University,
Syracuse, NY, USA

Tufts University School of Medicine,
Boston, MA, USA
e-mail: piesr@upstate.edu

H. S. Moffic et al. (eds.), *Eastern Religions, Spirituality, and Psychiatry*,
https://doi.org/10.1007/978-3-031-56744-5_23

"fit" into the structure and culture of American Judaism—possibly accounting, in part, for the prevalence of the "American JewBu."

The burden of the present chapter, however, is to elucidate how Buddhism and Judaism share certain *core values* of considerable importance in counseling and psychotherapy, regardless of their theological differences. (I will not be discussing specific Buddhist practices or techniques, such as meditation, breathing exercises, yoga, etc.). To put the matter differently, I want to suggest that a sort of "convergent evolution" has occurred within the cultures of Buddhism and Judaism, such that the two have come to share important spiritual, psychological, and ethical insights. (In my book, *The Three-Petalled Rose*, I also relate these two traditions to the philosophy of Stoicism—the "third petal" of the Rose). Implicit in my thesis is the claim that the *psychological insights* found in Buddhism and Judaism are essentially inseperable from the *spiritual and ethical values* of these two ancient traditions.

Core Principles in Buddhism and Judaism: Relevance to Psychotherapy

If one were forced to summarize the "essence" of rabbinic Judaism in a few words, one could hardly do better than to cite the maxim of Hillel the Elder (born ca. 110 BCE). Hillel—renowned for his patience—was goaded by a non-believer to summarize the entire Torah while he, the heathen, stood on one foot! Ever the unflappable teacher, Hillel replied, "That which is hateful to you do not do to another; that is the entire Torah, and the rest is its interpretation. [Now] go study" [4].

In Buddhism, we find a very similar version of what is commonly known as "the Golden Rule." Thus, the Buddha taught, "Whatever is disagreeable to yourself, do not do unto others" [5].

Of course, both Judaism and Buddhism embrace many other values that are beyond the scope of this chapter. For example, Buddhism is perhaps most closely associated with the "Four

Noble Truths" and the "Eightfold Path," as detailed in the chapter by Prof. Koenig. For both traditions, ethical behavior is both a moral imperative and an essential feature of *the spiritually fulfilled life*. In Judaism, this is understood as living as God intends us to live, following the dictates of the Torah. In Buddhism, the "good life" is that which adheres to the *Dharma* (Pali: *dhamma);* i.e., the teachings and doctrines of the Buddha, sometimes broadly understood as "duties to be performed in accordance with the laws of nature" [6]. For the Buddhist, as Koenig notes, "Following the Dhamma results in deliverance from all suffering, including the deliverance from the desire for deliverance itself, and ultimately, leads to Nirvana" (see Chap. 11 in this volume).

In my view, there are at least eight core principles shared by Judaism and Buddhism that point us toward the "good life," and which—not incidentally—serve important functions in counseling and psychotherapy. In brief, they are as follows:

1. It is important to think clearly and carefully about our everyday experience and how we choose to respond to it.
2. There is a direct connection between how much we suffer or flourish in life, and how clearly and rationally we think.
3. There is a realm of human concern outside the narrow interests of "self," and a common bond that unites all human beings.
4. This common bond imposes ethical obligations upon us, and by fulfilling these, we also live a fulfilled life.
5. Limiting our desires and attachments is essential to living the good life.
6. Appreciating our impermanence and mortality allows us to find real meaning in life.
7. Being grateful for what we have is essential to the fulfilled and flourishing life.
8. Self-mastery and the avoidance of anger or aggression are essential to the fulfilled and flourishing life.

The remainder of this chapter will expand upon these eight principles by means of specific

Judaic and Buddhist teachings and will explain their relevance to counseling and psychotherapy. And while these principles may be especially suited to working therapeutically with Jewish or Buddhist clients or patients, I view them as applicable to persons of *any* faith, or of no faith et al.; in short, as principles applicable to anyone seeking a more fulfilling emotional and spiritual life. Perhaps the Greek term *eudaimonia* best captures this goal and is often translated as "flourishing." After elaborating on the eight core principles, I will conclude with a composite clinical vignette that attempts to incorporate these insights and values into a psychotherapeutic context.

Thinking Clearly

Both Judaism and Buddhism maintain that our happiness and fulfillment in life are critically dependent on the quality of our thinking. Both traditions hold, in effect, that we create our own happiness by thinking "good" thoughts—and create our own misery by filling our minds with "bad" thoughts. More specifically, Judaism emphasizes rational understanding, without which we are spiritually and emotionally "lost." Thus, we find the Talmudic teaching of Rabbi Elazar that, "Any person in whom there is no knowledge is ultimately exiled" [7].

Perhaps the greatest "rationalist" philosopher of Judaism, Moses ben Maimon (Maimonides, 1138–1204) held that "Man has been endowed with intellectual faculties which enable him to think, consider and act…and to control every organ of his body, causing both the principal and secondary organs to perform their respective functions" [8].

So, too, in Buddhism, what and how we think is an important determinant of our "reality." Thus, the Buddhist text, the *Dhammapada* teaches us that "We are what we think . . . with our thoughts we make the world" [9]. The Thai Buddhist Monk, Ajahn Chah (1918–1992) put it this way: "When confusion is penetrated with understanding, what remains is peace" [10].

Suffering and Muddled Thinking

Conversely, in both rabbinical Judaism and Buddhism, irrational or muddled thinking is believed to cause emotional suffering. Thus, Maimonides understood *insanity* as essentially a condition of disordered thought. He defined the insane person as "…one whose mind has become disturbed so that his thinking is consistently confused in some domain…" [11]. And in his *Hygiene of the Soul,* Maimonides admonishes us that "… the thoughts that cause heart failure because of what may possibly happen in the future must be abolished…" [12]. Much of Maimonides' writing in this area anticipates modern-day CBT by some eight centuries. Similarly, echoing the views of many modern cognitive-behavioral therapists, Rabbi Dr. Joseph Gelberman tells us that, "Of all the tyrants in the world, our own attitudes are the fiercest warlords" [13].

So, too, in Buddhism, emotional well-being is shattered when we think irrationally or unrealistically, or allow anger to permeate our mental processes. The Buddhist monk, Chagdud Tulku taught that, "Hell is the reflection of [the] mind's delusion, of angry thoughts and intentions and the harmful words and actions they produce" [14]. He adds—once again, sounding much like our modern cognitive therapists—"It's our failure to understand the essential nature of an emotion as it arises that gets us into trouble. Once we do, the emotion tends to dissolve" [14]. Similarly, the Thai Buddhist Master, Ajahn Chah (1918–1992) has commented:

> We want to be free of suffering . . . but still we suffer. Why is this? It's because of wrong thinking. If our thinking is in harmony with the way things are, we will have well-being. [15]

The Common Bond that Unites All Human Beings

The Talmud tell us, "Beloved is the human being, since he was created in God's image…".[1] Importantly, there is nothing in the Talmud

---

[1] *Pirke Avot*, 3:18.

regarding how to be a "good Jew." Talmudic ethics focus solely on how to be a decent human being. Indeed, as Rabbi Michael Hattin points out

> The Torah was the first and only code to promulgate the revolutionary idea that al human beings, irrespective of race, color or creed, were descended from a single man and woman who were fashioned in the 'Divine Image.' This implied, by extension, that all members of humanity were related to each other by a common bond of blood and destiny…. [16]

So, too, in Buddhism, we find an analogous "common bond" that unites all of mankind. As B. Allen Wallace notes, all human beings "…are endowed with Buddha-nature…[defined as] the potential for full awakening, or as the essential perfection of each sentient being…" [17].

Furthermore, we are, as human beings, all linked to one another through the cycle of birth, aging, sickness, death, and rebirth—what Buddhists call *samsara*. More concretely, recalling the first of the "Four Noble Truths," the Buddhist Monk Ajahn Sumedho (1934–) has taught that Buddhism is not based "…on a metaphysical or doctrinal position, but on an existential experience common to all humanity—the experience of suffering" [18].

This Common Bond Imposes Ethical Obligations Upon Us

The common bond that unites all of humanity has important ethical implications in Judaism. As Rabbi Moshe Lieber has put it, "…we must treat [all] people properly because all people play a role in God's plans…they are all part of the Divine Scheme" [19]. Accordingly, Hillel's admonition, "Do not do to others what is hateful to you," applies to *all* persons, regardless of race, religion, or ethnicity. As Rabbi Michael Hattin puts it, "All people have a right to be treated with respect and honor by virtue of their 'Divine Image…'" [16].

Similarly, Buddhism teaches that we are all joined in the same web of creation and must treat one another with deep reverence and respect. Indeed, Buddhist teachers instruct us to see every

being as our mother! Thus, Chagdud Tulku states that, "…all beings, at one time or another, through countless lifetimes, have been our own mother…" [14]. This perspective helps us to counteract anger toward someone we might otherwise regard as a stranger. For Tulku, we must "…develop a noble attitude of compassion for all beings without distinction…realizing that all beings, equally, want happiness. Nobody wants to suffer" [14].

Limiting Our Desires and Attachments

Rabbinic and Talmudic Judaism are replete with admonitions to limit our desires. The rabbis, of course, knew full well of our nearly insatiable desires and longings. In one rabbinical commentary, we find this frank assessment: "No man departs from this world with [even] half his cravings satisfied. When he has attained a hundred, he desires two hundred".[2] But, as Rabbi Leonard B. Gewirtz puts it, "Since desires are limitless and man can never satisfy them all, he must learn to discriminate among them and to control them" [20]. Maimonides recognized the danger that lies in excessive craving and unbridled materialism:

> All the difficulties and troubles we meet [in daily life] are due to the desire for superfluous things… the more we desire to have the superfluous, the more we meet with difficulties. [8]

In contrast to such inordinate desires, the Talmud poses this question: "Who is rich?" and answers, "One who rejoices in his portion".[3] We'll say more on this presently, under principle 7 (gratitude).

Buddhism—perhaps even more than Judaism—cautions against excessive desire and attachment. Buddhism posits (in the second "Noble Truth") that human suffering is caused by *selfish craving*, known as *tanha*. One scholar—E. A. Burtt—defines *tanha* as asking of the Universe "…more than it is ready or even able to give" [21]. It is not that Buddhism is opposed to material possessions per se, or even to wealth; rather, it is our *inordinate*

---

[2] Midrash Rabbah, Koheles 1:34 and 3:12.
[3] *Pirke Avot* 4.1.

attachment to these things that Buddhism warns against. As Chagdud Tulka observes, "The loss of wealth in itself is not the source of suffering, only [our] attachment to having it" [14]. Similarly, Ajahn Chah observes that

> The extraordinary suffering is [that which] arises from what we call *upadana*: grasping on to things. This is like having an injection with a syringe filled with poison. [10]

For Buddhists, grasping and attachment are not limited to material objects, like cars, jewelry, etc. Buddhism also cautions against undue attachment to ideas, beliefs—and even to Buddhism itself! Perhaps this is one explanation for the puzzling and paradoxical statement by the ninth-century Chinese Buddhist monk Linji Yixuan, who famously told his disciples, "If you meet the Buddha on the road, kill him!" [22]

One antidote to excessive grasping is the realization that all things—including our mortal selves—eventually cease to exist. Thus, Aitken Roshi teaches that "Renunciation is not getting rid of the things of this world, but accepting that they pass away" [23]. This insight leads directly to the sixth principle.

Appreciating Our Impermanence and Mortality

Rabbinical and Talmudic Judaism stress the fleeting and contingent nature of life—not as a message of gloom, but as a spur to spiritual growth. Thus, the Talmud instructs us to "repent one day before your death".[4] But how does one know when that day comes? As Rabbi Moshe Lieber explains

> Does one ever know when he will die? Rather, he must always assume that today is the last day of his life and not push off his repentance. Hence, he will spend all his life in perpetual self-improvement. [19]

Judaism, to be clear, does not view death as evil or calamitous; rather, it is seen as a regular occurrence in the "seasons" of life. As the book of *Ecclesiastes* states, "A season is set for everything…a time for being born and a time for

dying…" (7:2). Furthermore, our mortality can be given meaning through acts of righteousness during our lives. Thus, the Talmud teaches that *"Tzedakah tahtzeel memavet"*—"Righteousness can save from death".[5] In practice, this means that one can extend *the life of the community* by means of righteousness and loving-kindness.

Buddhism, too, teaches us that life—like everything else—is temporary and fleeting, and that this inexorable fact provides the opportunity for spiritual growth. Thus, the *Dhammapada* teaches that

> Neither Father, sons, nor one's relations can stop the King of Death. When he comes with all his power, a man's relations cannot save him. A man who is virtuous and wise understands the meaning of this and swiftly strives with all his might to clear a path to Nirvana. [24]

Furthermore, by contemplating—and fully accepting—our own mortality, we can reduce our grasping and *attachment* to things (*upadana*). In so doing, we prepare ourselves to depart this life with equanimity.

Gratitude and the Flourishing Life

Gratitude (in Hebrew, *hakarat hatov*) is among the highest values in Judaism. Without gratitude and thankfulness, the flourishing life is not possible, according to the rabbis. Indeed, Jews are instructed to begin each day with a prayer of thankfulness, known as the *modeh ani*. Jews are grateful even for the integrity of their basic bodily functions, as this Talmudic blessing demonstrates:

> Praised are You, Lord our God…who with wisdom fashioned the human body, creating openings, arteries, glands and organs…should but one of them, by being blocked or opened, fail to function, it would be impossible to exist. Praised are You, Lord, healer of all flesh, who maintains our bodies in wonderous ways. [25]

A more homely version of the same sentiment is expressed in this Yiddish proverb: "If a Jew breaks a leg, he thanks God he did not break both legs. If he breaks both legs, he thanks God he did not break his neck" [26].

---

[4] *Pirke Avot* 2.15.

[5] *Bava Batra* 10a.

So, too, in Buddhism: gratitude [*katannuta*]is highly valued. A saying of the Buddha states:

> These two people are hard to find in the world… The one who is first to do a kindness; and the one who is grateful and thankful for a kindness done.[6]

In the Pali language, the word for "grateful"—*katannu*—literally means, "to have a sense of what was done" for us. Thus, Thanissaro Bhikkhu—the abbot of the Metta Forrest Monastery—describes the gratitude we owe to all those who have given us life and preserved our health and safety:

> The fact that you are alive to read this means that somebody chose, again and again, to help you when you were helpless. [27]

Self-Mastery and the Avoidance of Anger

Talmudic and rabbinic Judaism place high value on self-control, self-mastery, and avoidance of anger. Thus, *Pirke Avot* asks, "Who is mighty?" and answers, "One who conquers one's passions…one who is slow to anger is better than the mighty, and one who rules over one's spirit is better than one who conquers a city." (4:1) Though rabbinic writings generally stop short of advocating total elimination of anger, they insist on modulating, minimizing, and carefully channeling it. Indeed, the rabbis considered intense anger—what some would call *rage*—akin to idol-worship. Perhaps the Jewish sages sensed the element of *narcissism* in this emotion. As two scholars of Judaism explain

> Anger places the ego at the center, displacing God and others, and causing the alienation of relationships. [25]

Buddhism is, if anything, even more disparaging of anger. One saying of the Buddha states, "Holding on to anger is like drinking poison and expecting the other person to die." *The Dhammapada* instructs us to "Forsake anger [and] give up pride…" adding

> He who can control his rising anger as a coachman controls his carriage at full speed, this man I call a good driver…. [24]

The Buddhist approach to anger is summarized in this comment from Pema Chodron: "… patience is the antidote to anger and aggression… patience means getting smart: you stop and wait" [28]. There is a remarkable concordance between that statement and one from the Rozdoler Rabbi:

> When I feel angry against a person, I delay the expression of my anger. I say to myself: 'What will I lose if I postpone my anger?' [29]

Case Vignette

Having surveyed the eight principles or values common to both Judaism and Buddhism, we can now apply these in a composite case vignette, based on many outpatients I have evaluated and treated over the years:

Morrie is a 50-year-old divorced engineer who presents to his psychiatrist, Dr. M., with the chief complaint, "I feel like I'm getting cheated in life—like I'm never getting my due. And I can't stand working around idiots who are constantly pissing me off!" Morrie—the youngest of four sons—was raised in a secular Jewish household in which, as he put it, "You had to yell and scream to get anything—otherwise, one of my brothers would beat me to it." He describes his mother as "kind of a scared little mouse—she never stood up to Dad's bullying." Morrie described his father as, "King of the Castle—and if you didn't obey the King, you'd get the axe!" He denied any history of physical abuse, but noted, "My dad would yell at us like crazy. And he could kill you with one of his dirty looks!" Morrie was married for 25 years, but his marriage ended 5 years ago, at his wife's initiative. As Morrie put it, "Miriam said I was never 'there' for her, whatever that means. I guess she resented me putting so much time in at work. And I gotta admit, I would lose my temper with her more times than I like to remember. I mean, I never hit her or anything, but I could raise the roof sometimes." Morrie acknowledged that his colleagues at work also complained about his "temper," and his supervisor at the engineering firm had reprimanded him on two occasions for "losing it with one of the morons I have to work with."

Dr. M.—who was also raised in a secular Jewish family and has studied Eastern reli-

---

gions—worked with Morrie using a combination of Albert Ellis's *Rational Emotive Behavioral Therapy* (REBT) and principles derived from rabbinic Judaism and Buddhism. In his sessions with Morrie, Dr. M rarely identified these principles as specifically derived from Judaism or Buddhism; rather, they were worked into the framework of REBT and presented to Morrie simply as "useful ways to help you understand your feelings better—where they come from; how you can get better control of them; and how you can get along better with others."

Although therapy was focused mainly on helping Morrie manage his anger, Dr. M. also gently probed some of Morrie's tendency to disparage others as "morons," as well as his sense of having been "cheated in life." Therapy was aimed at helping Morrie examine how his anger was generated by semi-conscious, irrational thoughts and expectations, following principles of REBT; and also teaching him ways of distancing himself from the anger, using modifications of Buddhist techniques. Morrie's sense of being "cheated in life" was explored by learning more about his expectations of reward, and how they had been frustrated. He was also encouraged to talk about the "good things" in life that had come his way and to construct a weekly "gratitude check list," in which Morrie would list all the things for which he felt grateful that week. At first, Morrie resisted these explorations and exercises, preferring his customary stance of aggrieved victimhood at the hands of "morons." However, as therapy progressed and Morrie's trust in Dr. M. deepened, Morrie was able to see how, in many ways, he had much in his life for which to be grateful. He was also able to modulate and manage his anger more effectively by examining the thoughts that preceded his anger. Late in the course of therapy, Dr. M. was able to elicit some of Morrie's fears about aging and mortality. Morrie was gradually able to focus on what was most meaningful in his life, and to use life's transience as a launching point for prioritizing his needs and wishes. Finally—shifting to a more psychodynamic approach—Dr. M. was able to help Morrie see how his childhood experiences with competitive siblings; a harsh, demanding father; and a passive, unprotective mother helped shape some of his emotional responses in adult life.

The following dialogue is representative of the interchanges between Morrie and Dr. M. and reflects my own experience with patients having presentations similar to Morrie's:

Dr. M. So, tell me what was going through your mind when you yelled at your colleague, Frank, at work.

M I was thinking, "How could this idiot have screwed up the report we were working on so badly? He made complete mess of it and ought to get canned!"

Dr. M. OK, I can understand why you were upset. But "idiot" is pretty strong. And was one mistake really cause for firing this guy?

M Yeah, I'd say so!

Dr. M. Morrie, do you remember what it was like when your dad would yell at you? How it felt, I mean?

M Well, yeah. It was pretty awful. I felt like—like a bug being crushed.

Dr. M. And how do you think Frank felt when you yelled at him in front of your other workmates?

M Well, I guess…pretty bad. Embarrassed, I guess.

Dr. M. Well, it's hard to put ourselves in somebody else's shoes when we are really angry with that person, isn't it? And it's also hard to understand why we are getting so riled up at that moment.

M Yeah, I guess I just tend to shoot from the hip—or the lip!

Dr. M. A little like your dad?

M Yeah, I guess, much as I hate to admit it!

Dr. M. And when we are really furious with someone, it's hard to see that we are all fallible human beings. Making a mistake doesn't turn somebody into an idiot.

M I guess I see that now, but at the time…

Dr. M. Right, I get it, Morrie. None of thinks clearly when we are furious with someone. Now, tell me: what level of anger do you think you would have felt if you had said to yourself, "Well, Frank really screwed up, but we all screw up from time to time, and this is not the end of the world"?

M   Well, I guess I wouldn't have gotten so pissed off with the guy.

Dr. M. OK, so: the next time you feel like blowing up at somebody, Morrie, I'd like you to try something that may sound a little weird. Try picturing the person as a new-born baby, being held in his mother's arms. *[Note: this is based on a teaching from the Jewish mystic, Moses Cordovero, 1522–1570 (36)]*

M   Wait, *what*? Doc, that does sound pretty weird!

Dr. M. Yes, I get that, Morrie. But it's a way of putting a little distance between you and your anger. Also, when we picture someone in that way, we remind ourselves that, at one time, we were all just "babes in arms" [30]. We are really all in the same boat, simply in virtue of our humanity.

Conclusion

Judaism and Buddhism are ancient spiritual traditions with widely divergent metaphysical foundations, but with closely related ethical and psychological values. In both traditions, *ethics* and *psychology* are tightly interwoven, with clear implications for incorporating Judaic and Buddhist principles into psychotherapy. Perhaps the most obvious example is the high value both traditions place on *rational thinking* and the *mastery of one's emotions*. These are, in an important sense, *ethical imperatives* in Judaism and Buddhism—but they are also paths to psychological health and spiritual flourishing. Thus, Maimonides taught that, "It is the duty of man to subordinate all the faculties of

his soul to his reason" [31]. But it is precisely our use of reason that allows us to remain unperturbed in the face of life's "slings and arrows." Similarly, the Buddhist monk, Ajahn Chah, taught that, "When confusion is penetrated with understanding, what remains is peace" [10]. We might sum up these Judeo-Buddhist principles in the maxim, *"Rationality is the foundation of equanimity."* Indeed, in an important sense, both traditions paved the way for modern forms of cognitive-behavioral therapies, such as Rational Emotive Behavioral Therapy (which also drew heavily from the Stoic tradition).

Another foundational value common to Judaism and Buddhism is *gratitude,* without which a flourishing and fulfilled life is nearly impossible. This value is closely related to the admonition to *limit desires and cravings*—for without limiting our desires, it is nearly impossible to feel grateful. Thus, the eleventh century Jewish philosopher, Solomon ibn Gabirol taught that, "The person who seeks more than he needs hinders himself from enjoying what he has" [32].

Similarly, to repeat Rabbi Leonard B. Gewirtz' words,

> Since desires are limitless and man can never satisfy them all, he must learn to discriminate among them and to control them. [20]

These are quintessentially Buddhist values, as well. As the spiritual leader of Tibetan Buddhism, The Dalai Lama has put it,

> Even if you had the world at your feet, it would still not be enough. Desire is insatiable. Excessive desire is not only impossible to satisfy, it's also the source of torment…It's better to establish boundaries right from the start, and feel satisfied within those boundaries. [33]

Indeed, living happily within psychological and spiritual "boundaries" is arguably a fair synopsis of many Judaic and Buddhist teachings. Thus, there is the boundary between clear and muddled thinking; between an impulsive or foolish response and a thoughtful, considered one; between self-centeredness and an empathic connection to the rest of humanity; between a life of ethical responsibility and one of dissolute irresponsibility; between gratitude for what we have been given and bottomless craving for what we lack; and, finally—perhaps most importantly—between self-mastery and unbridled passion. To be sure, these boundary lines are not always sharp or carved in stone. All of us, from time to time, need help in discerning these demarcations. For some, psychotherapy helps provide a guiding light, illuminated by the wisdom of Judaic and Buddhist insights.

References

1. Sigalow E. American JewBu. Princeton University Press; 2019.
2. Ellis RM. 'Confession of a Buddhist Atheist' by Stephen Batchelor. (Book review). Middle Way Society. https://www.middlewaysociety.org/books/the-middle-way-in-buddhism-books/confession-of-a-buddhist-atheist-by-stephen-batchelor/. Accessed 01 Mar 23.
3. Segall SZ. Is Buddhism non-theistic? The Existential Buddhist. May 6, 2011. https://www.existential-buddhist.com/2011/05/is-buddhism-non-theistic/. Accessed 01 Mar 23.
4. Babylonian Talmud, Shabbat 31a. https://www.sefaria.org/Shabbat.31a.6?lang=bi&with=About&lang2=en
5. Vilaythong TO, Nosek BA, Lindner NM. "Do unto others": effects of priming the golden rule on Buddhists' and Christians' attitudes toward gay people. J Sci Study Relig. 2010;49(3):494–506. http://www.jstor.org/stable/40959032
6. O'Brien B. What does Buddha dharma mean? Learn Religions. March 28, 2018. https://www.learnreligions.com/what-is-the-buddha-dharma-449710
7. Babylonian Talmud, Sanhedrin 92a. https://www.sefaria.org/Sanhedrin.92a.14?lang=bi&with=all&lang2=en
8. Maimonides M. The guide for the perplexed. Translated by M. Friedlander. New York: Dover Publications; 1956, p. 118.
9. Dhammapada: The sayings of the Buddha. Translated by T. Byrom. Shambhala Pocket Classics; 1993.
10. Chah A. Living Dhamma. The Sangha, Bung Wai Forest Monastery; 1992.
11. Maimonides M. *Hilchot Edut* (9:9–10).
12. Savitz H. Maimonides' hygiene of the soul. Ann Med Hist. 1932;4(1):80–6.
13. Gelberman JH. Physician of the soul. Freedom: Crossing Press; 2000.
14. Tulku C. Gates to Buddhist practice. Padma Publishing; 1993.
15. Chah A. Everything arises, everything falls away. Shambhala; 2005.
16. Hattin M. Kedoshim: love your fellow as yourself. September 21, 2014. https://www.etzion.org.il/en/tanakh/torah/sefer-vayikra/parashat-kedoshim/kedoshim-love-your-fellow-yourself
17. Wallace BA, Wilhelm S. Tibetan Buddhism from the ground up. Boston: Wisdom Publications; 1993.
18. Sumedho A. Is Buddhism a religion? BuddhaSasana. https://www.budsas.org/ebud/ebdha164.htm
19. Lieber M. Pirke Avos Treasury. Edited by N. Scherman. Brooklyn: Mesorah Publications; 1995.
20. Gewirtz L. The Authentic Jew and His Judaism. An analysis of the basic concepts of the Jewish religion. Bloch Pub. Co; 1st Edition, 1961.
21. Burtt EA. The teachings of the compassionate Buddha. Mentor; 1982.
22. Schell B. If you meet the Buddha on the road, kill him. Daily Buddhism/The Five Minute Buddhist. December 6, 2008. https://www.dailybuddhism.com/archives/670
23. Aitken Roshi. https://rudyh.org/buddhist-quotes-buddhism-quotations.htm
24. The Dhammapada. Translated by Juan Mascaro. Penguin Classics, 1973.
25. Sherwin BL, Cohen SJ. Creating an ethical Jewish life. Jewish Lights; 2001.
26. Gribetz J. Wise words: Jewish thoughts and stories through the ages. Harper Perrennial; 2004.
27. Thanissaro Bhikkhu (Geoffrey DeGraff). Head & heart together: essays on the Buddhist path. 2010. https://www.accesstoinsight.org/lib/authors/thanissaro/headandheartbook.pdf
28. Pema Chodron. The answer to anger & aggression is patience. Lion's Roar. Undated. https://www.lionsroar.com/the-answer-to-anger-aggression-is-patience/
29. Cited by Dovid Lieberman. How free will works. Accessed at: https://drdavidlieberman.com/wp-content/uploads/2017/01/how_free_will_works_for_printer.305-440.pdf
30. Abramson HM. The Kabbalah of forgiveness. 2014. Retrieved from https://touroscholar.touro.edu/lcas_books/2
31. Maimonides M. Eight chapters, chapter 5.
32. Ibn Gabirol S. Mivhar Hapeninim (A choice of pearls). Chapter 10.
33. Dalai Lama. Quoted in: How to Find Inner Peace—the Buddhist Way, by Victor M. Parachin. Spirituality + Health. https://www.spiritualityhealth.com/inner-peace-the-buddhist-way

Fifty Years and Counting: Meditation Practice and Experience in the Context of a Psychiatric Career

James L. Fleming

I am grateful to have the opportunity to share my experience of a life long journey of meditation and spiritual development. It also happens to be a journey that helped give me a start on a career as a physician and psychiatrist. I hope readers will enjoy discovering as I have important connections between psychiatry and Eastern meditation and spirituality. I will also describe how meditation led me to some remarkable Christian experiences and how this affected my life. The offer from the editor to write this chapter is also relevant and timely for me: I have just launched a website and blog I've called "The Bible Psychiatrist" as I continue to work on a book by the same name.

Perhaps the best way to bring out the points I wish to cover is to tell the story chronologically, the story of how I experienced these parallel journeys. First, a little background. I was raised in a middle-class family in Wisconsin and found out quite early from my dear mother—who took me and my three sisters to a local Methodist church as kids—that prior to getting married, she made my father promise that any children resulting from their union would ***not*** be raised Catholic. Despite his deep faith and strong Irish connection to the Catholic Church. Sadly for my father, due to rigid rules about marrying outside of the Catholic

Church, he was "excommunicated" (or at least that is how he understood the consequences for him of how they married). I grew up as a regular attendee at the Methodist church sometimes with mom but never with dad and while I grew to learn of his devout faith in God, he showed no interest in becoming Methodist or in joining a Protestant church. This brief background becomes relevant to my story after learning to meditate in college.

From Track Star to Meditator

As a scholarship runner (track and cross-country) at the University of Wisconsin in 1971, I aspired to go to medical school. While always a good student in high school, I was not prepared for the rigors of a pre-med curriculum especially while also running intense two-a-day workouts. And unlike other scholarship athletes, we were expected to run both track and cross-country so had to train year-round. I was "stressed and depressed" and not making the kind of grades I would need to be admitted to medical school which was very competitive at that time. I'm sure I would have met criteria for trichotillomania as I pulled out chunks of hair trying to figure out answers to calculus questions. Some of my friends on the track team noticed my stress level and told me I ***had to*** learn TM (Transcendental Meditation, https://www.tm.org/) as they themselves had. I learned TM in late April 1972,

---

J. L. Fleming (✉)
Private Practice: Integrative Psychiatry,
Kansas City, MO, USA

H. S. Moffic et al. (eds.), *Eastern Religions, Spirituality, and Psychiatry*,
https://doi.org/10.1007/978-3-031-56744-5_24

and the results were remarkable: first, I felt more rested than ever before and showed immediate improvements in my track performance including a cutting 6 seconds off my mile time in the Big Ten meet, running a 4:04 mile which won my heat, getting beat only by another freshman who ran a half second faster and also won his heat. I recall being deeply rested before the race and specifically did not recall any "pain" during the actual race. I was truly impressed with this meditation stuff!

Next, I noticed I could focus and study without effort. With only a few weeks in the semester after I learned to meditate, it was too late to raise my grade point average (then a dismal 2.7) by the end of my freshman year, but after getting all "A"s in my first semester of my second year, my GPA steadily increased until graduation with only one B. Again, I was impressed! I certainly enjoyed the rejuvenation which reliably occurred during the actual meditation sessions, but the positive effects on my academic and athletic performance made the recommended practice of regular, twice daily meditation a "no brainer." In psychological terms, these self-reinforcing benefits of meditations became strong motivators for adherence to a regular, twice daily meditation schedule.

What About Enlightenment?

I had learned TM for the deep rest and clearer thinking supported by the scientific research presented during the introductory lecture and within a few short months I could definitely vouch for many of these benefits. But what about the promise of "higher states of consciousness," enlightenment, which was briefly discussed in the TM introductory and subsequent advanced lectures? I wasn't particularly interested in, but nor was I averse to, learning about this. But by the end of the cross-country season in the fall of my sophomore year, I started to have experiences of expanded consciousness that were—to put it mildly— overwhelming. I spoke with a TM teacher about these experiences who enthusiastically proclaimed: "this is Cosmic Consciousness!"

Well, even though his assessment was certainly very premature, whatever it was that I was experiencing was not blissful or even neutral but rather dysphoric. It also felt like a great burden that I hadn't really sign up for!

Stabilizing Pure Consciousness

I do believe I was having strong but temporary experiences of expanded consciousness which hadn't been integrated or stabilized yet. Eventually, the intensity of these experiences diminished and while I focused on my studies and track and cross-country participation, I also ended up pursuing more opportunities for more knowledge about development of consciousness along with extended meditation periods on weekend "residence courses" offered by the TM organization. From time to time I experienced the phenomenon of "witnessing," a sense of watching oneself similar to depersonalization (a type of dissociative experience) but once stabilized is experienced not as dysphoric but rather as a sense of stable separateness from the constantly changing world of relativity. Cosmic consciousness (abbreviated CC in the TM community) was synonymous with enlightenment and involves the simultaneous maintenance of "transcendental consciousness," also referred to as pure consciousness or pure awareness, along with the other three changing states of consciousness: waking, dreaming, and sleeping. I will return to the discussion of higher states of consciousness (yes, CC is not the pinnacle of the evolution of consciousness) but back to the story.

By the time I finished my undergraduate degree, I had gotten more involved with the TM organization and took training to become a "checker," i.e., one who leads meditators through a procedure known as checking which was aimed insuring correct meditation practice and experience. Being an effortless technique rather one involving effort or concentration, checking primarily ensures that the practitioner is allowing the process of meditation to occur without effort, i.e., without attempts to control or get rid of thoughts, resist outside noises or to try and produce any particular experience. One is also instructed to not resist sleep if it comes in meditation since this is assumed to provide a natural need for more rest. As I became more involved with TM I moved into the TM center, in a former fraternity house on the campus of the University of Wisconsin—Madison. I later became inspired to become a TM instructor and did so in 1977 for Phase I in residence in Iowa, phase II (fieldwork in Madison) and Phase III in Switzerland in 1978.

Enter the Spirit

While living at the TM center, I also started to have some spiritual experiences that were fundamentally different from anything I had previously experienced or heard or read about in association with TM. However in retrospect these experiences certainly fit with the stage of evolution which Maharishi referred to as "God Consciousness" (or GC), defined as appreciation of "the finest relative" (God) in every experience [1]. While development from waking state of consciousness to CC primarily occurred on a mental level, the process of development from CC to GC was said to one of "refinement of the heart." In actuality, these two phases develop simultaneously rather than sequentially, the different aspects of development being the more important factor.

How this all unfolded for me ended up having repercussions which still reverberate in my current life. Here is how it happened: the TM center was two blocks away from the University Catholic Center and several of the active TM teachers and meditators started going to Mass there. One Sunday, I was sitting in one of the balcony rows in the church and while the priest was consecrating the bread and wine and saying the Eucharistic prayers, I experienced something so powerful and meaningful that it simply can't be adequately described in words. But here is the essence: put plainly I experienced, rather suddenly, a very powerful, loving spiritual presence entering my consciousness which I understood as Christ purging my heart, "wringing it out" as it were, of all smallness and limitation and while

this presence did not speak in audible words, the intent of the message to me was crystal clear: I, (Christ) am real, I am here (in this Eucharist), you are loved, you are forgiven, I am "calling" or "choosing" you. The experience was the most powerful and "real" spiritual experience I had ever had up to that point. I have never forgotten that day and when I share the experience with others (which is not often), I am fond of mentioning that I think "the Lord" has a good sense of timing since that Sunday just happened to be the Feast of Corpus Christi (Body of Christ)! This was the beginning of other similar encounters over the subsequent 45 years. These encounters, which felt like unbidden, yet welcomed "visitations," in general have a very different quality from most experiences associated with my TM practice, although I am convinced that meditation opened my consciousness and "softened" my heart to allow these experiences to emerge. One of these visitations however was very directly connected to a particular meditation session and I think it is of interest to describe the different components of this experience.

Limits of Mind and Opening of the Heart

Sitting in meditation 1 day in my room at the TM center, I began to experience the usual settling down of my mind and physiology toward what Maharishi described variously as "pure consciousness," "transcendental consciousness," or the "simplest form of awareness" in the sense that it is consciousness in its pure form without an external object of awareness. What happened next however was something of a different order which I still find remarkable: it was as if the quiet state of awareness—which felt like being at the bottom of an elevator—suddenly lost its bottom and I felt myself swept up into what felt like a cosmic heart of compassion which was much deeper and more expansive than my own individual consciousness. As in the experience in church on the Feast of Corpus Christi, I felt the distinct presences of Christ's consciousness but this time, the intention was to show me the massive needs of many millions of people in Latin America and the clear message was that I was to have some important role in helping these populations. Now, suffice it to say this vision did not manifest in any major way that had any significant impact and if anything, the problems and suffering, especially in Central Americans increased as indicated by the massive increase in immigrants presenting at the U.S. southern border. But I think it's interesting, that I did subsequently travel to Puerto Rico, Mexico, Cuba, Brazil and—between 2004 and 2017—six times to Nicaragua, variously for medical mission trips, team building in poor communities, tree planting, and educational exchange with mental health professionals. At this point, readers may be asking how a meditation technique originating from the Vedic tradition of ancient India could produce distinctly Christian experiences. I would say the answer is two-fold: (1) the TM technique turns out to be just what is promoted to be: a "mechanical" mental technique which does not promote or provide any particular religious experiences but rather facilitates a neurophysiological state correlated with expansions of consciousness and (2) The character of experience of any individual TM practitioner (and presumably any non-sectarian meditation technique) is likely determined by the religious background and current religious context. This latter assertion would seem to be a testable hypothesis.

Despite these powerful, "Christ-conscious" experiences which started fairly early in my fifty year meditation career, most of my spiritual reading and study during that time, much of it on TM Teacher Training courses, was focused on Vedic literature such as the Bhagavad Gita rather than Christian literature. After the "Corpus Christi" experience, I did start taking classes in Catholicism and within less than a year became a confirmed Catholic, much to the chagrin of my mother![1] (see second paragraph). Almost 30 years later I would become an Oblate of St Benedict's Abbey in Atchison, KS and serve as a Cantor in Mass. Meanwhile I also married a fellow TM

teacher who later became a Unity Minister (Unity a form of "New Thought Christianity" arose in the early twentieth century as an alternative to conventional theology especially fundamentalism which was on the rise at that time). I have also been working on a book, The Bible Psychiatrist, based on 20 years of study of the Bible. I mention these activities to bring out the following points: not only did my practice of a meditation technique which originated from an Eastern source not dissuade my becoming involved in Christianity, I am sure it actually led to my "conversion" which literally means "to turn around" (in a spiritual sense). Subsequently, my meditation practice continued to enrich my Christian spiritual experience.

On Becoming a Psychiatrist

A nearly 4.0 GPA and fairly good MCAT scores were not enough for me to overcome the competitive 3:1 ratio of applicants to admittees to medical school in 1975. But not getting into med school at that time allowed me to pursue TM Teacher Training in Iowa, and then Switzerland. Shortly after returning from Switzerland, I enrolled in a graduate school program in physiology, hoping to do research on the "neurophysiology of higher states of consciousness," an area I had already begun to read about in the scientific literature. And while as a grad student, I did conduct a small pilot study in meditation practitioners using visual evoked potential (EEG), I was unable to find a faculty member interested in taking on a doctorate student in my area of interest. Also, since grad students shared some of the same classes as medical students, I was able to notice that they seemed to be having a lot more fun than the grad students. So I applied to med school again, and this time was admitted to the Medical College of Wisconsin, conveniently located in my home town of Milwaukee.

On TM Teacher Training, the many hours of meditation (4–6 h/day for a total of 9 months) as well as extensive study of the Vedic literature along with scientific research on the effects of meditation made the choice of psychiatry easy. In

---

[1] Thankfully, her dismay did not last and we continued to have a close relationship until her passing in April of 2022

fact, I knew on the first day of medical school that I would specialize in psychiatry. Having discovered the powerful potential of consciousness both experientially and from an intellectual standpoint, it seemed that any other choice would have been inadequate. Fortunately, the psychiatry residency program I participated in still had a strong focus on psychotherapy and the biopsychosocial model vs the trend at the time in many residencies toward a "bio-bio-bio" model (as one past President of the American Psychiatric Association described a concerning trend). Below, I describe several key connecting points between psychiatry and meditation but one point became evident early on in my residency, in particular in my second year when we had 7 hours per week of supervision, all but 1 hour of which was psychotherapy supervision and most of that was psychodynamic psychotherapy. What I noticed was that the largely non-directive, insight-oriented therapy we were practicing lent itself to frequent periods of silence in therapy sessions. These periods of silence reminded me of the silent state of mind in meditation and conversely, I think my meditation experience helped me appreciate and feel more comfortable with silence in therapy and allowed me to use it more effectively.

The Psychiatry-Meditation Connection

Here are some other connecting points between psychiatry and meditation as I experienced these two areas over the last 30 years:

1. The process of "stress release" or "normalization of the nervous system" which is said to occur in meditation as a result of providing a deep and unique state would seem to provide an important and unique means of healing. Much of what we do in psychiatry is akin to managing symptoms rather than facilitating healing, although skilled therapists can often help motivated patients undergo fundamental change resulting in personality change and greater fulfillment. For meditation, the changes occur more automatically without consciously trying to analyze or even attend to or even be mindful of particular issues or past experiences such traumatic events. Ironically, even though TM is mental technique, the resultant positive changes occur on a physiological level. This occurs by exposing the nervous system to a deep and unique form of rest and then stabilizing the changes that occur by engaging in our usual daily activities.

2. The concept of physiological change, presumably including in neural circuitry may be particularly useful in the treatment of Post-Traumatic Stress Disorder (PTSD) for which re-exposure to traumatic memories has been considered a key ingredient to symptom improvement. Unfortunately, this re-exposure can itself be stressful and the fear of having to re-live trauma can lead some people to avoid treatment. Given this dilemma, I found interesting a study originally published in Lancet Psychiatry in late 2018 which reported Veterans with PTSD who participated in TM sessions over a 12-week period showed symptom improvements similar to those who participated in prolonged exposure therapy sessions [2]. This suggests that exposure to past trauma may not be necessary for improvement and recovery.

3. With regular meditation over the course of months and years, fundamental improvements in self-image, resiliency, and competency tend to occur. Theoretically, this makes sense: if we are contacting a deeper, more stable sense of our own being, this should make us less vulnerable to many challenges with which life confronts us. Perhaps the best example of an unstable sense occurs in patients with borderline personality disorder (BPD). It is as though the individual sense of self is defined by outside situations especially other people and this leads to inevitable disappointments and rapid shifts from idealization to devaluation of others. While I am unaware of any case studies or other research on the use of TM per se in BPD, an interesting study published in 2021 looked at mindfulness, an important component of many types of meditation as well as in dialectical behavioral therapy, the

"gold standard" for treatment of BPD [3]. The authors compared mindfulness-based DBT skills training to interpersonal-based skills training and found that the mindfulness approach was more effective in reducing BPD symptoms, particularly emotional dysregulation.

4. I would hypothesize that TM practice in patients with BPD as well as other disorders would enhance effectiveness of standard psychotherapeutic strategies. I would assume other techniques could have similar effects and the literature certainly supports the effectiveness of mindfulness-based stress reduction techniques. However, I believe it would be a mistake to lump all meditation and relaxation techniques into the same category or assume they all have equal efficacy for various symptoms and conditions. For example, meta-analysis showed Transcendental Meditation (TM) to be significantly more effective than ordinary rest in producing a physiological state consistent with decreased stress (e.g., decrease blood lactate and respiratory rate) [4]. Another meta-analysis compared TM with several other forms of meditation and relaxation and found that TM was significantly more effective at increasing measures of self-actualization and psychological health [5].

5. Teaching our patients a simple meditation technique can provide an entry into important new self-care strategies. One cognitive-behavioral principle I find very useful is the idea (backed up by extensive experience of many meditation practitioners including myself) that expanded consciousness greatly strengthens our ability to cope with virtually any stressor. Small or limited awareness is easily overwhelmed by even moderate stressors; when consciousness is expanded, it becomes like a wide-angle lens which on the one hand makes the "size" of the stressor less, but at the same time allows us see or think of more options to deal with it. With practice, these strategies can also help reduce reliance on controlled substances for stress, anxiety, insomnia, etc.

6. Of course, in order for us to teach meditation, we need to be quite familiar with the experience of meditation and its use in our lives and then we must be able to effectively communicate the "how" of meditation to our patients at the appropriate time. I've had the advantage of many years of meditation practice as well as the benefit of being a trained meditation instructor. In addition, in about 1998, Maharishi spoke to meditating doctors and encouraged us to begin teaching our patients a very simple meditation technique which he called "the simplest form of awareness." Unlike the regular TM course which takes about 8 h over the course of 5 days, this technique can be taught in a few minutes. I have adopted this simple strategy and incorporated some other elements of TM into a technique I have called "Effortless Meditation." I introduce the concept and—if acceptable to the patient—the experience of this meditation early on in treatment for most of my patients in private practice. We then review their practice in subsequent sessions. Many of my patients have incorporated this type of meditation into their daily routine, often with modifications individualized to the patient.

7. Complementary to experience gained in meditation, intellectual understanding gained by listening to trusted teachers and/or reading revered literature is generally believed to be important if not essential to one's personal development and spiritual growth. I believe these resources can also be helpful in clinical work with patients. One of the most revered scriptures for Hindus which is also easily accessible to others is the Bhagavad Gita (Gita). I personally never tire of reading it and have mainly relied on Maharishi's translation and commentary on the first six Chapters [6]. I am especially fond of Chapter 2 which contains Lord Krishna's explanation of the immortality of the soul to the great warrior Arjuna, just as a great battle is about to begin. Early on the Gita, Arjuna becomes acutely conflicted and is so distressed that he feels completely unable to fulfill his "dharma" (duty) as a military commander which is to

lead the forces of good into battle thereby rescuing society from forces of evil. When Krishna asks him to look at the assembled armies arrayed in battle formation, he is distressed when he sees his own teachers as well as kinsmen and in short order he descends into a state of panic and paralysis. An amazing dialogue about the nature of reality, of dharma and of enlightenment ensues and becomes the basis for the remainder of the Gita.

I can think of at least two important applications in psychiatry of this crucial dialogue from Chapter 2 of the Gita:

A. Military and others (such as frontline healthcare workers), due to their duties, can at times become highly conflicted as Arjuna was when they must take extreme actions: for soldiers, killing an enemy and for frontline health workers, being unable to provide adequate care to patients in a pandemic and having to allow some patients to languish or die. Helping warriors/caregivers remember the ultimate, immortal essence of the people upon whom severe consequences are wrought can help mitigate against *moral injury*, which is capable of producing post-traumatic symptomatology, *not due to what one has **seen** but rather due to what one has **done or not done**.*

B. At some point in our lives—a point at which I have arrived in recent years—most of us become aware in a very concrete fashion of our own mortality. It's remarkable how young people are able to put off any real cognizance of the transient nature of each human life. That's probably a good thing: otherwise, we might not be very motivated to marry, have children, pursue a career, work to improve society and our natural environment, etc. But when faced with death, either of friends and loved ones or our own impending death, it can be helpful to our mental health, even essential, to have a sense of immortality of the soul. Otherwise, given the infinite expanse of time after we vanish with this earthly sphere, what would be the point of anything we do or experi-

ence? Religious faith often fulfills the sense of purpose to our lives because of the belief that our existence does not end when the body stops functioning but rather endures in some important way. Various religions make different assertions and give different degrees of explanations about this issue. While subscribing to Christian faith and doctrine, I actually find the detailed description of the persistence of the soul from the Bhagavad Gita to be much more intellectually satisfying than simple assertions of faith or expositions of religious doctrine. I hope others will find this passage from Chapter 2 of the Gita as enriching and reassuring as I have. I will leave it each reader to decide whether and how they would utilize this knowledge. Readers may also want to see an interesting article from the psychiatric literature in 2014 which reviews some cognitive-behavioral aspects of the interaction between Arjuna and Krishna while also briefly addressing the role of the Gita in contemporary Indian psychiatry [7].

Enlightenment on the Battle Field of Life

The following section begins after Arjuna declares that he "will not fight" due to his sense of profound conflict which has severely weakened his nature and created in his mind "confusion about dharma" (duty). He also surrenders to Lord Krishna for guidance. Then, despite the profound desperateness of the situation, with the great warrior "sorrowing in the midst of the two armies," Lord Krishna, in his unshakeable Absolute nature, addressing Arjuna "smilingly" speaks these words:

> You grieve for those for whom there should be no grief, yet speak as do the wise. Wise men grieve neither for the dead nor for the living.
> There was never a time when I was not, nor you, nor these rulers of men. Nor will there ever be a time when all of us shall cease to be.
> As the dweller in the body passes into childhood, youth and old age, so also does he pass into another body. This does not bewilder the wise. (v. 11–13)

These bodies are known to have an end; the dweller in the body is eternal, imperishable, infinite. Therefore, O Bharata, fight! (v. 18)

He is never born, nor does he ever die; nor once having been does he cease to be. Unborn, eternal, everlasting, ancient, he is not slain when the body is slain. (v. 20)

Weapons cannot cleave him, nor fire burn him; water cannot wet him, wind dry him away. He is uncleavable; he cannot be burned; he cannot be wetted nor yet can he be dried. He is eternal, all pervading, stable, immovable, ever the same. He is declared to be unmanifest, unthinkable, unchangeable; therefore knowing him as such you should not grieve. (v. 23–25)

Creatures are unmanifest in the beginning, manifest in the middle state and unmanifest again at the end, O Bharata! What grief is there in this? (v. 28)

Ah, so rich are these words! Obviously, there is much more to be discussed here. I have just scratched the surface of potential psychiatric applications of the wisdom of such profound literature as the Bhagavad Gita. But I hope the sharing of my spiritual journey and insights gained from meditation, study, and clinical experience has been informative and inspiring.

In Gratitude

I would like to end in the traditional Indian manner of giving gratitude and honoring one's guru (spiritual teacher), in this case, Maharishi Mahesh Yogi, who made available the technique of Transcendental Meditation which has allowed me so many wonderful opportunities: spiritual, personal, and professional, and without which, I'm not sure I would have otherwise had. But Maharishi's preferred way for his students to express gratitude was to acknowledge his own teacher, Swami Brahmananda Saraswati who at the later part of this life served as the Shankaracharya (teacher in the tradition of the great master Shankara) of Jyotir Math, Himalayas. And we also do this in the traditional way, simply by saying: "Jai Guru Dev."

References

1. Maharishi Mahesh Yogi. The science of being and art of living (Revised and updated edition, 2001), Plume, Penguin Group; 1963.
2. Zagorski N. Transcendental meditation may be as effective as exposure therapy for PTSD. Psychiatric News, Jan 3, 2019 (https://psychnews.psychiatryonline.org/doi/10.1176/appi.pn.2019.12b12). (Original abstract: https://www.thelancet.com/journals/lanpsy/article/PIIS2215-0366(18)30384-5/fulltext).
3. Schmidt C, et al. Mindfulness in borderline personality disorder: decentering mediates the effectiveness. Psicothema. 2021;33(3):407–14. https://doi.org/10.7334/psicothema2020.437.
4. Dillbeck M, et al. Decreased physiological stress markers through the transcendental meditation technique compared with ordinary rest. Am Psychol. 1987;42:879–81.
5. Alexander CN, et al. Transcendental meditation, self-actualization and psychological health: a conceptual overview and statistical meta-analysis. J Soc Behav Pers. 1991;6(5):189–247.
6. Maharishi Mahesh Yogi on the Bhagavad Gita. A translation and commentary chapters 1–6. Penguin Books; 1969.
7. Pandurangi A, et al. Psychotherapy in the Bhagavad Gita, the Hindu spiritual text. Am J Psychiatry. 2014;171:8.

Looking at the West Looking at the East: The Radical Western Search for Self Through the Faith of Imagined Others

Vincenzo Di Nicola

"Doctor Di Nicola's Report": Looking at the West Looking at the East

In "Doctor Brodie's Report," a *faux* anthropological tale written by the Argentine master Jorge Luis Borges [1], David Brodie, D.D., a Scottish Presbyterian missionary to the "backlying regions of Brazil," encounters the Yahoos and catalogs their ways, as missionaries, adventurers, and anthropologists used to do. The conceit is that the narrative, missing its first page, is found among the leaves of *The Arabian Nights,* itself a symbol of what Edward Said [2] called *orientalism* and I see, more simply, as the West looking at the East.

From this brief but vivid narrative, two observations stand out in the court of memory, to invoke Augustine's lovely phrase in his *Confessions*. In one, Doctor Brodie refuses the offer of sexual relations with the queen of the Yahoos, usually granted only to witch doctors, writing, "My cloth and my ethics … forbade me

V. Di Nicola (✉)
University of Montreal, Montréal, QC, Canada

The George Washington University,
Washington, DC, USA

World Association of Social Psychiatry (WASP),
Paris, France

Institut universitaire en santé mentale de Montréal
(IUSMM), Montréal, QC, Canada

that honor" [1, p. 137]. Raymond Prince [3], my mentor in Social and Transcultural Psychiatry at McGill University, reported just such an encounter with a witch of the Yoruba tribe in Nigeria in which he declined to imbibe a potion offered to him for fear that it contained human body parts, as a prelude to sexual intimacy with his Yoruba informant.

As Dr. Brodie continues the narrative of his cross-cultural encounter, the missionary looks for links between his own cosmology and that of his hosts, seeing parallels with his own:

> Only too well do I know the Yahoos to be a barbarous nation … but it would be unjust to overlook certain traits which redeem them. They have institutions of their own; they enjoy a king; they employ a language based upon abstract concepts; they believe, like the Hebrews and the Greeks, in the divine nature of poetry; and they surmise that the soul survives the death of the body. They also uphold the truth of punishments and rewards. After their fashion, they stand for civilization much as we ourselves do, in spite of our many transgressions. [1, pp. 145–146]

In a later encounter in the jungle with "black men who knew how to plough, to sow, and to pray, and with whom I made myself understood in Portuguese," he meets a "Romish missionary" (Protestants, in rejecting the authority of the Pope, challenged the universality of Catholicism by locating it in Rome) and despite recalling with "distinct pleasure" their theological debates, Doctor Brodie "had no success in turning him to *the true faith of Jesus*" [p. 145, italics added]. Decades later, I remain struck by the respect the missionary showed for other ways, gently refusing sexual intimacy as an undeserved privilege, and remaining steadfast in his own faith ("the true faith of Jesus"), despite his curiosity about others ("the Romish missionary").

Published in 1970 and mimicking nineteenth century travel narratives of missionaries, like the field reports of the Jesuits from New France or Brazil, Borges' parable gives us a glimpse of what it means to encounter differences, along with the limits of such encounters. Today, of course, all of this would be read under the rubric of colonization and cultural appropriation. Understood.

George Steiner was a polymath who grew up speaking several European languages simultaneously and dedicated his career to comparative cultural, linguistic, and literary studies. His masterwork *After Babel* [4] presents translation as the key concept and tool of intercultural communication. Here is Steiner [4] on the double-edged sword of twentieth century anthropological curiosity and exploitation:

> The notion of travelling to far places in order to study alien peoples and cultures, is unique to Western man; it springs from the predatory genius of the Greeks; no primitive peoples have ever come to study us. This is, on the one hand, a disinterested, intellectually inspired impulse. It is one of our glories. But it is, on the other, part and parcel of exploitation.... *The Western obsession with inquiry, with analysis, with the classification of all living forms, is itself a mode of subjugation, of psychological and technical mastery.* [4, p. 251, italics added]

Such are the risks. Nonetheless, let's take a page or two from both Borges and Said and imagine a traveler looking at other cultures and other societies (as we say in sociocultural psychiatry) and other "worlds" (as philosopher Alain Badiou would say) [5]. And allow me to call it, "Doctor Di Nicola's Report."

In this imagined voyage, I want to turn the philosophical notion of *le regard* or "the gaze," inside out. The gaze usually indicates an awareness and perception of the other. I propose to look at my fellow Westerners looking East, just as Doctor Brodie does in meeting another missionary of a different confession while both of them are looking at other cultures, other societies, and other religions—in short, other *worlds.* In our case, the other worlds are symbolically located in the East, although as I have written in my own travel narratives, I am not sure we ever really leave home [6] (see "At the Sufi Tavern" in this volume [7]). Nobelist V.S. Naipaul pithily couches this paradox in the title of his novel, *The Enigma of Arrival* [8]. In fact, we rarely arrive at our destination because we barely leave home. At best, like a snail bound to its shell, we take it with us wherever we go. And yet, we are restless: we move, we migrate, we conquer, we colonize. American philosopher of movement and migration Thomas Nail holds that we are all migrants and calls for a new psychology and a new politics of movement—*kinopsychology* and *kinopolitics* [9, 10].

And that's why my subtitle is, "The Radical Western Search for Self Through the Faith of Imagined Others." We imagine other faiths, other peoples, but it is more often a search for some sort of original self—a "genuine self" or "true self"—that is *discovered* or *constructed*, depending on the preferred framework [11]. The fact that we are often looking for ourselves through others in exotic, idealized or romanticized places means that we have to come to terms with human migration not only in economic and geopolitical terms but also as a search for meaning.

This chapter offers two perspectives on looking *elsewhere* for what life means *here.* These questions arise from a lifelong career in sociocultural psychiatry [6, 11, 12] and from work in the humanities, including philosophy and theology [13–15].

The first approach to Westerners looking to other traditions, notably Eastern religions, has been described (and criticized) as seeking what is *global and universal.* This approach deploys what we learned about the "classical school" of Social and Transcultural Psychiatry founded by psychiatrist Raymond Prince [3] and associates at McGill University in the 1950s to explore the religious and spiritual turn to the East. Is looking to another faith parallel to learning a new language, moving to a new country, or adopting a new gender identity? What do we know about changing languages, culture, gender, and other aspects of identity and its vicissitudes, including adaptation and the traumas that impede it, that might help us understand the motivation, the process, and the impacts of the religious turn? Another way of putting this is to ask whether what we have understood about psychology and psychiatry is "universal" as we used to say in the social sciences, "transcultural" as Transcultural Psychiatry put it, or "global" as the Global Mental Health movement now expresses it? Or do we Westerners have more to learn from other traditions than we have to teach them?

And that is the second perspective, associated with the "New Cross-cultural Psychiatry" established by anthropologist-psychiatrist Arthur Kleinman [16] at Harvard University in the 1970s, which asks what is *local and particular* about other worlds—cultures, languages, gender constructions, and religious traditions that makes it hard to understand them or import them to our world? [17] Are people so anchored in their mythologies and symbols, rituals, and practices as to be *rooted in place*? Can we empathize with other traditions enough to truly enter them and *can we transplant* them by retaining what is essential in new soil? From the universal to the particular, what is lost and what is gained in the encounters with other faiths?

The Search for Meaning

And what has all this to do with religion?

One way of looking at religion is this: aside from its claims to divine revelation or transcendental truth, socially, culturally, and historically *religion creates a community and a tradition built around an understanding of the world and our place in it; of forces both natural and divine and how to deal with them; and how to understand other people and our obligations to them.* The ambiguities and uncertainties of the world inspire the sense of awe and wonder that make some of us philosophers, and the search for meaning that make others believers.

Sojourning here in southern Brazil, presumably not far from Doctor Brodie's fictional Yahoos, and possibly a century or more later, there are fewer such encounters with the unknown. This country is now marked by a *creole culture*, blending origins and creations among the indigenous peoples, the European colonizers, and the slaves transported from Africa, all of which is celebrated in a *syncretic faith*, mixing Catholicism and more recently Evangelical Protestantism, with the belief systems that the African slaves brought with them. Now reconstructed as *Candomblé*, *Macumba* and *Umbanda*, these cosmologies have the same *deuses* (gods, in Portuguese) or *orixás* (an African word) in their pantheon as we encounter in Cuba's *Santería* or Haiti's *Voudoun*—originating in Yoruba, Bantu and Gbe cultures of West Africa. A celebrated Brazilian writer Jorge Amado, for example, nominally a Christian, also entered the world of *Candomblé*, the Afro-Brazilian religion of his native Bahia [18].

A Saída do São Sebastião In Salvador da Bahia, I had my first encounter with this Afro-Brazilian religion at a *terreiro do Candomblé*. Although it was not a folklore show typical of tourist sites, this *terreiro* or temple, located outside Salvador in a rural *favela* where the poverty was palpable, attracted both the curious and the studious. As the ceremony began, a young woman from Belgium was tittering nervously beside me and speaking to her friends in French about how phony it all was. *How can a spirit enter someone just because he shaved his head and they splatter some chicken blood and feathers all over it?* I asked her if she was Catholic which she acknowledged. And do you believe in the sacraments like communion? Again, she acknowledged that she did. Do you have an explanation for the transubstantiation of the wine into blood and the unleavened communion wafer into the body of Christ, I asked her? Few Catholics even think about it. Yet, is this so very different from what Catholics practice every time they go to Mass, I wondered aloud? American anthropologist Gregory Bateson [19] called such beliefs "metaphors that are meant"—where the bread IS the body, the wine IS the blood.

Later, I learned the real meaning of syncretism—the African *orixás* have their counterparts in both Greek mythology and Catholic saints, such as *Oxóssi, orixá* of hunting and forest, who is syncretized as *São Sebastião*, the Christian martyr who died with three arrows in the chest during the persecution of the Roman Emperor Diocletian. And the young man, in a trance, leaping into the air, with blood and feathers staining his white sacramental garments, resembled no one in my ken so much as St. Sebastian and, in my worldview, I wondered what kind of martyrdom this augured for him. The *saída* (which literally means "exit" in Portuguese) of the *orixá* or saint in fact marked his own *entrance* into the faith. And for him this meant a belief system, a community, and a new world. Unlike the young Belgium sceptic, I could only admire his courage and envy his journey.

Salman Rushdie [20], who knows something about religion and what it can do, is an Indian Muslim whose writing came afoul of the Mullahs of the Islamic Republic of Iran. Listen to his truth:

> In writing "The Satanic Verses," I think I was writing for the first time from the whole of myself. The English part, the Indian part. The part of me that loves London, and the part that longs for Bombay. And at my typewriter, alone, I could indulge this. But most of the time, people will ask me – will ask anyone like me – are you Indian? Pakistani? English? What is being expressed is a discomfort with a plural identity. And what I am saying to you – and saying in the novel – is that we have got to come to terms with this [20, p. 24].

We are all each other's guests. There is no middle kingdom, no master race, and no privileged starting point or hallowed end; just bits and fragments from here and there. But the world won't let this lie still and continues to express a discomfort with the pluriverse we have become. Yes, *we are here*, as Salman Rushdie affirms—*and we are always moving there*, as Thomas Nail argues.

Naming a Destination: *The Conference of the Birds*

> We are increasingly becoming a world of migrants, made up of bits and fragments from here, there. We are here. And we have never really left anywhere we have been.
> —Salman Rushdie [20, p. 24]

In the Sufi poem "The Conference of the Birds" written by Attar (Shaykh Farīd-Ud-Dīn Attar, 1145–1220) [21] in modern-day Turkey, the birds go as far as China to seek the Simorgh to lead them. After a long journey in which only thirty birds survive (*simorgh* means thirty birds in Persian), they gaze into the lake, only to see their own reflection. Like Attar's birds, Westerners looking for enlightenment, redemption or salvation in the East, the land of the imagined other and their idealized faith, may travel far, crossing seven valleys and many trials and tribulations—only to discover their own reflections.

Some say, "You can't go home again" (American novelist Thomas Wolfe). Others say, "You can and *must* go home again" (American family therapist James Framo). I say, *You never leave home and like a snail bound to its shell, you carry it with you wherever you go* [6].

By Way of Not Concluding: *The School of Suspicion*

Through narrative irony, the history of migrations [9, 10], and the epistemological ambiguities and uncertainties of knowing anyone or anything for sure, we Westerners have exploded the idea of knowing yourself and finding yourself through others.

In fact, as a social psychiatrist and philosopher, I would argue that such a search and this way of constructing psychology are misguided. We don't know—and can't know—ourselves easily anyways. Especially if that means that we may find our identities already forged, prepackaged and prepaid like so much processed food. The nineteenth century triumvirate of Friedrich Nietzsche, Sigmund Freud and Karl Marx that Paul Ricoeur [22] called *maîtres de soupçon*, "masters of suspicion" has put paid to this fantasy for us in the West. Collectively, the writings and followers of this *école de soupçon* or "school of suspicion" are not going to allow a simple-minded return to appearances which are inevitably deceptive, imbued as they are with hidden, forgotten and latent meanings, so that all our work is a *deconstruction* of the traces that haunt our investigations of the past, shadow the present and are continually projected into the future [23]. In my therapeutic work, I call this temporal triad of traces the *nostalgic past*, the *present imperfect*, and the *counterfactual future*. Our only escape is to imaginatively construct a future that does not conform to the so-called facts of the past and the supposed realities of our present.

Behind appearances are the disavowed, hidden, and repressed, but never completely erased, traces of the past, personal, and collective [23]. The only real question for us is not whether they are real but whether they belong to the realm of philosophy or of psychiatry. The most haunting passage for me as a social psychiatrist and philosopher in the considerable *oeuvre* of Michel Foucault [24] is this:

> It is of little importance on exactly which day in the autumn of 1888 Nietzsche went mad for good, and after which his texts no longer afford philosophy but psychiatry: all of them, including the postcard to Strindberg, belong to Nietzsche and all are related to *The Birth of Tragedy*. But we must not think of this continuity in terms of a system, of a thematics, or even of an existence: Nietzsche's madness – that is, the dissolution of his thought – is that by which his thought opens out onto the modern world. What made it impossible made it immediate for us; what took it from Nietzsche offers it to us. [24, pp. 287–88]

Excursus: In the Magic Theatre of the East: "For Madmen Only"

In Hermann Hesse's novel, *Steppenwolf* (1927) [25], Harry Haller (HH)—obviously a stand-in for the empirical author—confronts a midlife crisis. The novel tells the reader that a manuscript called, "Harry Haller's Records (For Madmen Only)," has been left haphazardly with a near-stranger who has the book published. HH is a university professor who was known in one field then turned to the study of Eastern religions and now finds himself an outsider in his own society, given to brusque and rude reactions even among old friends, rejecting their bourgeois sentimentality. In a serendipitous encounter, he comes across a book—"Treatise on the Steppenwolf"– which speaks to HH by name and describes his dual nature—a cultured and spiritual self, contrasted with a more animalistic, primitive part, "a wolf of the steppes." Contemplating suicide as his fiftieth birthday approaches, unable to reconcile his dual nature, HH walks all night and comes to rest at a dance hall where he meets the young Hermine who intuits his existential crisis. HH is intrigued and postpones his suicide for a second meeting with her. Hermine, a younger, feminine and more integrated version of himself, introduces HH to all that he considers bourgeois, and by association, corrupt and base—dancing, marijuana, a lover, and the sensuous Pablo, a musician. Pablo introduced HH to the "Magic Theatre"—"For Madmen Only"—in which HH experiences his full self through the fantasies that have haunted him, achieving what psychoanalyst R.D. Laing called "ontological security" [26].

Hermann Hesse (1877–1962), the empirical author, experienced psychiatry and psychoanalysis personally with a schizophrenic son and his own earlier dismissal from military service leading to psychotherapy and a friendship with Carl Jung. The parallels with HH, the ascribed or model author of *Steppenwolf*, are deep. For our purposes, I have always thought that the search elsewhere—in the East for both the empirical author and the ascribed author—is a stand-in for the search for self, a more integrated, balanced self to be found by looking within in one's own backyard, as it were, rather than voyaging afar. Are the experiences of The Magic Theatre only for madmen in the West? Short of madness, can we find them in the East? Many Westerners have thought so.

HH wasn't the first Westerner on this journey to the East and he wasn't the last. Another one, closer to our work, was Ronald David Laing (1927–1989) who spent time in Sri Lanka and India to study meditation and learn Sanskrit. We see this reflected in Laing's writing, especially *Knots* in which he describes his poetic schemas of relationships as the "webs of Maya" and refers to Buddha's metaphor of the finger and the moon [27] (see "*Excursus:* The Finger and the Moon").

So much for August Comte's nineteenth century *positivism* but perhaps more disappointingly for some of us in psychology, psychiatry, and psychotherapy, so much too for Edmund Husserl's *subjective phenomenology* and his followers, from Karl Jaspers to Ludwig Binswanger [14], as the science of grasping "things as they are." Wallace Stevens put it poetically in his fine poem, "The Man With The Blue Guitar" [28]. Someone in the audience (representing the empiricist and positivist scientist) complains:

> … '*You have a blue guitar,*
> *You do not play things as they are.*'

To which the guitarist (and the philosopher of deconstruction) answers:

> … '*Things as they are*
> *Are changed upon the blue guitar.*'

Knowledge and perception are as performative and prescriptive as they are archaeological and descriptive. In a world of new social realities, from social media to online avatars and porous identities, we can no longer rely on the verities of Alfred Korzybski's [29] *general semantics*, notably his famous dictum, "The map is *not* the territory." Michel Foucault [30] cited a short story by Jorge Luis Borges about a map the size of the territory it was supposed to represent [31]. As Borges (1946/1975) tells it, and Foucault revels in its reversal of representation, sometimes the Chinese emperor's men still get lost in the Badlands where pieces of the map are isomorphic with the territory.

Excursus: **The Finger and the Moon**

> The finger is not the moon.
> —The Buddha

Among observant Jews, the Torah is so sacred that its parchment rolled into scrolls cannot be touched so it is housed in well-crafted casings and dressed like a regal "bride," adorned with a

silver "breastplate" and "crown." Readers of the sacred scroll use a pointer called a *yad* (from Hebrew for hand) to track their reading of the text. The pointer, often made of silver, ends in a small hand with its index finger extended.

Several thoughts come to mind. First, religious folks happily get lost in their rituals and fetishize the trappings. If the divine is a sacred light, they reason, its earthly emanations are also illuminated by that light. The Buddha taught us not to mistake the finger pointing at the moon for the moon itself. Alfred Korzybski [29] formulated the same insight as a premise of general semantics: *The map is not the territory.*

Second, Jacques Derrida called his philosophical method *deconstruction* [23]. In brilliant archaeological digs into the roots and received meanings of words, Derrida carefully unearthed hidden meanings, lost nuances and forgotten connections among words and thoughts, the most celebrated being the φάρμακον (*phármakon*) or "Plato's pharmacy" in which he unpacked the meaning of Plato's narrative about his teacher Socrates in a dialogue with Phaedrus about the indeterminacy of translation [23]. The pharmakon is about *polysemy*, the multiple meanings of words. It can ambiguously point to the binary "poison" or "remedy," but it can also signify "scapegoat" and highlights the undecidability of words. I connect this also to Socrates' death by hemlock in which it is both a poison, ending his life, and an escape or cure from the untenable demands of the Athenian court that found him guilty of corrupting the youth. And in the end, its real meaning is revealed in this context, where Socrates is a scapegoat for other social and political dynamics of Athens.

Finally, with his deconstructive method, I see Derrida himself as a *yad*, a pointer in a recursive iteration of meanings, almost without end, and never quite getting there. During my philosophical investigations for my doctorate, I asked Derrida's son, Piero Alferi, who was one of my teachers, about this interpretation. He was delighted and told me that his father collected such *yads*. And so, for me, the circle is complete: from pointer to text to reader to interpretation—and back. The reader becomes the pointer, the text becomes the interpretation, and the interpretation is inseparable from the reader. The finger IS the moon; the map IS the territory.

Identity is always constructed through the mirror of attachment and early family relations [6, 32, 33]. As pediatrician and psychoanalyst Donald Winnicott wrote, before the so-called mirror phase (a reference to psychoanalyst Jacques Lacan's early work on identity formation) is the mother's face [34]. Finding yourself through others? We are only a personal collection of others to start with. The idea of swapping this set of faces from our first circle of intimates for another is attractive for some people—precisely perhaps those who are motivated by curiosity or dissatisfaction to move, to migrate, and to explore [35].

So, why not subvert all the verities?

The map IS the territory.

The journey IS the destination.

The bread IS the body and the wine IS the blood.

The finger IS the moon.

Home IS where your heart is.

Scottish psychiatrist-psychoanalyst Ronald David Laing wrote a classic psychiatric study called *The Divided Self* [36] followed by *Self and Others* [37]. In all his work, Laing addressed the paradox of the self and its divisions, attempting to heal them with his social phenomenology [26]. Now, at its heart, German philosopher Edmund Husserl's phenomenology is radically centered on the subjective experience of the individual. Calling for a *social* phenomenology is to reach beyond the individual self to social *others* in Laing's language. He never quite achieved it, in spite of many different projects, from a therapeutic community in London to poetic distillations of the "knots" of relationships [27]. Laing never quite gets to *self with others*, either in his work or in his own life (his son lamented that his father was a famous family psychiatrist who couldn't talk to his own family). And a bolder formulation

still would be *self through others*, which is the heart of attachment theory and a cornerstone of social psychiatry.

Laing did get something absolutely right. In a documentary episode of the Canadian television series, "Cities" [38] about his native Glasgow, Laing concluded in his soft Scottish accent …

> I once asked a man from Liverpool why he was living in London and he said it was because he wanted to be near the center of reality… Well, no Glasgow man would ever dream of leaving Glasgow in order to find the center of reality *elsewhere*. The center of reality is where one's heart is.

So much for colonization, so much for cultural appropriation!

And so ends my report.
Respectfully submitted,
Doctor Vincenzo Di Nicola, MD, PhD
Santa Maria, Rio Grande do Sul, Brazil
May 2023

Postscript: "If We Wanted Home Truths We Should Have Stayed Home"

> Whoever sees you from where he is, sees only himself.
> —Muhyiddin ibn 'Arabi [39, p. 210]

Either we encounter alterity and radical difference and prepare to lose ourselves or we stay home. Whether we call numinous encounters a "religious conversion" [40], a "search for the absolute" [39, p. 17], "limit-experiences" [24], "madness" [41], or the quasi-psychiatric "Jerusalem syndrome" and "Stendhal syndrome" that I described in another chapter ("At the Sufi Tavern" [7])—such experiences are inherently disorienting. And that may be a good thing. But if we take our starting points with us, we don't really get anywhere.

On the one hand, I believe that most of us, most of the time don't really leave home and we confuse the reassuring welcome of a new place with home. A famous American hotelier's slogan was, "The best surprise is no surprise." That may be appealing for people who hate to travel or do so often for business so that familiarity is comforting but genuine encounters with other cultures require something else altogether. It goes by different names: in literature the Russian formalists called it "defamiliarization," in psychoanalysis Freud described "the uncanny," and in theatre Bertolt Brecht employed the "estrangement effect," but the common thread is of a shocking encounter that renews our perceptions, like modern art that was brilliantly captured as "the shock of the new" [42].

Whether it's about anthropological encounters, religious pilgrimages or going "on mission" for the international community, America's preeminent cultural anthropologist, Clifford Geertz, distilled an insightful kicker: "If we wanted home truths, we should have stayed home" [43]. Now, if we really want to enter other worlds, if we have the cognitive skills to do it and moral strength to stand it, be sure that you will be changed by your journey and the destination. In a very real sense, as I testified about my own journey to meet my estranged father in Brazil [6] and as I describe my numinous encounters in another chapter in this volume ("At the Sufi Tavern" [7]), you don't come back to the same place from a real encounter because the defamiliarization, the uncanniness, the estrangement means you are no longer the same person.

"Light from the East": The Event

So, do Western psychology and psychiatry have adequate theories for this?

In spite of more than a century of Emil Kraepelin's "comparative psychiatry" (1904) [44] and 75 years of McGill University's Social and Transcultural Psychiatry (where I found my voice as a psychiatrist 40 years ago), the short answer is no. In that span, "transcultural psychiatry" morphed first into "cultural psychiatry," then into Global Mental Health, and has now branched into such progressive concerns as EDI (equity, diversity, inclusion). Cultural anthropology and cultural psychiatry now offer two things: first, seemingly endless variations on how *others* are different from us (ethnographies) and, second, *self-criticisms* about the structural or systemic

factors in place in our own worlds that create filters and persistent blind spots in our intercultural encounters and perceptions (EDI).

What they fail to address is what it would be like to have *genuine intercultural—and for our purposes interfaith—encounters*, what "genuine" could possibly mean, and how we would emerge from such encounters. Hence, I believe that cultural psychiatry is at an *asymptote*—the point of diminishing returns—and I invested 30 years in my own model of cultural family therapy [6, 11, 33]. After consulting widely across many different cultures and with many religious groups, I have tested its strengths and confronted its limits. There is little appetite either in Western psychiatry or in society generally for coaching people through cultural adaptations in new or rapidly changing societies. We have fetishized others as genuine and inherently authentic and are reluctant to help them integrate into our own rapidly changing and complex Western societies. What's more, we're apologetic about it. This leaves little room for the possibility of migration across borders, rapid change within societies, religious conversion, or revolution as an *Event* in people's lives.

Here in the Canadian province of Quebec, for example, we had a "national" commission—meaning *provincial* and this tells you everything you need to know about Quebec politics—into "reasonable accommodations" with our cultural communities. Nothing came of it. My comment was that no one could define what is "reasonable" and I suggested that we replace it with "reciprocal accommodations." It's a two-way street, after all.

Is such a theory possible? Yes, a theory that understands the nature of change and how new things come into the world. We have such a theory in the work of French philosopher Alain Badiou on the Event [5]. In foundational work on the *theory of the subject* [45], refocusing philosophy on *ontology* or being [5], Badiou offers a way to define the radical rupture with the ordinary world that occurs when an Event takes place, how it defines us as subjects of that Event, and through our fidelity to such a life-defining occurrence, how the change that comes with the Event offers a map for a new life and a new world. Badiou has put this in evidence in studies on everything from mathematics and politics to theatre and love, and critically relevant for this volume, on Saint Paul as the "foundation of universalism" [46].

The Event is nothing less than a theory of rupture, radical change, and revolution. If you want home truths, stay home, but if you really want to engage with another world, from Afro-Brazilian *Candomblé* to Middle Eastern Sufism to the traditions of Buddhism, Hinduism, and Shintoism and the panoply of cosmologies in the vast universe of what we fetishize as the Far East, be sure that you're in for a revolution. And what I learned from my own world-altering conversion and engagement with Judaism is that when you open one door, you close another. What does that mean? That means your answer to a total society from the newfound perspective of your faith, your coherent, organizing vision of living a life, doesn't encompass all the others. I try to preserve the familiar warmth of my Catholic childhood and the mature Jewish wisdom of my adult years, along with Sufism's bracing search for the absolute, through an abiding love for these human communities, albeit not in the same moment, not at the same place. I live a kind of personal "Rashomon effect," named for Kurosawa's classic Japanese movie in which several narratives of the same incident—a sexual assault and a murder—are related, each of them compelling yet contradictory [11].

What strikes me about people who live their faith deeply is that they do so without either apology or chauvinistic pride. When I was invited to a Vatican health conference, I was struck by the deep clarity and humility of Pope John Paul II. And how the physicians and health scholars were drawn to him from all faiths and cultures. That's why religion isn't only theology and spirituality isn't only a personal matter—it's a culture, an entire world. And why it's so hard to integrate a new one without profound structural changes in yourself and your social relations. To my fellow Westerners turning their gaze eastward, I am saying that we are rooted in place by custom and habit and that our search elsewhere is often for a substitute home that masks our origins and distorts our perceptions of other places and beliefs.

Here is the Tibetan Dalai Lama on "How to Be a Buddhist in Today's World" [47]:

> If you study the Buddha's teachings, you may find that some of them are in harmony with your views on societal values, science and consumerism—and some of them are not. That is fine. Continue to investigate and reflect on what you discover. In this way, whatever conclusion you reach will be based on reason, not simply on tradition, peer pressure or blind faith.

During a visit to Britain, the Dalai Lama went so far to say "that he did not wish to encourage people to convert to Buddhism. Instead, he emphasized the importance of staying with the religion in which one was raised" [48]. Other concerns range from "cultural appropriation" of other traditions to the "psychiatrization" [49] and "instrumentalization" of Eastern thought by isolating such practices as meditation from their cultural and religious roots [50] for instrumental ends such as symptom relief.

Every cultural community, every faith tradition has within it adequate resources to guide its members in their search for meaning, as we defined it above: *religion creates a community and a tradition built around an understanding of the world and our place in it; of forces both natural and divine and how to deal with them; and how to understand other people and our obligations to them.* We may nonetheless be ignorant of the depth, richness, and relevance of those resources.

Some of us are moved to find more congenial, more satisfying answers to life's challenges elsewhere. And it is the very interaction between the familiar and the strange that may be at the heart of the human story of migration [9, 10]. In his imaginative reconstruction of Marco Polo's voyages to the Mongol Empire in East Asia, Italo Calvino [51] offers this insight:

> Arriving at each new city, the traveler finds again a past of his that he did not know he had: the foreignness of what you no longer are or no longer possess lies in wait for you in foreign, unpossessed places.

Yet, looking elsewhere comes at a price and the more sincere and genuine the search, the more edifying the discovery, the more likely that it will trigger a tsunami of change—a veritable personal revolution that we call an Event.

References

1. Borges JL. Doctor Brodie's report. In: Doctor Brodie's report, trans. N.T. di Giovanni. New York: Bantam, 1973. p. 133–46.
2. Said EW. Orientalism. New York: Pantheon Books; 1978.
3. Prince R. Why this ecstasy: reflections on my life with madmen. Montreal: Avmor Art and Cultural Foundation; 2010.
4. Steiner G. Real presences: is there anything in what we say? London: Faber & Faber; 2010.
5. Badiou A. Being and event, trans. O. Feltham. London: Continuum; 2005.
6. Di Nicola V. A stranger in the family: culture, families, and therapy. Foreword by M. Andolfi, MD. New York/London: WW Norton & Co.; 1997.
7. Di Nicola V. At the Sufi Tavern: adventures in African and eastern spirituality. In: Moffic HS, et al., editors. Eastern religions, spirituality, and psychiatry. New York: Springer Nature; 2024.
8. Naipaul VS. The enigma of arrival. New York: Viking Press; 1987.
9. Nail T. The figure of the migrant. Stanford: Stanford University Press; 2015.
10. Nail T. Theory of the border. Oxford: Oxford University Press; 2016.
11. Di Nicola V. Letters to a young therapist: relational practices for the coming community. Foreword by M Andolfi, MD. New York/Dresden: Atropos Press; 2011.
12. Di Nicola V. Luminaries in social psychiatry—the *Gurū-Chelā* relationship revisited: the contemporary relevance of the work of Indian psychiatrist Jaswant Singh Neki. World Soc Psychiatry. 2022;4(3):182–6.
13. Di Nicola V. Letter to young psychiatrists. "Small answers"—lessons for the left hand. Washington Psychiatr Mag. Summer 2017;12–14.
14. Di Nicola V, Stoyanov D. Psychiatry in crisis: at the crossroads of social science, the humanities, and neuroscience. Foreword by K.W.M. Fulford, MD, Afterword by A. Frances, MD. Cham: Springer Nature; 2021.
15. Di Nicola V. On vit déjà dans l'avenir de l'illusion de Freud: La foi au risque de la psychanalyse ou la psychanalyse au risque de la foi? [We are already living in the future of Freud's illusion: faith confronted by psychoanalysis or psychoanalysis confronted by faith?], 1ère Colloque Inaugural de la Moroccan Association of Dynamic Psychiatry (MADP) [1st inaugural conference of MADP], Oujda, Morocco, March 11–12, 2022.
16. Kleinman AM. Depression, somatization and the *"new cross-cultural psychiatry"*. Soc Sci Med. 1977;11(1):3–10. https://doi.org/10.1016/0037-7856(77)90138-X. PMID 887955.
17. Geertz C. Local knowledge: further essays in interpretive anthropology. New York: Basic Books; 1983.
18. Trindade-Serra OJ. Jorge Amado, Sincretismo e Candomblé: Duas Travessias [Jorge Amado, syncretism and Candomblé: two crossings]. Rev Antropol. 1995;38(1):101–68. (In Portuguese).
19. Bateson G. Steps to an ecology of mind: collected essays in anthropology, psychiatry, evolution, and epistemology. Chicago: University of Chicago Press; 1972.
20. Marzorati G. Salman Rushdie: Fiction's embattled infidel. N Y Times Mag. January 29, 1989, Section 6.
21. Attar F. Conference of the birds, trans. S. Wolpé. New York/London: W.W. Norton & Co.; 2017.
22. Ricoeur P. Freud and philosophy: an essay on interpretation, trans. D. Savage. New Haven: Yale University Press; 1970 (French original, 1965).
23. Derrida J. Plato's pharmacy. In: Dissemination, trans. B. Johnson. Chicago: University of Chicago Press; 1981. p. 63–171.
24. Foucault M. Madness and civilization: a history of insanity in the age of reason, abridged, trans. R. Howard. London: Tavistock, 1964.
25. Hesse, H. Steppenwolf, trans. B. Creighton. New York: Holt, Rinehart and Winston, 1963. (German original, 1927).
26. Laing RD. The use of existential phenomenology in psychotherapy. In: Zeig JK, editor. The evolution of psychotherapy. New York: Brunner/Mazel; 1987. p. 203–10.
27. Laing RD. Knots. London: Tavistock Publications; 1970.
28. Stevens W. The man with the blue guitar and other poems. New York: Alfred A. Knopf; 1937.
29. Korzybski A. Science and sanity: an introduction to non-Aristotelian systems and general semantics. Lakeville: The International Non-Aristotelian Library Pub. Co.; 1933.
30. Foucault M. The order of things: an archaeology of the human sciences, trans. A. Sheridan. New York: Pantheon, 1970.
31. Borges JL. On exactitude in science. In: A universal history of infamy, trans. N.T. di Giovanni. London: Penguin Books, 1975. (Spanish original, 1946).
32. Di Nicola V. "A person is a person through other persons": a manifesto for 21st century social psychiatry. In: Gogineni RR, Pumariega AJ, Kallivayalil R, Kastrup M, Rothe EM, editors. The WASP textbook on social psychiatry: historical, developmental, cultural, and clinical perspectives. New York: Oxford University Press; 2023. p. 44–67. https://doi.org/10.1093/med/9780197521359.003.0005.
33. Di Nicola V, Song S. Family matters: the family as a resource for the mental, social, and rela-

tional well-being of migrants, asylum seekers, and other displaced populations. In: Gogineni RR, Pumariega AJ, Kallivayalil R, Kastrup M, Rothe EM, editors. The WASP textbook on social psychiatry: historical, developmental, cultural, and clinical perspectives. New York: Oxford University Press; 2023. p. 244–55. https://doi.org/10.1093/med/9780197521359.003.0005.

34. Nussbaum MC. Dr. true self, review of F. Robert Rodman, Winnicott: life and work. In: Philosophical interventions: 1986–2011. Oxford: Oxford University Press; 2011. p. 274–84.

35. Grinberg L, Grinberg R. Psychoanalytic perspectives on migration and exile, trans. N. Festinger. New Haven: Yale University Press; 1989.

36. Laing RD. The divided self: an existential study in sanity and madness. London: Tavistock Publications; 1960.

37. Laing RD. The self and others. London: Tavistock Publications; 1961.

38. Laing RD. "R.D. Laing's Glasgow." Documentary in the "Cities" series, Director J. McGreevy. Toronto: Canadian Broadcasting Corporation Cities, 1979. Available at: https://www.youtube.com/watch?v=Nuf-402VpRs. Last Accessed 25 May 2023.

39. Adonis. Sufism and surrealism, trans. J. Cumberbatch. London: SAQI Books, 2005.

40. James W. The varieties of religious experience: a study in human nature, being the Gifford lectures on natural religion delivered at Edinburgh in 1901–1902. London: Longmans, Green & Co.; 1902.

41. Kusters W. A philosophy of madness: the experience of psychotic thinking, trans. N. Forest-Flier. Cambridge, MA: MIT Press, 2020.

42. Hughes R. The shock of the new: art and the century of change. London: Thames & Hudson; 1980.

43. Geertz C. Anti anti-relativism. In: Available light: anthropological reflections on philosophical topics. Princeton: Princeton University Press; 2001. p. 42–67.

44. Jilek WG. Emil Kraepelin and comparative socio-cultural psychiatry. Eur Arch Psychiatry Clin Neurosci. 1995;245:231–8. https://doi.org/10.1007/BF02191802.

45. Badiou, A. Theory of the subject, trans. B. Bosteels. New York: Continuum, 2009.

46. Badiou, A. Saint Paul: the foundation of universalism, trans. R. Bassier. Stanford: Stanford University Press, 2003.

47. Dalai Lama, Tenzin Gyatso. How to be a Buddhist in today's world. Wall Street J. July 6, 2017. Available from: https://www.dalailama.com/messages/religious-harmony-1/how-to-be-a-buddhist-in-todays-world. Last accessed 25 May 2023.

48. Batchelor S. Faith & reason: no more Buddhists, says Dalai Lama. Independent (UK Edition). Saturday 29 May 1999. Available from: https://www.independent.co.uk/news/people/faith-reason-no-more-buddhists-says-dalai-lama-1096508.html. Last accessed 25 May 2023.

49. Mills C. Decolonizing global mental health: the psychiatrization of the majority world. London/New York: Routledge; 2014.

50. Kelly BD. Buddhist psychology, psychotherapy and the brain: a critical introduction. Transcult Psychiatry. 2008;45(1):5–30. https://doi.org/10.1177/1363461507087996.

51. Calvino I. Invisible cities, trans. W. Weaver. New York: Harcourt Brace Jovanovich; 1978.

Part IV

Social Psychiatric Perspectives

At the Sufi Tavern: Adventures in African and Eastern Spirituality

Vincenzo Di Nicola

The Said, the Unsaid, and the Unsayable

> If you do not witness what cannot be said, you will shatter what can be said.
> —al-Niffari (cited by Adonis, 2005, p. 212) [1]

A running thread throughout Western culture of the twentieth century concerned what can be said and what cannot be said. This was as true for the humanities and the social sciences as it was for philosophy. Here are two examples from philosophy and *belles-lettres* as bookends. The concluding proposition of Ludwig Wittgenstein's *Tractatus Logico-Philosophicus* [2], the most famous philosophical text of the twentieth century, asserts:

> Whereof one cannot speak, one must consign to silence.

Wittgenstein is easily misunderstood here. What he is saying is that we should aim to be clear on those things about which it is possible to be clear: factual statements about the world and about our perceptions of the world. What he is

V. Di Nicola (✉)
University of Montreal, Montréal, QC, Canada

The George Washington University, Washington, DC, USA

World Association of Social Psychiatry (WASP), Paris, France

Institut universitaire en santé mentale de Montréal (IUSMM), Montréal, QC, Canada

not saying is that these other things that lack clarity are unimportant. In fact, he made it clear that those other things, about which we must *as philosophers* remain silent, are by far more important: aesthetics, religion, and transcendent truths. In *Culture and Value*, Wittgenstein [3] asked: "Is what I am doing [my work in philosophy] really worth the effort? Yes, but only if a light shines on it from above."

In a celebrated essay on silence, Susan Sontag ([4], p. 6) observed that:

> The art of our time is noisy with appeals for silence. A coquettish, even cheerful nihilism. One recognizes the imperative of silence, but goes on speaking anyway.

Sontag's essay on silence is an answer to Wittgenstein, insisting on the necessity to speak—and to do so clearly and intelligibly. She turns Wittgenstein on his head, essentially asserting in her anxious activism, *Whereof we cannot be silent, thereof we must speak* [5].

Silence may be explored in psychoanalysis—whether in the reticence of the analyst or the resistance of the analysand. It was spoken in the sparkling poetry of Polish Nobelist Wisława Szymborska ([6], p. 261):

> When I pronounce the word Future,
> the first syllable already belongs to the past.
> When I pronounce the word Silence,
> I destroy it.

And yet, a deeper truth about human existence is dialectical—we experience things that we don't quite have words for in any language and yet, at least some of us, philosophers and psychotherapists alike, want to express. Now, in every culture around the world, East and West, North and South, before psychiatry and psychoanalysis and even before philosophy, religion was there first. In fact, the theme that cuts across world religions concerns *the said, the unsaid, and the unsayable*. At the heart of Judaism's *mysterium tremendum* (the idea of the Holy) is the notion that we cannot truly know the divine and we cannot pronounce its name. To Jews, God is unsayable. In Hebrew, pious Jews refer simply to *HaShem*, "the Name." Islam's most profound assertion, the *Shahada*, a testimony, is stated as a negation, starting with *la*, Arabic for "no" …

> *La ilaha illa Allah*
> There is no God but God (Allah)

"I Have Understood Everything That You Have *Not* Said"

Transcultural Pediatrics Clinic, Maisonneuve-Rosemont Hospital, Montreal, Quebec, June 2005

Let us see how this applies in our work as psychotherapists. In the transcultural pediatrics clinic that I co-founded in Montreal, a therapist from Haiti told the mother of a family we were seeing in Creole, the common language of the people of Haiti: "I have understood everything that you have *not* said."

This is a very complex message! What is going on?

The mother was from Haiti as is my colleague, the psychotherapist. He understood from her discourse that she was *voudouisante*—that is, one who practices *Voudoun* (to be distinguished from the "Voodoo" of Louisiana), an African diasporic religion that developed in Haiti, *syncretically* combining traditional elements of West and Central African cultures, such as the Yoruba, with the Roman Catholicism imported by the French colonists. Due to the attitudes of the French colonists and their Haitian successors even after independence, *Voudoun* was proscribed in favor of the official state religion, Catholicism. While it is no longer proscribed, traditions die hard and many Haitians keep their beliefs and practices more or less secret. For a certain class of Haitians, practicing *Voudoun* is somewhere between the unsaid and the unsayable. The practices are simply unavowed, unsaid, while their actual beliefs– such as thinking that someone is *envouté* (bewitched) or a *chwal* (horse in Creole from *cheval* in French, meaning possessed)– are unsayable.

So, my Haitian colleague, seizing the fact that the mother made oblique references to her son's mental state in French colonialist terms (the said), understood that the *Voudoun* practices that she had pursued to help him were to be left unsaid, and her beliefs about his state, that he was *envouté* or a *chwal*, were altogether unsayable.

As Elbert Hubbard wrote, "He who does not understand your silence will probably not understand your words." [1] The Haitian psychotherapist attended to both the words that were said and the resonating silence of what was left unsaid. By empathically joining her, he offered an act of empathy. Could it also be understood as a provocation? A challenge? Could we call it an interpretation? More basically, what kind of interaction is this? Is it better understood as a clinical encounter or a cultural one? And what is more important here, is it therapy or religion? We can only guess but we must make the effort. As the father in one of the most memorable cases in my book on cultural family therapy, *A Stranger in the Family*, ([7], p. 243) qualified when I tried to reframe their predicament as questions about a cultural encounter between the Middle East (Syria/Lebanon) and the West (Canada), "Human questions, *human* questions!"

Empathy, provocation, interpretation—all of these are possible, yet if we stay close to the lived experience of the mother and her family—that R.D. Laing called *social phenomenology* [8]— what the Haitian psychotherapist offered was a testimony. And this testimony was an acknowledgment aimed at liberating her from the burden of keeping her religious practices and beliefs secret, voicing the unsaid and allowing us to open space for the unsayable in therapy.

At the Sufi Tavern

> Every era has to reinvent the project of "spirituality" for itself.
> —Susan Sontag [4], p. 1

At the Sufi Center, Montreal, Quebec, October 2006

We are all strangers here. And Sufism, a mystical branch of Islam, is an alien, Eastern presence in this outpost of Western civilization. When people asked about the Sufi Center in Montreal, Shaykh Farhat, our Tunisian Sufi mentor, encouraged his followers to engage them warmly and positively. Rather than complain about Islamophobia in Montreal, the Shaykh exhorted them to live their faith and show themselves: *We are Sufis, this is Islam.* And in lighter moments, the Shaykh would say, *Tell them it's a Sufi tavern.* It's a self-deprecating joke since practicing Muslims do not drink alcohol (ironically, an Arabic word, *al-kuhul*). And yet, like all ironies, it reveals a deeper truth: Sufism is intoxicating (Fig. 26.1).

An African Night at the Sufi Center—March 2007

The Ivorians, the Malis (*maliens* in French, playfully teased by the others with a French pun on their name, *malins,* meaning crafty, cunning), and the Senegalese Sufis transport me to Africa. The prayers are louder that night, the revelers more ebullient, the communal meal more voraciously eaten, and the dancing that continued well into the night was altogether more vibrant.

I got drunk from vertigo just watching them spin …

Then, late into the night, Shaykh Farhat arrives and invites me to dance …

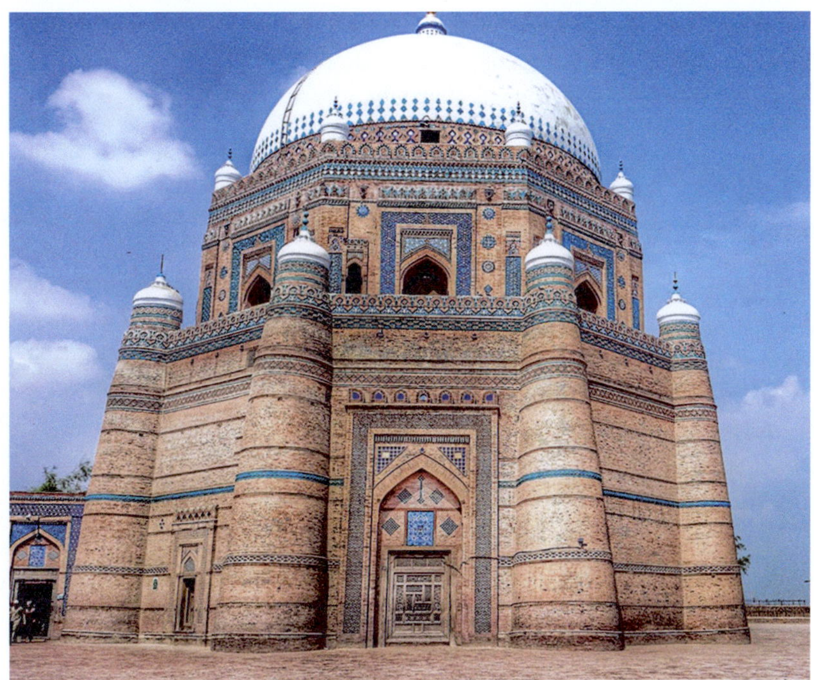

Fig. 26.1 The Tomb of Shah Rukn-e-Alam (built 1324 A.D.) is located in Multan, Pakistan. Known for its multitude of Sufi shrines, Multan is nicknamed as *The City of Saints*. (Source: https://en.wikipedia.org/wiki/Sufism#/media/File:Tomb_of_Shah_Rukn-e-Alam_2014-07-31.jpg)

"I get vertigo," I warn him.

"I will support you," he replies.

And he does. And I spin. And … well, did I experience vertigo? Did I enter another dimension?

First, it's important to understand how were we chosen for this honor—and honor it was, granted by the Shaykh. The Shaykh would point to someone, indicating his turn to dance, to spin. All men with one exception: a young Turkish woman, the only woman there who turned, who was spinning … deliberately, slowly, with great control, and then with abandon. It reminded me of the Calvinistic notion of the "elect" … Who could dance and who could merely watch?

> O body swayed to music, o brightening glance
> How can we know the dancer from the dance?
> —W.B. Yeats [9]

And I knew that this verse, waiting inside me since my youth–I could see it on the printed page of my copy of Yeats' poem—was finally coming to life in front of my eyes.

Second, the significance of dance among the Sufis is that it is a state of non-speech ([1], p. 211). The Turkish girl spun elegantly, effortlessly, and wordlessly. Her body silhouetted against the light as her dress billowed out from her spinning, her glance brightening the room, occasionally falling on my face … or was it just a coincidence? No, another turn, and there it was again. We are elementary particles circling an atomic nucleus … she's an electron to my proton—whirling around the Shaykh as our nucleus ([10], p. 14).

And I'm charmed in rapture, losing track of time, perhaps even my strange identity, and both the dancer and the dance lose their boundaries and etch themselves into my neural patterns … as I start crying …

"Knowing What You Are Not Supposed to Know, Feeling What You Are Not Supposed to Feel"

99 Names for Crying ([11], p 147)
>And I think of the 99 names of Allah.
>which start with Allah the Compassionate, Allah the Merciful …
>and the 99 names of Allah become the 99 names of his tears,
>this other man who lives my life,
>and I tell him that he is …
>*Crying for release, crying for pity, crying in pain, crying for relief,*
>*crying in compassion, crying because you have no permission to cry,*
>*crying because you have not cried enough, and because it is too late …*
>*and crying in anticipation of the pain you will surely feel for love …*
>*And your tears are a prayer for those who have no tears.*
>*and for those who have no prayers …*
>*Crying for knowing what you are not supposed to know.*
>*and crying for feeling what you are not supposed to feel …*

The final lines of my Sufi poem ([11], p. 147) were inspired by a very insightful article by John Bowlby, the psychiatrist-psychoanalyst who created attachment theory [12].

Such numinous moments are like pearls strewn by chance in our paths … and we can do no better than "to *dance* on the feet of chance" to invoke Friedrich Nietzsche at his most irreverent in *Thus Spake Zarathustra* (cited in [13], p. 290). I experienced such a moment during the time of my engagement with Judaism in Jerusalem (Fig. 26.2) [14].

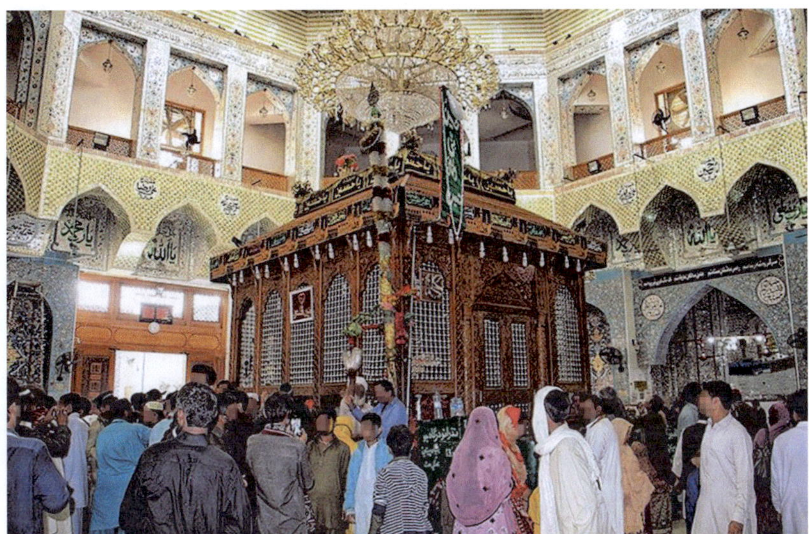

Fig. 26.2 Muslim pilgrims gathered around the *ḍarīḥ* covering the grave (*qabr*) of the thirteenth-century Sufi saint Lal Shahbaz Qalandar, a shrine located in Sehwan Sharif, Pakistan. (Source: https://commons.wikimedia.org/wiki/File:Shrine_Lal_Shahbaz_Qalandar,_Sehwan_Shareed,_Pakistan.jpg)

Jerusalem Syndrome

At the Damascus Gate, the sun casting its oblique light over the Jerusalem stone rendering it like the song, "Yerushalayim Shel Zahav"/"*Jerusalem of Gold," Jerusalem, Israel, August 1979.*

A young man with *payot*—the long sidelocks particular to observant Jewish men—who is with the Chabad-Lubavitchers approaches me and asks me in a Brooklyn accent in English, "Did you bind *tefillin* today?"

"What's tefillin?"

"Phylacteries."

"Well, that's clear," I turn to say to my Israeli girlfriend. Then, turning back, I ask him, "What's a phylactery?"

She steps aside to let me have my moment as the Chabadnik shows me little leather boxes with long leather straps which he winds around his left arm.

"Right-handed or left-handed?" he asks.

"Left."

"It's worn on the other side of your writing hand," he explained, reaching for my right arm. In spite of being older, a medical student, I submit passively, like a *yeshivah bocher*—a young Talmud student.

He binds my arm with leather straps, carefully lacing them so that the phylactery—a little leather box encasing a holy scripture—is placed on my arm while another is placed on my forehead.

Then he recites a *brachah* or prayer. He points to a book he is holding, "Can you read Hebrew?"

"Like a child," I say.

"That's enough," he says.

I recite the *brachah* in my halting Hebrew.

I feel faint. The setting sun on the ancient stones, this strange new experience, the leather straps impinging on the venous return to my heart … was there an explanation for feeling faint? Or am I confusing and conflating biology and belief?

No matter. My sense of self or whatever was left of it, was melting into the stones.

I am not sure that I ever, entirely came back to my senses.

Psychiatrists there call it "Jerusalem Syndrome." [15] Usually reserved for overly pious Jews and madmen. "For madmen only," Hermann Hesse wrote of the Magic Theatre in his novel, *Steppenwolf* [16] about a man who becomes alienated from human society. So be it—I was among the mad. And let it be a cleansing madness [17].

"After Three Days, Forget Everything"

At the Sufi Center, Montreal, Quebec, April 2007

One evening when the Catholic Pope was in the news, Ali an Iranian Sufi whom I had met as the chef at Rumi Restaurant, a short walk from the Sufi Center, asked me for my opinion of John Paul II since he knew that I was raised a Catholic and had met the Pope. Although I tried to give a balanced view, I thought later that maybe he could take offense at my explanation. The next time I saw Ali, I asked him for forgiveness if my thoughts about the Pope gave offense. And Ali, replied, *I don't know what you are referring to.* And I recalled our conversation. Again, he said he had no recollection. As I tried to explain yet again, he interjected, *The Prophet said after three days, forget everything.* I calculated: our conversation had taken place a week before. And as Shaykh Farhat often said, with an open-handed gesture toward the Sufi temple and the Sufis around him, *This is Sufism, this is Islam.*

There are doubts and scholarly debates about the origins of Sufism. What is consensual is that Sufism is part of Islam, representing the "inward dimension of Islam," which is characterized by asceticism, mysticism, and esotericism. There are the Sufis texts themselves which tell their history and there are *orientalist* readings of Sufism [18], which I call the West looking at the East (see another chapter in this volume) [19]. It cannot be any other way. There is no sure reconstruction of the past, it's always a contemporary reading for our needs, here and now. And the strength of tradition is precisely its capacity to give answers adapted to the present. As Augustine, the North African theologian of Christianity, replied when asked about the different practices in Milan and Rome of the Roman Empire, *When in Rome, do as the Romans do.*

Sontag's ([4], p. 1) update on that is wider one for a global culture: *Every era has to reinvent the project of "spirituality" for itself.* For Sontag, that project for her era was in the arts. Her essay on the aesthetics of silence was a late sign of Nietzsche's pronouncement of the death of God and an early sign of a postmodern culture where everything would be questioned, in the form of criticism (slouching toward nihilism) or irony (in a deflating satire).

Westerners, in my view, come to Sufism through an orientalist gesture that universalizes it [18]. They see its origins predating Islam. They read with enthusiasm that St. Francis of Assisi was a Sufi and that St. Teresa of Ávila, a Carmelite Nun who was born to Jewish conversos during the Spanish Inquisition after centuries of Islamic rule, and who wrote *Interior Castle* [20] one of the most celebrated texts of mystical theology, which owes its depth to the Jewish mystical tradition of the Kabbalah and to Sufism.

Now, this aspect of the life of Teresa of Ávila holds the key to my understanding of Sufism. Here is a bravado feat of association. There is a connecting link in these three historical phenomena:

- The Jewish conversos and Marranos of Portugal and Spain scattered around the world.
- Philosopher Leo Strauss' notion of exoteric versus esoteric writing [21]·
- Sufism as a form of arcane and secret knowledge.

Persecution and the Art of Writing— Believing and Writing in a Dangerous Time

When the Spanish Inquisition expelled Portuguese and Spanish Jews from the Iberian peninsula to Italy, North Africa, and the Ottoman Empire, their search for safety and security led to the transformation of the Jewish mystical tradition called Kabbalah into a messianic doctrine. Kabbalists imagined two aspects of God—a *concealed* God whose essence is transcendent, and a *revealed* God who is immanent, manifesting himself to humanity.

This dichotomy of what is revealed and what is concealed is repeated in Strauss' notion of *exo-*

teric writing (accessible for the many) and *esoteric* writing (hidden for the initiated few) and in Sufism's view of *appearances* (outward knowledge) versus *illumination* (intuitive knowledge which reason cannot access). We saw it in the interventions of the Haitian therapist with the Haitian mother who is a hidden *voudouisante*—"the said and the unsaid." And, finally, in an oblique reference to Hesse's *Steppenwolf* (elaborated in more detail in another chapter in this volume, "Looking at the West Looking at the East") [19], there is knowledge and experience available only to the select few, "For Madmen Only."

Relevant for our considerations about the relation between religion and psychiatry, throughout his work as a Jewish German philosopher, Leo Strauss stressed the tensions between "Jerusalem and Athens" or revelation and philosophy and whether one can be reduced to the other [20]. This is the stake for a dialogue between psychiatry and religion: *Will psychiatry adopt positivism, determinism and materialism in its attitude towards religion?*

Strauss argued that esoteric writing by premodern philosophers was a way to preserve the truth not from the crowd (who didn't read much anyway before modern times) but from those who did read and were empowered to defend the status quo. Esoteric writing was a form of self-censorship in dangerous times, artfully concealing the truth through textual subterfuges. According to Strauss, modern rationalism implodes upon itself: what starts as a modern quest for delineating scientific standards in the name of certain knowledge (represented by positivism, determinism, and materialism) leads to the conclusion that there are neither such standards nor such truths (represented for Strauss by the metaphysics of German philosopher Martin Heidegger and for us by the social construction of knowledge and cultural relativism).

Strauss believed that the enlightenment critique of religion ultimately meant the self-destruction of rationalism because the philosophical conclusion that scientific knowledge is "the highest form of knowledge" would lead to a "depreciation of pre-scientific knowledge." In this, Strauss was prescient and visionary. Strauss rejected above all the Enlightenment's view of the "self-sufficiency of reason." By being on the side of Enlightenment, of the self-sufficiency of reason, translated today as Evidence-Based Medicine (EBM), psychiatry depreciates what religion represents—revelation and illumination—meaning reality beyond appearances, truths beyond empiricism, values beyond materialism.

What Sufism (and other numinous experiences that I am describing here) represents is precisely the possibility that there are human experiences beyond our ken along with a radical doubt that the consensual reality to which modernity reduces all experience is the whole of the truth. In the end, from positivism to phenomenology, modernity clearly believes that a science of appearances is an understanding of reality. I have contested that in my Sufi-inspired "Slow Thought Manifesto" [22] and in our book on *Psychiatry in Crisis* [23]. Furthermore, I believe with Strauss that a psychiatry deprived of the capacity to value what religion and spirituality represent (and not for the weak pretext of diversity) is an impoverished psychiatry that doesn't deal with a core, fundamental aspect of human nature—and one quite different from mental illness as it is conceived today as deficit or dysfunction. What religion and spirituality, especially in their mystical varieties, represent are not such limitations but possibilities. As American philosopher of religion William James affirmed, "We believe all that we can. We would believe everything if we could." [24]

Here is a final provocation pitting science against belief. Since I cannot do the higher mathematics of theoretical physics, a statement that *neutrinos* (neutral subatomic particles with a mass close to zero and half-integral spin, which rarely react with normal matter, and are the most abundant particles in the universe) *are bombarding us* is as verifiable (within my means) as the Sufi belief that *djinn* (mostly invisible non-human beings) *circulate among us unnoticed*. I have to take both of these matters, if I take them at all, on faith.

The Shortest Shadow

Stat crux dum volvitur orbis.
The Cross is steady while the world turns.
—From The Order of the Carthusians [25]

From a shopping center in Santa Maria to a Carthusian Convent in Ivorá, Rio Grande do Sul, Brazil, September 2013.

In my meanderings between faith and what philosopher Simon Critchley calls the "faith of the faithless," [26] I have traversed the three Abrahamic faiths and some of their avatars. Sometimes, I was sure I was on the right path. More often, I lost sight of the path altogether in a "dark wood" as Dante Alighieri, Italy's great poet, described his mid-life crisis in the opening lines of *La Divina Commedia,* or *The Divine Comedy* (composed in Italian, 1308–1321).

In a true tale, much like Paul Auster's *The Red Notebook* [27], I find the path again. Auster is a master of the chance encounter, leaving people at a loss—characters and readers alike. We are at the *Convento da Cartuxa de Nossa Senhora Medianeira* in Ivorá near the city of Santa Maria in the southern Brazilian state of Rio Grande do Sul. "The Carthusian Convent of Our Lady of Mediation." The *Ordem dos Cartuxos*—the Order of the Carthusians—is an enclosed religious order whose Latin motto is, *Stat crux dum volvitur orbis,* "The Cross is steady while the world turns." [25]

How we got there is a story in itself. At a modern shopping center in Santa Maria, we are at a dress shop and while my fiancée Letícia is trying on clothes, I found myself in a dialogue with the shop owner. Complimenting me on my idiomatic Portuguese in spite of my foreign accent, she listens as I explain that I am a stranger and curious about exploring the countryside. She tells me that there is a monastery nearby, in a breathtakingly beautiful setting, set atop the *serra* or highland overlooking the plateau where Santa Maria is located.

When I express interest in visiting it, she informs me that the Carthusians are a cloistered community of monks who take a vow of silence. But maybe she could arrange something. The monks produce honey and specialty wines that she helps to market. And there was something that she needed to deliver to them. She would arrange a meeting with her contact there who could show us around, if would we deliver something to the monks.

Coming out of the changing room, Letícia was intrigued. As we work out the details, she and the shop owner discover a social connection—a cousin of Letícia's. The next day, map in hand (since the GPS is unreliable on the *serra*) and the package we are to deliver safely stored in the trunk of our rented car, we set out for Ivorá and the monastery. We drive by it several times, unsure if we are really there. Set atop the highland on a level plain, the monastery is surrounded by so much fenced-off land that we could not be sure we had arrived. There was no grand entrance and only the simplest of signs indicating its presence, pointing to a small dirt road leading to the monastery.

The monk who met us at the appointed time was in fact a priest and the Prior of the order, greeting us in fluent but slightly accented Portuguese, like my own. He showed Letícia and I around the foregrounds of the Carthusian monastery and then offered us something to drink in a small, dark and cool visitors' alcove, away from the burning noonday sun when the "shortest shadow" falls, as Nietzsche declared [28].

Could we visit the monastery itself? On two conditions: I could visit the monks' quarters, the refectory and the chapel with him but Letícia had to wait outside. And the second condition? Within the monastery, I had to respect the vow of silence and not interact with the monks I met. After consulting with Letícia, she encouraged me to go in.

We went in, the Prior and I, to visit the cells and the chapel. Inside the chapel, we sat down face to face and without ceremony, he asked me, *Why are you here?* As I hesitated, he started talking about himself. He was Belgian and had lived and worked in sub-Saharan Africa, in Italy, in Israel, and now in Brazil. I told him I'm Italian, working in French in Montreal, that I had also briefly lived in Israel, and had family in Brazil where I had met Letícia. He looked at me intently, without averting his gaze and plunged into his reading of me … *You are older than she … you have a past … you have doubts … that is why you are here* … the spaces between his probes were little eternities in which I could live alternative histories.

Although we had started in Brazilian Portuguese, our exchange now migrated to continental French, peppered with the occasional modern Hebrew phrase and liturgical Latin, and ambled back to Portuguese. He talked about the Carthusian Order and their convents—*chartreuses* in French. I wondered aloud about Stendhal's stirring novel, *La Chartreuse de Parme—The Charterhouse of Parma* [29]—about love across borders, secret and forbidden, desired yet incomplete. He knew it of course: he was a worldly man who had retired from the world. And his sagacious nod made it suddenly seem so serendipitously revealing. Was I living a version of the notorious *Stendhal syndrome*—an exquisite response to an aesthetic or religious experience? [30, 31]

As we talked, time stood still. Not so much that it lasted long but that the conversation entered a timeless dimension where past, present, and future lost their boundaries, like Haitian Créole that has no tenses. There were moments when I swear I heard phrases in Spanish and Italian in a kind of *grammelot*, the language pastiche of the *commedia dell'arte* [32]. Think of a wiser version of the character Salvatore, speaking a language soup of Latin, Italian and Provençale in Umberto Eco's *The Name of the Rose* [33], but remaining wild somehow and untamable—and you have him. A veritable *Steppenwolf!*

In this inverse confession where the Carthusian Prior divined my reasons and my fears, the burning light of the noonday sun was mimicked by his polyglot discourse entombed in the silence of the monastery. This shortest of shadows nevertheless revealed that my project of "two becoming one" with Letícia was precisely upside down. Not the unity of all truth embraced by the sun, but its moment of splitting at noonday, "the shortest shadow," when "one turns into two" (Friedrich Nietzsche's notion, brilliantly elaborated by Slovenian philosopher Alenka Zupančič) [28]. Me and my shadow. In this case, where I recognize my multiplicity, my otherness in the light of

my new relationship. And to accept her uniqueness and difference.

On the clock, the encounter, as I reckoned after we left, had lasted some 45–50 minutes, like the famous "50-minute hour" of psychoanalysis. But it felt like some strange story from Jorge Luis Borges—"The Aleph" [34] perhaps, or Ambrose Bierce's memorable story, "An Occurrence at Owl Creek" (1890)—where entire episodes, memories, even lifetimes are lived in mere seconds and where time loses all meaning.

I did not return to Letícia the same man, since I was two—me and my shadow, which opens space for the other. And she knew nothing of my inverse confession with the Prior of the Carthusian Convent, nor of who knows what "mediation" occurred there. We were married the following year after all and now have a daughter, Anita Sofia.

And what is the moral of this true tale? That we need to arm ourselves against today's antinomies of dogged determinism and excessive rationalism (both often in the guise of scientism). So, there are two connected lessons to be drawn for our purposes. Just as *chance* is a fence against a dogged determinism, *mysticism* is a shield against the excessive rationalism of our times. As for chance, I follow French philosopher Alain Badiou [35] rather than his countryman, Nobelist in Medicine Jacques Monod, whose *Chance and Necessity* [36]—a staple of my youthful reading—is biological reductionism in the name of so-called objective knowledge. As a philosopher of psychiatry, my answer to Monod would be: *Chance, yes, but not necessity*, the latter of which many consider a kind of scientific heresy and a distortion of Darwin's evolution. If I believe in anything it is in *pure contingency*—chance, randomness and, sometimes, *serendipity* or the happy accident.

And as for mysticism, like Wittgenstein I prefer clarity and precision where it is possible, but also like him, I recognize that there are things that are not reducible to simplification. Mysticism is related to subjectivity, to personal experience. I see it as a shield to protect us from the Western war against subjectivity in *technopoly* [37], which is clearly also opposed to religion and spirituality except where it can be harnessed by industry to make their workers "more productive." Nothing is more profane to me than this *instrumentalization* of the sacred.

Both Letícia and Giuseppe, my late Italian father in Brazil, believed in destiny. My father's favorite opera was Giuseppe Verdi's *La forza del destino*, "The Force of Destiny" (Italian original, 1862). I hold by chance. Meaning is not given but conferred. My worldview is not deterministic, neither directed by a dark fate nor drawn to a bright destiny [38]. Things happen by pure contingency, not forgetting the forces that shape but do not determine them, and out of these accidents and happenstances of life, we make meaning.

That is why Paul Auster's work appeals to me. In *The Red Notebook* [27], he collected true tales of pure serendipity out of which he constructs awe and mystery with a pinch of suspicion. I am open to the possibility that there is another reality, a deeper, more authentic one under the illusions of appearances and the dogma of received wisdom. As a Catholic, I was raised on Augustine and Aquinas who brought a rational Hellenism to faith. When I engaged with Judaism and Jewish history through my conversion, I read the great rabbi, physician and philosopher, Maimonides' *Guide for the Perplexed* (written in Classical Arabic in Hebrew writing, 1190) which similarly tried to reconcile Aristotle with Rabbinic Judaism. In my studies in Sufism with Shaykh Farhat and Shaykh Omar in Montreal, I read the scholarly texts of the Sufis. But in the end, it is Augustine's *Confessions*, not his theology that persist in the "court of memory" as he called it. It is St. Francis and St. Teresa that remain after the residue of the Catholic Church settles down. It is the Jewish heretic Spinoza's appeal to reason balanced by emotion and the Kabbalah that persist, along with the searing testimony of the Shoah by Primo Levi and Jewish poets like Osip Mandelstam, Paul Celan, and Yehuda Amichai. And it is through great poets that Sufism abides: Adonis [1], in his brilliant exploration of *Sufism and Surrealism* (to which we could add psychoanalysis as a third sensibility) to grasp through reason and metaphor the unreason of mysticism. And it is the Sufi poets Rumi [39] and Rabi'a of Basra from the East who bring Sufism closer to home by revealing its heart through friendship and love.

Dénouement—*Chez Mambo Fabiola*

Mambo Fabiola's Voudoun Ounfò, Montréal-Nord, May 2014

After I gave a talk on cultural family therapy at the third Haitian Mental Health Summit [40], organized by Rebâti Santé Mentale and sponsored by my psychiatry department at the Université de Montréal, my wife Letícia and I joined my Haitian colleagues and the head of the department at a Haitian restaurant to celebrate. We were then invited to an evening at a *Voudoun ounfò* or temple in Montreal North.

When I told our host, the priestess or *mambo* Fabiola, that Letícia and I had been recently married in Brazil, she nodded appreciatively, encircled us with a big hug and said, "Let's see what we can do. I will arrange something for you." Intrigued, we sat down in the front of several rows of folding chairs in what was essentially a basement apartment, transformed into a temple, overflowing with believers and visitors.

With the rhythmic beating of drums, the atmosphere changed from friendly introductions to intense anticipation. What followed is best conveyed in a series of moments and images.

It was spiritual, it was religious, it was a prayer meeting. It was Catholic and *Voudoun*, it was syncretic.

It had a pace and a structure that I recognized—from the Catholic Mass of my childhood and my experience in the *terreiro do Candomblé* on the outskirts of Salvador da Bahia in Brazil 20 years earlier. And it was led by women. Mambo Fabiola and her fellow *mambos* were all women.

Throughout the long night, we felt the heat rising and the drums, as much through our feet through the floor as through our ears, pounding into our bodies. I whispered to Emmanuel, my departmental chair, how can they make such a ruckus and not have the police shut us down?

C'est Montréal-Nord, mon cher, c'est Haïti ici! It's Montreal North, my dear, we're in Haiti here!

I was transported back to my training days in transcultural psychiatry at McGill University, imagining realities beyond our own and adaptations we called "culture-bound syndromes" which has been criticized as exoticizing other peoples and their practices. Yet here were nurses, physicians, health care workers of all kinds that worked daily in our midst in our city, and this made it both more intimate and more intimidating. When Fabiola went into a trance, I was startled to attention. She was clearly in an altered state of being. Looking at the front row of worshippers and visitors, she passed me over sitting beside my new wife and chose Emmanuel, (who was single), to join her in a sensual dance during which her co-celebrants, the other *mambos*, threw a large colorful sheet over the two of them and the scene became more earthy and frankly erotic.

And the drums, always the drums banged out by the men … as the beat went on!

In this trance state, which I had no doubt now included my friend Emmanuel, I could discern elements of a culture-bound syndrome from Southeast Asia called "Latah"—where the graceful dancing of the *voudouissants* was punctuated by herky-jerky startle movements [41]. The role of the persons in a trance intrigued me—their actions, gestures, and facial expressions.

The drummers were like a Greek chorus, at times leading, at times responding, always part of whatever was happening in syncopated rhythms of this exquisite partnership between female *mambos* and male drummers.

Coda: "Where Is Here?" Emmanuel had explained that we were in *Montréal-Nord,* suggesting that it was a *quartier* of *Haïti.* Let's unpack this. In this territory of the land and peoples of Tiohtià:ke, colonized by the French who renamed it *Montréal* and who had also colonized *Haïti,* on a French island surrounded by a sea of English, we two psychiatrists from Europe (Emmanuel from France and myself from Italy) were celebrating with fellow immigrants from Haiti their own New World religion, *Voudoun,* a syncretic mix of what their ancestors had brought with them from West Africa and French Catholicism. Beside me was my wife Letícia, a fifth-generation Italian from Brazil which has a large population of African descendants who practice their own versions of Afro-Brazilian religions like *Candomblé* in Bahia. These are uniting, joining practices and worldviews—mixing and matching and melding into something new and different, strange yet familiar, inviting and intimidating all at once.

It's midnight of a moonlit night; time of the longest shadows. Letícia and I are still pulsating to the pounding of the drums, dancing, and wilting like hothouse flowers in the heat of the overcrowded temple. We are tired, but strangely alert. Mambo Fabiola hasn't forgotten us. She brings us together in front of the *Voudoun* congregation to bless our union. After a social celebration in Brazil and a civil ceremony in Montreal, Letícia and I can well and truly say we have been "joined" in a *Voudoun* marriage ritual *chez mambo Fabiola.* And where was this taking place, you may well ask? Tiohtià:ke or Montréal? Port-au-Prince (Haïti) or perhaps Porto Alegre (Brazil)? West Africa or Bahia? Canadian literary critic Northrop Frye ([42], p. 220) had a lasting insight about this:

> It seems to me that Canadian sensibility has been profoundly disturbed, not so much by our famous problem of identity … as by a series of paradoxes in what confronts that identity. It is less perplexed by the question "Who am I?" than by some such riddle as "Where is here?"

What these adventures in non-Western religion and spirituality open up for us is a redefinition of the sayable and the unsayable, what is known and what is not, and the feeling of being at home or feeling estranged. *The East that we seek—that we feel we need—is here, at our side.* As it always was. And what religion does, certainly what mystical beliefs and spiritual practices do, is to anchor you in place through a community of believers, and then, surprisingly, gracefully liberates you to transcend it, totally.

References

1. Adonis. Sufism and surrealism, trans. Cumberbatch J. London: SAQI Books; 2005.
2. Wittgenstein L. Tractatus Logico-Philosophicus, trans. Ogden CK, Moore GE, Ramsay FP. London: Routledge & Kegan Paul; 1922. (Original German, 1921).
3. Wittgenstein L. In: von Wright GH, editor. Culture and value. rev ed. London: Wiley-Blackwell; 1998. (Original German, 1977).
4. Sontag S. The aesthetics of silence. In: Styles of radical will. New York: Farrar, Straus & Giroux; 1969. p. 1–19.
5. Crispin DM. "Whereof one cannot be silent, thereof we must speak": Susan Sontag's "Silences," IIIIXIII Four By Three Magazine, Sept 9, 2016. http://christine-jakobson.squarespace.com/issue/susan-sontags-silences. Last accessed 3 June 2023.
6. Szymborska W. The three oddest words. In: Baranczak S, Cavanaugh, C, translators. Poems new and collected: 1957–1997. San Diego: Harcourt/A Harvest Book; 1999. p. 261.
7. Di Nicola V. A stranger in the family: culture, families, and therapy. Foreword by Andolfi M. New York/London: W.W. Norton & Co.; 1997.
8. Laing RD. The use of existential phenomenology in psychotherapy. In: Zeig JK, editor. The evolution of psychotherapy. New York: Brunner/Mazel; 1987. p. 203–10.
9. Yeats WB. Among school children. In: Finneran RJ, editor. The poems of W.B. Yeats: a new edition. London: UK: Macmillan Publishing Company; 1933.
10. Di Nicola V. The Sufi Tavern. In: Two kinds of people: poems from mile end, with photography by Donoyan A and an Afterword by Vaubel S. Singapore: Delere Press; 2023, p. 14.
11. Di Nicola V. 99 names for crying. In: The unsecured present: 3-day novels and pomes 4 pilgrims. Foreword by Jorgensen J, Afterword by Zummer T. New York/Dresden: Atropos Press; 2012, p. 147.
12. Bowlby J. On knowing what you are not supposed to know and feeling what you are not supposed to feel. Can J Psychiatr. 1979;24(5):403–8.
13. Sloterdijk P. In: Klein B, editor. Selected exaggerations. Conversations and interviews 1993–2012, trans. Margolis K. Cambridge, UK: Polity Press; 2016.
14. Di Nicola V. Letter to young psychiatrists. "Small answers"—lessons for the left hand. Washington Psychiatrist Magazine. 2017;Summer:12–4.
15. Bar-El Y, Durst R, Katz G, Zislin J, Strauss Z, Knobler HY. Jerusalem Syndrome. Br J Psychiatry. 2000;176:86–90.
16. Hesse H. Steppenwolf, trans. Creighton B. New York: Holt, Rinehart and Winston; 1963.
17. Kusters W. A philosophy of madness: the experience of psychotic thinking, trans. Forest-Flier N. Cambridge, MA: MIT Press; 2020.
18. Said EW. Orientalism. New York: Pantheon Books; 1978.
19. Di Nicola V. Looking at the west looking at the east: the radical Western search for self through the faith of imagined others. In: Moffic HS, et al., editors. Eastern religions, spirituality, and psychiatry. New York: Springer Nature; 2024.
20. Teresa of Ávila, Saint. Interior Castle, trans. and ed. Peers EA. Garden City: Doubleday; 1961. (Spanish original, 1588).
21. Strauss L. Persecution and the art of writing. Chicago: University of Chicago Press; 1988.
22. Di Nicola V. Take your time: seven pillars of a slow thought manifesto. Aeon (online magazine). February 27, 2018. https://aeon.co/essays/take-your-time-the-seven-pillars-of-a-slow-thought-manifesto. Last accessed 3 June 2023.
23. Di Nicola V, Stoyanov D. Psychiatry in crisis: at the crossroads of social science, the humanities, and neuroscience. Foreword by Fulford KWM, Afterword by Frances A. Cham: Springer Nature; 2021.
24. James W. The will to believe and other essays in popular philosophy. Cambridge, UK: Cambridge University Press; 2014. (Original, 1897)
25. Wikipedia contributors. Carthusians. Wikipedia, The Free Encyclopedia. August 22, 2023, 01:21 UTC. https://en.wikipedia.org/w/index.php?title=Carthusians&oldid=1171583994. Last accessed 3 June 2023.
26. Critchley S. The faith of the faithless: experiments in political theology. London: Verso; 2014.
27. Auster P. The red notebook: true stories. New York: New Directions; 2002.
28. Zupančič A. The shortest shadow: Nietzsche's philosophy of the two. Cambridge, MA: MIT; 2003.
29. Stendhal M-HB. The charterhouse of Parma, trans. Howard R. New York: The Modern Library; 1999. (French original, 1839).
30. Innocenti C, Fioravanti G, Spiti R, La Faravelli C. Sindrome di Stendhal fra psicoanalisi e neuroscienze [Stendhal syndrome between psychoanalysis and neuroscience]. Riv Psichiatr. 2014;49(2):61–6. (In Italian)
31. Nicholson TRJ, Pariante C, McLoughlin D. Stendhal syndrome: a case of cultural overload. Br Med J Case Rep. 2009:bcr0620080317. https://doi.org/10.1136/bcr.06.2008.0317.
32. Fo D. The tricks of the trade, trans. Farrell J, editor and with notes by Hood S. New York: Routledge/A Theatre Arts Book; 1991.
33. Eco U. The name of the rose, trans. Weaver W. New York: Harcourt Brace Jovanovich; 1983. (Italian original, 1980).
34. Borges JL. The Aleph. In: Borges JL, A personal anthology, trans., ed. & with a Foreword by Kerrigan A. New York: Grove Press; 1967, pp. 138–154. (Original Spanish, 1949).
35. Badiou A. Saint Paul: the foundation of universalism, trans. Bassier R. Stanford: Stanford University Press; 2003.

36. Monod J. Chance and necessity: an essay on the natural philosophy of modern biology, trans. Wainhouse A. New York: Alfred A. Knopf; 1971.
37. Postman N. Technopoly: the surrender of culture to technology. New York: Vintage Books; 1993.
38. Di Nicola V. Intimate strangers—there is no dark fate or bright destiny, only things that happen. Aeon (online magazine). April 13, 2020. https://aeon.co/essays/there-is-no-dark-fate-or-bright-destiny-only-things-that-happen. Last accessed 3 June 2023.
39. Rumi J. The essential Rumi, trans. Barks C with Moyne J, Nicholson R. Edison: Castle Books; 1997.
40. Di Nicola V. "Dèyè chak timoun gen yon fanmi e yon kilti/Behind every child is a family & a culture: cultural family therapy with Haitian families," Rebâti Santé Mentale, 3rd Haitian mental health summit, Montreal, May 30, 2014.
41. Winzeler R. Latah in South-East Asia: the history and ethnography of a culture-bound syndrome. Cambridge, UK: Cambridge University Press; 1995.
42. Frye N. The bush garden: essays on the Canadian imagination. Toronto: House of Anansi; 1971.

Roy Abraham Kallivayalil and P. N. Suresh Kumar

"The essence of all religions is one. Only their approaches are different"

— Mahatma Gandhi

Kerala is home to people of various religions. The caste system became prevalent in Kerala later than any other parts of India after fourth and fifth century AD. This diversity has led to a rich tapestry of religious practices and traditions. According to 2011 census of India figures, 54.73% of Kerala's population are Hindus, 26.56% are Muslims, 18.38% are Christians, and the remaining 0.33% follow other religions or have no religion [1].

The mythological legends regarding the origin of Kerala are Hindu in nature. Kerala produced several saints and movements. Hindus represent the biggest religious group in all districts except Malappuram, where they are outnumbered by Muslims [2]. Various tribal people in Kerala have retained the religious beliefs of their ancestors. In comparison with the rest of India, Kerala experiences relatively little sectarianism [3].

Hinduism

Several saints and movements existed. Adi Shankara was a Hindu philosopher who contributed to Hinduism and propagated philosophy of Advaita. He was instrumental in establishing four mathas at Sringeri, Dwarka, Puri, and Jyotirmath.

Melpathur Narayana Bhattathiri was another religious figure who composed Narayaniyam, a collection of verses in praise of Lord Krishna. Temples in Kerala follow elaborate rituals and traditionally only priests from the Nambudiri caste could be appointed as priests in major temples. But in 2017 as per the state government's decision, the priests from the historically backward caste communities are now being appointed as priests. Malayali Hindus practice ceremonies such as "Chorunu" (first feeding of rice to a child) and "Vidyārambham" (beginning of education, writing the first letter) [4]. Interesting the Hindu tradition of "Vidyaramabam" is observed by many other religions of Kerala as well, under-

R. A. Kallivayalil (✉)
Department of Psychiatry, Pushpagiri Institute of Medical Sciences, Thiruvalla and Mar Sleeva Medicity, Palai, Kottayam, Kerala, India

P. N. S. Kumar
Chethana – Center for Neuropsychiatry, Kozhikode, Kerala, India

scoring the secular fabric of the State. Sri Narayana Guru, Chattampi Swamikal, Ayyankali and Mannathu Padmanabhan are considered the most prominent modern day reformers who have contributed greatly to the social advancement of modern Kerala.

Islam

Islam is the second-largest practiced religion in Kerala (26.56%), only surpassed by Hinduism. The Muslim population in Kerala state is 8,873,472 [5]. Most of the Muslims in Kerala follow the Shāfiī School (Sunni Islam), followed by Salafi movement. Muslims in Kerala share a common language (Malayalam) with the rest of the non-Muslim population and have a culture commonly regarded as the Malayali culture. A number of different communities, some of them having distant ethnic roots, exist as status groups in Kerala [6].

Kerala has been a major spice exporter since 3000 BCE and it is still referred to as the "Garden of Spices" or as the "Spice Garden of India." [7] Kerala's spices attracted ancient Arabs, Babylonians, Assyrians, and Egyptians to the Malabar Coast in the third and second millennia BCE.

Islam arrived in Kerala, a part of the spice and silk traders from the Middle East. Kerala Muslims are generally referred to as the Mappilas. The Muslims were a major financial power to be reckoned with in the old kingdoms of Kerala and had great political influence in the Hindu royal courts [8].

The arrival of the Portuguese traders in Malabar Coast in the late fifteenth century checked the then well-established and wealthy Muslim community's progress [9]. Portuguese began to expand their territories and ruled the seas between Ormus and the Malabar Coast and south to Ceylon (now Sri Lanka). By the mid-eighteenth century, the majority of the Muslims of Kerala became landless laborers, poor fishermen, and petty traders, and the community was in "a psychological retreat." [9] The subsequent rule of English East India Company allegedly brought the land-less Muslim peasants of Malabar District into a condition of destitution, and this led to a series of uprisings (against the Hindu landlords and British administration). The series of violence eventually exploded as the infamous Mappila Uprising (1921–22).

A large number of Muslims of Kerala found extensive employment in the Persian Gulf Countries in the following years [10]. This widespread participation in the "Gulf Rush" produced huge economic and social benefits for the community. Great influx of funds from the earnings of the employed followed. Issues such as widespread poverty, unemployment, and educational backwardness began to change [11].

Christianity

Christianity is followed by 18.38% of the population of Kerala [12]. The Christianity in Kerala has long traditions from first century AD many of which is similar to the Malabari Jews, the latter has settled in Kerala since the King Solomon. According to traditional accounts, [13] Saint Thomas, the Apostle of Christ visited Muziris in Kerala in the first century around 52 AD and proselytized some of the then settled Cochin Jewish families and some Upper castes, they became the present "Mar Thoma Suriyani Nasrani" or Saint Thomas Syrian Christians. The first Roman Catholic Diocese in India was founded at Quilon in the year 1329 with the Catalan Dominican friar Jordanus Catalani as first Bishop("Index – Quilon DIocese") (www. quilondiocese.com).

The 2011 Indian census found a total of 6,411,269 Christians in Kerala, with their various denominations as stated: Saint Thomas Christians (Syrian Christians) constituted 70.73% of the Christians of Kerala, followed by Latin Catholics at 13.3%, Pentecostals at 4.3%, CSI at 4.5%, Dalit Christians at 2.6%, and other Protestant groups at 5.9% [12]. The Syrian Christians fostered education grately in Kerala. Pioneers like Kuriakose Elias Chavara, who was one of the most prominent reformers in Kerala, insisted on a having a school along with the Syrian Catholic Churches in Kerala. These schools were open to students from all castes, creeds, and religions—a revolutionary idea at that time. Chavara also started one of the earliest Sanskrit schools at

Mannanam, near Kottayam. Syrian Christians found education as imperative for social advancement. Consequently, highly educated Syrian Christians reached high positions in administration under the Central and State governments. They were also pioneers in agriculture especially rubber in Kerala. Around the time of Indian independence in 1947 large sections of the community migrated to the high ranges and also to Malabar in search of fertile lands for agriculture. Although they suffered many hardships, their efforts led to the economic advancement of the community, making Syrian Christians one of the most prosperous in Kerala.

Judaism

Judaism arrived in Kerala with spice traders, possibly as early as the seventh century BC [14]. The Portuguese did not look favorably on the Jews. They allegedly destroyed the Jewish settlement in Kodungallur and ransacked the Jewish town in Cochin and partially destroyed the famous Cochin Synagogue in 1661. However, the Dutch were more tolerant and allowed the Jews to pursue their normal life and trade in Cochin. Since the 1960s, only a few hundred Jews (mostly white Jews) remained in Kerala with only two synagogues open for service: the Pardesi Synagogue in Mattancherry built in 1567 and the synagogue in Parur [15].

Jainism

Jainism, one of the three most ancient Indian religious traditions still in existence, has very small presence (0.01%) in Kerala, in south India. According to the 2011 India Census, Kerala only has around 4500 Jains, most of them in the city of Cochin, Calicut and in the Wynad district. The so-called Rules of the Tirukkunavay Temple provided model and precedent for all other Jain temples of Kerala [16]. A number of images of Mahavira, Padmavati, and Parsvanatha have been recovered from Kerala. Some of the Jain temples in Kerala were taken over by the Hindus at a later stage.

Buddhism

Buddhism probably flourished for 200 years (650–850) in Kerala. The Paliyam Copper Plate of the Ay King, Varaguna (885–925 AD) shows that the Buddhists benefited from royal patronage in the tenth century [17]. The religion's popularity declined following the onset of Advaita Vedanta propagated by sage Shankaracharya.

Parsi (Zoroastrianism)

There were a number of Parsi families settled in Kerala, particularly around Kozhikode and Thalassery area. They practiced Zoroastrianism and even built the 160-year-old dadgah (fire temple) at S. M. Street, Kozhikode which is still in existence. They were mostly wealthy families who immigrated during the eighteenth century from Gujarat and Bombay. The community included famous families such as the Hirjis or Marshalls [18].

Tribal and Other Religious Faiths

Various groups classified as tribes in Kerala still dominate various remote and hilly areas of Kerala (Idukki—People and culture—Tribes). They have retained various rituals and practices of their ancestors despite influences of mainstream religions.

Religious Diversity

Kerala has a long history of religious syncretism, where different religious practices often blend together. This is particularly evident in art, architecture, festivals, and rituals that may have elements from multiple faiths [19].

Religious festivals are a significant part of Kerala's culture. They bring people of all backgrounds together and include events like Onam (a Hindu harvest festival), Eid, Christmas, and other celebrations that are widely observed and enjoyed by people of various faiths. Kerala has a multitude of temples, mosques, churches, and other places of worship, each with its own unique architecture and cultural significance. These places often serve as social centers and foster a sense of community. In Kerala, there is generally a history of peaceful coexistence and tolerance among different religious communities. Interfaith marriages and interactions are not uncommon, and people from various religions often participate in each other's family and cultural events. Religion can influence social and economic aspects, such as educational institutions run by religious communities and charitable work done by religious organizations.

Religious Harmony in Kerala.

Kerala is a secular state with a diverse population that has peacefully coexisted for centuries, influenced by trade and adopting different religions at different times. Kerala's history of religious tolerance and interdependence between Hindus, Muslims, and Christians was shaped by trade and the support of local rulers. The interdependence between Hindu, Muslim, and Christian communities in trading and agriculture in Kerala has historically led to peaceful coexistence, cultural integration, and the adoption of local practices. Kerala's religious sites were once similar, but the arrival of the Portuguese in the fifteenth century led to their differentiation.

Despite minor communal incidents, Kerala is considered a truly secular state where Hindus, Muslims, and Christians have been living together peacefully for centuries. The interdependence between Hindus and Muslims in Kerala, where Hindu carpenters built ships for Muslim traders, exemplifies the religious tolerance and cooperation that existed in the region. Stanford professor Saumitra Jha's study reveals that trading hubs where Hindus and Muslims work together have a lower incidence of communal riots, highlighting the importance of economic collaboration in maintaining religious harmony (Rational Expressions, Inc. 2023). The religious harmony in Kerala was maintained during the 2002 riots because Hindus and Muslims showed solidarity by exchanging bangles and actively rejecting violence. The belief that Lord Ayyappa had close friends from both the Muslim and Christian communities highlights the inclusive nature of religious practices in Kerala. Kerala's high Human Development Index indicates that social and political factors contribute to religious harmony in the region ((Rational Expressions, Inc. 2023).

Religious beliefs and practices serve as coping mechanisms during times of stress, grief, or illness. Rituals, prayers, and community support provide comfort and solace, helping individuals navigate difficult life situations. Religions in Kerala, like elsewhere, provide moral and ethical guidelines for individuals. These frameworks can influence decision-making, interpersonal relationships, and societal behavior, shaping the psychosocial fabric of the community.

Religious practices such as meditation, prayer, and mindfulness, which are often integral to religious traditions in Kerala, have positive impact psychological well-being. These practices are believed to reduce stress, enhance emotional resilience, and promote a sense of inner peace.

Political Influence

Religious communities often have a voice in the political landscape of Kerala. Different religious groups may have their political affiliations and play a role in shaping state policies. The remittances sent from the Gulf to Kerala played a significant role in the state's economy, with 10% of the population contributing Rs. 1 lakh crore. ($10 billion)

Influence on Mental Health Services

Religious beliefs and practices in Kerala have influenced attitudes toward mental health and the utilization of mental health services. Some individuals seek religious or spiritual interventions alongside or instead of conventional mental health treatment.

Education as a Vehicle for Advancement

The people of Kerala, irrespective of their religious affiliation, has realized the value education and found it the most important tool for social advancement. Today with a 95% literacy rate and 93% female literacy, the State is a model for India. Initially Christians were in the forefront for promoting education. Later Hindus and Muslims too came forward to promote education significantly. Besides religious establishments, all these communities run arts, science, engineering, medical, and other educational institutions. Many people believe, one of the secrets of Kerala's communal harmony is its high level of literacy.

Conclusion

A study of the major religions of Kerala—Hinduism, Islam, and Christianity and the smaller Jewish, Jain, and other communities takes one to the conclusion, one of Kerala's main strengths has been its religious harmony. People of all faiths here live in peace and harmony practising their faiths but at the same time deeply respectful to the traditions and religious practices of others. It's rich heritage that should never be lost!

References

1. Population by religious communities—Census of India.
2. Kalathil MJ. In: Nair PR, Shaji H, editors. Withering Valli: alienation, degradation, and enslavement of tribal women in Attappady (PDF). Kerala research programme on local level development. Thiruvananthapuram: Centre for Development Studies; 2004. ISBN 978-8187621690.
3. Heller P. Social capital as a product of class mobilization and state intervention: industrial workers in Kerala, India. University of California; (2003). pp. 49–50.
4. India News—IBNLive. Ibnlive.in.com.
5. Nandakumar T. 54.72% of population in Kerala are Hindus The Hindu August 26, 2015.
6. Kunhali V. "Muslim communities in Kerala to 1798" PhD dissertation Aligarh Muslim University (1986).
7. Pradeep Kumar, Kaavya. "Of Kerala, Egypt, and the spice link". The Hindu, 28 January; 2014.
8. Menon AS. The legacy of Kerala (Reprinted ed.). Department of Public Relations, Government of Kerala; 1982. ISBN 978-8–12643-798-6.
9. Nossiter, Thomas Johnson (January 1982). Communism in Kerala: A Study in Political Adaptation. ISBN 9780520046672.
10. Arab states of the Persian Gulf, Wikipedia.
11. Miller ER. Mappila Muslim Culture. Albany: State University of New York Press; 2015. p. xi.
12. 2011 Census of India. C-1 Population By Religious Community. Office of the Registrar General & Census Commissioner, India Ministry of Home Affairs, Government of India.
13. Edin Michael. www.catholic.cafe/. 12 February 2020) Saint Thomas the Apostle visited Muziris in Kerala in the first century around 52 AD and proselytized some of the then settled Cochin Jewish families (History | Payyappilly Palakkappilly Nasrani. www.payyappilly.org
14. Katz 2000; Koder 1973; Thomas Puthiakunnel 1973; David de Beth Hillel, 1832; Lord, James Henry 1977.
15. Paradesi Synagogue, Wikipedia.
16. Narayanan MGS. Political and social conditions of Kerala under the Cēra Perumāḷs of Makōtai (c. AD 800–AD 1124). Thrissur (Kerala): CosmoBooks; 2013. pp. 340–342.
17. A social history of India S. N. Sadasivan APH Publishing, 2000.
18. Kozhikode's Parsi legacy. The Hindu.
19. Census of India, 1931, VOLUME XXVIII, Travancore, Part-I Report (PDF). Thiruvananthapuram: Government of Travancore. 1932. pp. 327, 331.

Caste in Religion and in Health Inequality

28

Emily Diamond

Introduction

Many years ago, I went to the doctor and took a brief questionnaire. I don't recall the answers I gave, but I remember its brevity and some of the questions asked. Some years later, on the other side of graduate school, I learned it was likely the Adverse Childhood Experiences survey, what many now call the ACEs [1]. I learned how based on this handful of questions, researchers were finding that as the number of childhood adversities goes up, so too does the risk for many of the main causes of early mortality.

In ACEs, there is something powerful and easy for the public to understand about the connection between trauma, adversity, and later health. So powerful have the correlations been that many states and counties have Adverse Childhood Experience surveys, as does the CDC in the US, and the World Health Organization.

To better understand these findings, I started my own adversity study, called the Health Path Project. I wanted to conduct a study that would help me see on a more granular level how these findings came about and in some basic way,

understand the impact on participants' children. I thought it would be interesting to be able to compare the national data I was getting to data coming from other countries. I started with my own country, the US, and currently have nearly 3000 participants.

In one question, I said that there were things that sometimes hold people back from enjoying the freedoms and respect that others enjoy. I asked if there were aspects of their identity that they felt were barriers to this. The top five things on that list were their age, economic disadvantage, ethnic background, gender, and having a physical or mental illness. Very powerful for me were the least common responses. For this group, what was holding them back were the religion or faith community to which they belonged, the region or place from which they came, their job, being a refugee, and their caste identity. It was moving for me because I wasn't aware of any general trauma studies in the US that were asking about caste. By adding it, I could begin to hear that signal in my data.

I began to learn how the most common things and the least common things intersect, like being a woman from a lower caste. The chapter will discuss the nature of castes in different contexts and also the intersection between the most common things on the list and the least common things.

The chapter will end with a section on how to capture relevant clinical data at the outset of men-

E. Diamond (✉)
The Wright Institute, Berkeley, CA, USA

The Health Inequality Studies Group,
Berkeley, CA, USA
e-mail: ediamond@wi.edu

tal health treatment that is likely not to cause offense. Also included is a section on the guiding principles or priorities I developed while studying caste; while there is trauma-informed therapy and clinical research, caste requires its own set of principles.

Do We Have Caste in the United States?

In the US, we have become used to talking about color, but caste has been put forth eloquently by many for more than a century as a factor in the oppression of Black Americans. The American civil rights leader Martin Luther King visited India in early 1959 and met with Prime Minister Nehru, who helped to lead India's independence movement and became its first post-colonial Prime Minister. Many years later in a sermon King gave at Ebenezer Baptist Church on Independence Day, 1965, a church with a focus on social justice, he said this to the congregation:

> *I remember when Mrs. King and I were in India, we journeyed down one afternoon to the southernmost part of India, the state of Kerala, the city of Trivandrum. That afternoon I was to speak in one of the schools, what we would call high schools in our country, and it was a school attended by and large by students who were the children of former untouchables ....*
>
> *The principal introduced me and then as he came to the conclusion of his introduction, he says, "Young people, I would like to present to you a fellow untouchable from the United States of America." And for a moment I was a bit shocked and peeved that I would be referred to as an untouchable ....*
>
> *I started thinking about the fact: twenty million of my brothers and sisters were still smothering in an airtight cage of poverty in an affluent society. I started thinking about the fact: these twenty million brothers and sisters were still by and large housed in rat-infested, unendurable slums in the big cities of our nation, still attending inadequate schools faced with improper recreational facilities. And I said to myself, "Yes, I am an untouchable, and every Negro in the United States of America is an untouchable." [2]*

The Study of Hierarchy, Caste and Health

If you want to study adversity and health disparity, wherever you are, the expedient way to do this is to study heritable hierarchy, the mechanisms by which the same families maintain it, and the societal institutions that are supporting it. Many castes and hierarchies are maintained through the practice of endogamy, where people either must or are strongly encouraged to marry within their caste, often in marriages arranged by their parents or elders. In many places, marriage is seen as bringing two suitable families together, not simply two individuals. Parents have disowned their children for wanting to marry someone of another caste, and at times have done violence in order to prevent it. In some cases, inter-caste marriages are seen as potentially harming the future marriage possibilities of the other children in the family.

The study of caste and hierarchy helps me to understand who is allowed to live where, what occupations are reserved for whom, what you can eat with what wages, and who gets the best medical care. When someone seeks care for their troubles, the study of hierarchy lets me know if that person is likely to get that care from someone who has walked in their shoes. If the person seeks mental healthcare, it tells me if the stories that shape that life are likely to be shared by the person doing the treating. How strong a hierarchy is can be measured not just by how many centuries or millennia it has been in place, but by the relative movement of families between those ranks.

To study caste is to also study a culture's metaphysical ideas about what or who is clean and pure, and what or who is defiled or dirty. This is why where there is caste, one can often see rules around where those seen as the lowest caste can live, who can rent an apartment where, and who can touch what. Historically, a person who was "polluted" could "contaminate" another person just by looking at them [3]. Through metaphysical association, this will attach to the person's children too, this is what makes castes hereditary. It puts manacles on children's futures even before they're born.

As castes are hereditary ranking systems, caste systems will always have some way to identify who is in what caste. This can be by last name, it can be by neighborhood, or it's often by occupation. It can also be done by official family registries that the government keeps. When caste also overlaps with racism, it can be by color. Often a combination of methods is used. In historic times, sometimes the lowest caste wasn't allowed a last name, wasn't allowed to wear certain types of clothes that others wore, and so identification was made in different ways.

The Difficulty of Discussing Caste

For me, broaching the topic of caste is painful. For example, in the Japanese context, someone told me, *tell your reader we don't do that anymore, it ended with our new constitution in WWII, we are all equal* now. There is what you know to be an issue internally in a culture, and there is what you want people on the *outside* of your culture to know.

I have also heard that by talking about it, it can make the situation worse. As a clinical researcher who focuses on health disparities, not talking about is not an option.

If you think about the prejudice that has been endured, the cultural stereotypes, the cultural misunderstandings, the ethnic violence, putting aside the history of imperialism, and war, it makes sense why it's difficult to discuss.

Sometimes listening to someone talk about their caste experience can be hard because it's something that the listener has little knowledge of. Sometimes listening is hard because it's a situation the listener knows all too well. Sometimes it's uncomfortable because it forces the person to look anew at how others are experiencing the world beyond the soft confines of their personal experience.

Caste discussions are difficult for the same reason that talking about something like racism is hard, it's a major societal issue but the details of its pain, the laws around it, its history, and the amazing people involved in its fight can be very regional. Furthermore, the more entrenched the institution, the more hopeless it can appear.

I've brought caste up to my students because history matters, history always has one hand gripping the ankle of the present. I also bring it up because a career in mental health is training in the art of listening to notes that are sometimes barely audible, and the more one knows, the better the chance of hearing them. I bring it up because if they see me being able to talk openly about something, then maybe they can be brave too, because all cultures by dint of having a long history, leave various legacies, some good and some bad.

This bravery is needed because mental health is the rare space within modern society to think aloud about those things that are hardest to say. People may want to think together about how to talk to children about their family's history. There could be inter-caste issues in a relationship or between generations. College students may feel that there are caste issues in their educational setting and in their social lives. Caste may be arising at work, in their spiritual lives, and also in their healthcare, and I have not yet seen it appear as an issue on an intake. There is also caste-related violence.

Japan's Caste

My mother sometimes talks of her best friend from her childhood in Japan who was one of the *Burakumin*. *Burakumin* is a word made in the nineteenth century to mean people who live in *those* villages or hamlets, meaning ghettoized in segregated neighborhoods. It is a replacement word for the earlier word, *eta*, which means filth. More exactly, it means an abundance of filth. There were historically other words too, like *hinin*, meaning non-human [4]. Regardless of the word, and there have been many, they refer to a caste [5] within a Japan that mostly prefers to see itself as having one large middle class [5].

Jobs relating to death and refuse are necessary to societies. Despite that fact, it might have been that through an earlier more orthodox form of

Japan's native religion, Shintoism, or Buddhism, which arrived and began to be practiced in the sixth century CE, these jobs were categorized as "unclean," and a hereditary caste was created out of it [6]. The other traditional occupations of Burakumin are tanning of hides, leather working, working in abattoirs, or being butchers. This spared those who did not do this work and their children too. It also elevated the status of religion by making them the arbiter of social status and sometimes legal status. In some cases, temples may have earned more because beliefs around pollution and purity will require rituals of cleaning and purification, and these will come with monetary gifts to the priest who presides over them. In some other accounts of the origin of *Burakumin*, they were the more recent immigrants to the Japanese islands. Very likely it was a combination of factors.

Discrimination is an ongoing issue—for example, a father who works in an abattoir might go to great extent to hide his occupation from his child, so his child can be spared the bullying and ostracization that is a real potential [7].

In some older maps, there are designated areas for Burakumin, meaning they are in ghettos in a formal sense. Whether identified by their occupation, or a region of town where they lived, they would be identifiable for the next centuries. It also meant that people rarely married into that group. Just how many still exist in Japan is not certain, but that there is a problem is certain. When Google Maps offered users a layer where they could superimpose a historic map with areas clearly marked for *"eta"* onto a current map, there was an outcry that it could cause harm to Burkamin [8].

Caste in India

The Burakumin are somewhat similar to those who we know as *untouchables* in India, now referred to as *Dalit*. This is a word that can have several meanings, but in this case means, *oppressed* [9]. The term *untouchable* persists because while less frequent than in the past, the practices of untouchability and caste can still exist, though it is officially against the law in India through the Protection of Civil Rights Act, passed in 1955.

Hinduism refers to beliefs and practices that very likely varied by region and pre-date the written texts that emerged some 3000 years ago. The caste system within it is at least that old and is the oldest I have come across. While caste, as understood and practiced across many South Asian countries can differ, since Hinduism is the religion of about 80% of India [10], and India is the most populous country in the world with about 17.5% of the world's population, with millions part of the great Indian diaspora, it is a good place to start.

In Hinduism, there are *varna* [11]. This is a Sanskrit word and can mean caste, hue, color, and tribe [12]. Sanskrit is an ancient South Asian language in the Indo-European language group in which the original sacred texts of Hinduism and Buddhism were written. In two such sacred texts, the *Rigveda* and *the Mahabharata,* the former which may be one of the oldest texts written in any Indo-European language, the word similarly covers these meanings.

At the top of this caste system are Brahmins, traditionally the caste of scholars, teachers, and religious leaders. They currently make up 4% of the Indian population [13]. One level below this caste are the Kshatriyas, who are the traditional rulers, administrators, and the warrior class. Next are the Vaishyas, the agriculturalists, merchants, and farmers. Next down are the Shudras, the artisans, laborers, and those who are servants [11]. There are also thousands of sub-castes associated with more specific occupations and with different regions. Implicitly, there is a fifth varna, and they are Dalits. They are those below this major four-tiered system. This is not simply a system of occupational divisions, and the reason is because a determining factor for which varna one is in, is *karma.*

Karma and Caste

Karma is a broad metaphysical belief held in Hinduism as well as Buddhism and Jainism, that actions in life leave an indelible impression, and those actions have consequences that affect the person's future lives [14]. It's like the phrase, *as you sow, so shall you reap*, except that it applies to the fate of the soul over successive incarnations. Related to this is the idea of *dharma*, another Sanskrit word that has no exact English translation and many uses [15]. In Hinduism, dharma often refers to the laws that govern individual conduct, and *Svadarhma* has to do with those rules or laws as they apply to one's caste or varna. Embodied in these words are ideas of living one's life in accordance with divine law or righteously. So dharma and karma work together to maintain the order of society. On an individual level, one's soul may move up or down this latticework of hierarchies and caste.

Interestingly, in a 2021 survey of nearly 30,000 people in India, 77% of Hindus believed in karma, but so did 77% of Muslims [16], implying that this is a belief that has moved beyond its origins.

A Focus on Dalit

The word *untouchable* is more than a label for the lowest caste, the Dalit. It describes many practices, such as those seen in caste-based crimes, for example, when a Dalit child is beaten or killed for drinking out of the water reserved for those of a higher caste. These are both illegal under current Indian law but reflect the practice of untouchability. This untouchability can extend to who is allowed entry into a house, whether a non-Dalit midwife will attend to the birth of a Dalit woman, whether an apartment manager will rent an apartment to a Dalit family, and in rural areas, it can extend to whether people are willing to share a common well. It can determine whether upper caste people feel comfortable sharing the same plates and food as Dalit, and whether they will attend the wedding celebration of a Dalit they work with, and more.

Overlapping with the varna is another Hindu system of jātis, coming from the Sanskrit word, *jāta*, or "born." People are also born into their jātis, often marry within it, and spend their religious, spiritual, and social lives within it. It sculpts how people relate to others, in other jātis. These are understood as being castes too and how

you identify yourself to others is dependent on who the other person is [17].

It would not be realistic to think that frictions and struggles in the home country do not ripple out in myriad ways throughout the great diaspora. There are approximately 18 million Indians in the great diaspora, with varying degrees of ties to their homeland, with many sending remittances home. In the US, there are 4.2 million people of Indian origin [18].

Other Caste Systems of Asia and Those Systems Moving Abroad

Casteism exists throughout Asia. As discussed earlier, there is a caste system in Japan. There is another in Korea, and in China there is the *hukou* system, which is a family registry system that codifies urban and rural citizenship and creates differential wages and possibilities for both groups [19]. There is also a caste system in Pakistan [20]. It is easy to see which countries have active caste systems simply by looking up the country and putting in the word "*caste.*" The last centuries have seen sufficient movement of people around the world that casteism from the Eurasian continent has moved abroad, albeit with some changes, and at times mixing with other pre-existing systems of hierarchy.

Girls and Women in the Hierarchy

The economist Amartya Sen, as a child, was witness to an extraordinary famine in his native Bengal which killed more than 3 million people. Later he wrote about inequality as the root cause of the staggering loss of life. Then he wanted to look further at inequality. He knew that boys and girls are born at roughly equal rates, so by looking at population statistics, he could see how many missing girls and women there are. That number is 100 million. These losses are most concentrated in countries across Asia, the Middle East, and Africa where customary hierarchy makes females worth less [21]. This number is consistent with subsequent research which has found similar numbers.

Factors behind this 100 million missing girls and women include sex selection prior to birth; infanticide; and failure to invest in girls' nutrition, safety, health, education, and healthcare. Girls become economically costly to families due to the very powerlessness to which they have been consigned. These factors lead to child marriages, higher rates of death in childbirth, greater mortality from illness and injury, and eventually to the monumental loss of girls and women.

Colorism

Tending to fall more heavily on women than men, there is also a preference for pale or whiter skin that constitutes the colorism that one can see across many countries and has been a part of Asian countries prior to contact or colonization by Europeans. In China, there is evidence that skin whitening was practiced as early as 200 BCE [22]. On the other side of the Eurasian continent, for whiter skin, the men and women of ancient Greece covered their faces in white lead masks, and ancient Romans also used a lead mixture to whiten their skin. In Europe, skin whitening was practiced in the Middle Ages to the Renaissance, a period spanning the fifth century to the seventeenth century [22]. It's currently a multi-billion dollar global industry extending far beyond the Eurasian continent to North America, South America, Australia, and Africa. This process now includes lasers and is at times no less toxic than it was in the past when arsenic and mercury were used.

Here is a portion of a painting by an unknown artist in a popular theme called *Raga Hindola*, painted between 1590 and 1595 (Fig. 28.1). *Raga* refers to the melodic framework from which musicians can build. The word *hindola* means *swing*. Here you can see women pushing a couple on a swing and trees in bloom. There was a tradition of child brides which may be why the female figure is small. She also has the pinched waist and white skin that has been preferrable for several centuries across the Eurasian continent, and everywhere that people from the continent came to inhabit.

Color, caste, and gender are the kinds of layered oppression experienced across the various contexts of a woman's life, private and public, such that it may be difficult for her to experience full dignity, possibility, equality, and freedom. Dalit poetry is a rich repository of various intersections. Some of the nuances of this woman's poem are likely lost on me, but in *Nature's Fountainhead*, by Sukurtharani [23] there is

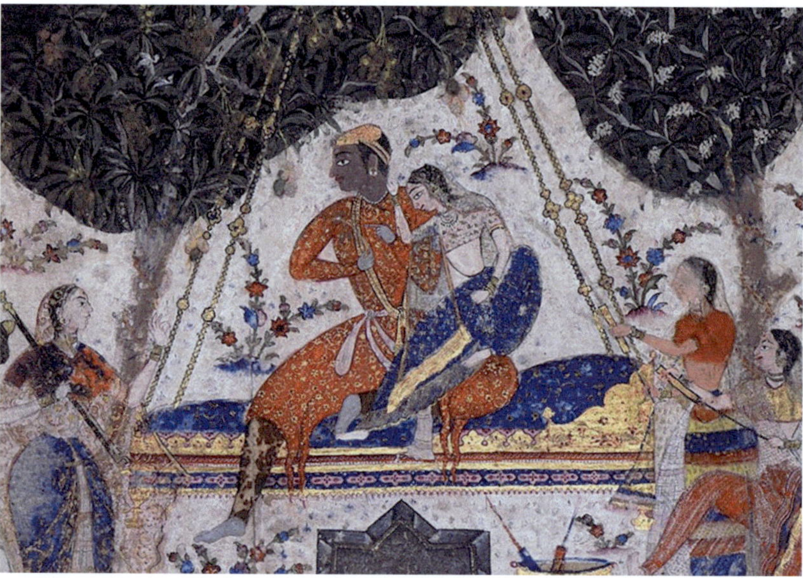

Fig. 28.1 *Raga Hindola*, by an unknown artist, circa 1590s, Wikimedia

power in her lines. As the last name can be caste-identifying, like many others she chooses to go by a single name. The second stanza refers to being set on fire, which has been a part of domestic violence in South Asia. This is referred to by the term *bride burning* in the English health literature, though burning a woman by throwing acid or setting her alight can also happen to women as part of community violence [24]. This poem was translated from the original Tamil by the translator, Lakshmi Holmströmm, MBE.

Say you bury me alive.
I will become a green grass-field
and lie outspread, a fertile land.
You may set me on fire;
I will become a flaming bird
and fly about in the wide, wide space.
You may wave a magic wand
and shut me up, a genie in a bottle;
I will vaporize as mercury
and stand upright towards the sky.
You may dissolve me into the wind
like water immersed into water;
from its every direction
I will emerge, like blown breath.
You may frame me, like a picture,
and hang me on your wall;
I will pour down, away past you,
like a river in sudden flood.
I myself will become
earth
fire
sky
wind
water.
The more you confine me, the more I will spill
*   over,*
Nature's fountainhead.

The Persistence of Caste

While India's 1949 Constitution prohibits caste-based discrimination, those who are at the bottom of this ranking system are still more likely to lack the same educational opportunities, to endure more caste-based crimes, and to experience more

health issues compared with those in the upper castes.

Castes may seem foreign to many, but where there is generational poverty one can see some of the same issues of greater exposure to environmental hazards, illness, and crime victimization, as well as the bodily and psychic consequences of despair. I see this in my data, as does every researcher I know of who works on trauma, adversity, and health.

As in the United States, which has used affirmative action to help bring historically under-represented and marginalized groups into colleges and jobs, there is a similar system in India. In a survey of nearly 30,000 Indian adults in 17 different languages in India, the majority of Indian adults said they are a member of a Scheduled Caste, often referred to as Dalits (25%), Scheduled Tribe (9%), or Other Backward Class (35%) [25]. Caste identification also extends to those who say they belong to religions that do not traditionally have castes. In fact, a majority of people identify as a member of a caste, regardless of their religious background [26].

In the same survey, with little variation between castes, 64% of Indians said it was very important to stop women in their community from marrying into other castes, and 62% said it was important to stop men [26]. This is a major reason for its persistence but there are others. In modern times, for castes to persist, usually all the major institutions—marriage, education, medicine, religion, arts, entertainment, journalism, research, law enforcement, judiciary, and voting—will have all played some role in keeping it as it is. If one institution pulls away from supporting it, like a building that has been overbuilt for safety, it will continue to stand.

Caste, Hierarchy, and the Immigrant Experience

In what ways might this matter in the closed conversations of mental health treatment, taking place thousands of miles away be relevant? My mother is an immigrant and from seeing her adjust to life in the US, I see a double immigration process. One task is to learn how to integrate and navigate through a new culture and raise your children within it. The person may be referred to by new names like Asian, South Asian, East Asian, API, POC, or BIPOC, or some hyphenated amalgam of labels. They may feel confused, or compelled to embrace or accept these new labels that are foreign, and not of their choosing.

The second immigration challenge which is less talked about is how to integrate and navigate relationships with people from the same cultural group. It might involve school, finding a partner, getting a job, starting a family, and perhaps selecting a temple or spiritual community to belong to. This group is also heterogeneous, but in the eyes of the wider community, is often identified as being more homogenous than it really is.

Here is a wonderful passage by a professor in the US, interacting with a student about Dalit history. It is also about being part of a new history.

> *I gave her an assignment to find out about Dalit diaspora. After spending two weeks in the library she told me, "There is nothing on the Dalit diaspora, what can I do?" I said, "No, there is a lot of material and you have to find it." She came with the hypothesis that Dalits are not very professional or they don't represent professional backgounds in North America. I asked her why. She said, "bechare woh to gareeb hai [they are very poor]. After they come to North America they don't have money. They don't have power." And I said, "No, no, this is not true. There are Dalits who are professionals, who are engineers, doctors, you can find Dalits everywhere in every city." She said, "No, no, no, it's not true." When she insisted, I said, "There is one sitting in front of you." And she said, "You.".. .She burst into tears and said, "I can't imagine a Dalit can be a distinguished professor. This is a shock to me." I said, "This is not shocking and there are many people who have received education and are doing good jobs like others." [27]*

What that paragraph is also about is something that comes up in caste literature and narratives on non-visible identities. It is about when and how one outs oneself. If casteism can drive people to secrecy about their jobs, make them switch religions, immigrate, or change last names, then part of one's history is about the process of coming out, and the stories of being unexpectedly outed.

A South Asian child in the US may not know much about caste or know how it relates to them, but the adults in that child's life may have practiced caste. Often all it will take is for adults to inquire about their last name for a child to have an indelibly confusing and hurtful experience. So mental health clinicians can help families think aloud about how to help the next generation create lasting and meaningful friendships in a positive context. They can also provide a place to talk about how to heal from traumas and indignities brought over and to heal when those wounds are re-opened. It is also a place to try to keep discrimination, whatever its source, from becoming internalized. What I see in my data is that across several kinds of trauma and adversity, if it's experienced in childhood, it's more likely to occur again in adulthood. So while childhood trauma is a risk factor for later poorer mental and physical health, this is in part because childhood trauma is a set up for experiencing adult trauma.

I still remember a professor asking our class to think through where our values came from. This is such a beautiful question because many of us are picking it up much as we do the grammar of language, it's often out of our awareness. The behaviors and actions that arise out of them are reflexive. Mental healthcare offers an opportunity to think aloud about where our values come from, which ones we may want to keep, and which others we want to retire. Importantly it is an opportunity to talk about generational differences, particularly because respecting the older generation can be an important cultural value for many. This way, our actions in life, no matter how big or small can be in keeping with the values we have intentionally made. More than that, it teaches us that there is always the opportunity to think them through again.

Adjusting to Change

Certainly, no religion I know is practiced exactly as it was even a century ago, or as its oldest members recall it being practiced. In this way, religions, sects within religions, and spiritual systems can be seen as living, being shaped by each generation over the course of centuries or millennia. There are discussions to be had about how these changes happen, who leads them, why the change is happening, what is most important to people, and what they would like the next generation to have. Simultaneous to these conversations are changes happening within the wider society that will reverberate through all the institutions of society, religion included. No religion stands apart from its context.

Customs, both secular and religious, change with immigration. In Japan, my recollection is that on meeting new people, it felt customary to say where you were from and who you were. These bits of information were collected as a part of meeting people, like GPS coordinates of the family. If you are practicing in a culture where identity is more about who the individual is, then you can help people acclimate to this. I have lived in my neighborhood for many years, and I mostly know my neighbors and what they do, but certainly not what their parents or grandparents did or what kind of position they had in another time or country. Yet we have celebrated many things together, shared sadness, marked milestones, and looked after one another for years. With climate change upon us, we think of our safety and survival together.

Two Systems: Faith Systems and the Power Structure of Faiths

What has been interesting to me in studying religions around the world, both historic faith systems and those that are still practiced is that they can have female gods and deities, while the female population can be struggling for equality. In Shintoism, Japan's native religion, the Japanese islands were thought to have been formed by a goddess, and yet it's a culture where gender equality has been elusive. There are powerful goddesses in the pantheon of Hinduism too. Certainly, they existed in the Greek and Roman traditions. In the spiritual care of people, sometimes it's valuable to distinguish the values one holds dear, the parts of it that one draws solace or resilience from, separate from the governance and administration of the faith.

Challenges and Recommendations for Closing Health Disparities

Disparities in health that show up in adults often start at birth or childhood, and so it is powerfully the responsibility of medicine and mental health to think about how to create a healthy start to life. In my study, when I asked people about getting the healthcare they needed, many of the poorest said they didn't go because they feared being turned away. Many went without medication and needed treatments because they couldn't afford them. Many also wanted greater integration between their physical healthcare and their mental healthcare. Studying the sources of despair and health inequality, it is easy to see why this would be the case. Our healthcare system is siloed, while our problems are not.

This work has not been made easy by the history of psychiatry or psychology, which focuses on illnesses and conditions of individuals almost exclusively. Its history is to see problems in people, even when those problems are set in a societal context of war, structural disenfranchisement, or pervasive bias and inequality. While the ICD-11 now has the diagnosis of complex post-traumatic stress disorder (6B41), for someone living with caste trauma, class trauma, or multi-generational poverty, it's their *present*.

Capturing the Needed Clinical Information

A good intake helps orient the clinician to the person they are about to work with. In general, this helps the clinician, like a mariner, to navigate by finding in the sky, the constellations. It can also function to help clinicians avoid being blind to issues that can be the reason for early dropout [28]. In time-limited treatments, this can be a serious problem. The other function of a good intake is for the person seeking help to understand through the questions, the breadth of what can be discussed, and therefore to some degree what is permissible to talk about, and what knowledge the clinician has. Many people tire of having to identify aspects of their identity to others in order to facilitate any relationship. They are likely to feel differently if asked by a clinician what issues they would like to think aloud about, in the process of developing a problem list together.

This can be organized in tiers. One can ask people to circle or indicate any societal or community issues that are troubling them. These can be such things as workplace harassment, unemployment, community and neighborhood violence, environmental issues, immigration issues, issues at school, bullying, trouble accessing appropriate medical care, issues having to do with people in their religious or faith community, or with societal racism, sexism, casteism, ableism, and ageism.

Next people can indicate issues that one would consider more home-based, or closer to home. Examples include generational problems, family estrangement, problems with their intimate partner, gender roles, domestic violence, addiction in the home, housemate issues, issues with children, caregiving, being homebound, problems with friends and family, confronting homelessness, and issues of blended families (inter-religious, inter-caste, bi-cultural, multi-generational, families with adoptions, step-families, etc.).

The next tier concerns how they feel and how they are currently doing. Among the options could be sleep or eating issues, anxiety, depression, suicidality, grief, trauma, panic, mood disorders, body-image issues, stage-of-life issues, burnout, sexuality, gender identity questions, and questions around faith and spirituality.

Then there are more medical issues. Is the person wanting discussions of past diagnoses or perhaps current diagnoses? Is there a need for assessment, or a needed discussion of medications, side effects, and dosage issues? Perhaps they want to explore how their conditions or diagnoses exacerbate each other or interrelate.

A good thing about asking people to check which things they would like to talk about is that you will not offend anyone by asking a question. You will only be giving people an opportunity to register an issue. It should be made clear that they can revisit that list anytime they want and add things they did not see on it the first time.

Offering lists accomplishes several things that are typically missing. First, it directly speaks to the broad societal issues that may be at issue and helps to make a mental health encounter a place where they can be discussed. Secondly, although there is still an enormous stigma for some around getting mental health care, people seeing this list are very likely to see that many things troubling them are not issues of personal failure. Thirdly this strategy brings climate and environmental issues into a bio-psycho-social model that has long needed to incorporate the physical environment. The fourth thing is that it may help both the practitioner and patient find how these spheres we inhabit impact each other. A fifth thing is that it directly invites people to add things to it, so that they can co-create that list with you. For those who have endured the condition of having too little control over their own lives, it's nice to be able to offer this. Lastly, it may help you see areas that are going well, so you can build upon areas of strength and resilience.

I use a version of this format in the Health Path Project. I also ask participants to create two wish lists for me. One is for what they want in order to increase their health and resilience, and the other is for what they want for their community, in order for it to be a healthier place to live.

Developing a Caste-Informed Framework

Much has been written about trauma-informed clinical work and research. In learning about castes and casteism, there is a need for something different. Here are several guideposts I came to through my work.

Trauma and adversity risk studies need to include descent-based trauma.

Mental health in this interconnected world needs to include caste or descent-based adversity in training and clinical work.

When I can, I advocate for (1) the need to get regular care from someone who is sensitive to descent-based discrimination and adversity, (2) the importance of early intervention, (3) the profound need to try and limit experiences of trauma and adversity, because early adversity predisposes one to later adversity.

How we hurt each other is a large part of the study of history. This education is available, and something that's my responsibility to learn, it's not the burden of people who are hurting. The forms that caste-based discrimination takes are varied, some of it is subtle and some of it is violent and lethal. The more I know, the more I'm not pressing someone to explain something that may cause them shame or pain to talk about.

How castes form can be lost to history, they may have originated in religion, or they can be part of racism or other forms of strategic multigenerational stigmatization. In talking about caste with people, knowing this past is helpful. We cannot disentangle ourselves from a history we don't know.

I've come to learn about different countries and different barriers to reporting caste-based discrimination and crimes. Knowing these issues has helped me understand some of the persistence of caste discrimination, and what those who experience casteism contend with. This is my responsibility to understand.

Trauma, illness, mental health struggles, bereavement, and stigma are among several things that often lead people to turn to spirituality and faith, and it's also the place where people can feel forsaken and conflicted. While we may not be able to know a person's religion as they know it, we can often learn enough to have important conversations about it. At times, an outsider's perspective may be valuable.

Our identities are layered, and there is a need to think not just of caste but all the other aspects of identity, such as being a woman, a gender minority, someone with a mental health condition, or a physical disability. This is the multiplicity we inhabit, and the context in which discrimination and violence are happening. Though harder, learning to see casteism in this context is an imperative.

The worlds we're connected to, especially when we're immigrants can be vast. A person can have siblings and family members across several countries. If crimes against a caste are going up in the country where someone's family resides, then worry, sorrow, and indignation, will reverberate thousands of miles to the rest of the family. To care about caste issues locally is to care about them globally.

Studying caste has underlined for me how the greatest wealth of a society is its children, so by extension, their early experiences of disenfranchisement, their self-conceptualization, dignity, and their safe passage through life are priorities.

There are historical figures who fought for the dignity and full inclusion of others, and some are on the front lines now. They are the people who inspire others on this journey from trauma to healing. There is a responsibility to learn about them and from them.

Years ago, when I was in high school, psychiatric hospitals around the country were being closed down in the hopes that community care would suffice. Patients were being loaded onto buses and dropped off in cities with amenable climates and liberal politics in the hopes that they would have a soft landing into homelessness. I remember one such person telling me that the hardest thing to endure was that no one looked at him. On the streets, people averted their eyes as though he didn't exist. He said no one would touch him. I wondered at the time whether this meant we would develop a caste within our society that one did not touch or meet the gaze of. A generation has passed since then. Understanding castes is of profound importance because we may be seeing new ones forming in many of the major cities of the world.

Casteism is not for one person to overcome, it's for the culture to unyoke itself from.

The Work That Lies Ahead

I write this on the 60th anniversary of Martin Luther King's speech in which he said, "I have a dream." As we know, the dream of equality is far from realized. From time to time, the system will allow someone to rise to prominence. Those at the bottom know from centuries of experience that this does not mean that they or their children will make it through the gauntlet of internal doubts and external barriers. So in whatever country we work, the work continues.

Looking at the responses from people in my study who said they don't feel they have the freedoms or get the respect that others have, when asked what they wanted in order to make their community a healthier place, it was often a greater sense that they are part of one caring community. They wanted less division. Mental health is in a difficult position where the equality that people know would be healing is not something that can be provided. Societies as a whole must provide that equality. This doesn't mean that the issues cannot be discussed, the feelings of frustration at the slow place of change can't be talked about, and that caring respect can't be experienced.

Certainly, people everywhere, no matter their faith or country may have internalized long-standing and disabling cultural messages around such things as worth, capability, dignity, beauty, aging, and gender roles. Mental health treatment has a valuable role in trying to disentangle the person from these ideas. I have had students who have struggled for these reasons. Before they leave for Internship, I make sure they know how I see them, because I remember that as I wrote my college application essay, stuck on what I should say about myself, I asked my father for help. He put some words down on a piece of paper to tell me how he sees me, and I still have it. We have the ability in our private and professional lives to make sure that among all the things young people hear about themselves, they are also hearing the things that will enable them to stay strong and perhaps to hold ambitions for themselves that they didn't know they could or should.

It is the work of a lifetime to understand how we can create a society where all children can flourish. It is for their sake, but it is also inextricably connected to ours. We do not have societal health so long as we have children whose mental health and futures are tied to the births of their forebears, or whose possibilities are already in jeopardy through early experiences of adversity. Their real possibility is the metric of our humanity.

In my study of the history of mental health, I often think that the great revolution of psychology is that no story is unspeakable.

References

1. Anda RF, Felitti VJ, Bremner JD, Walker JD, Whitfield C, Perry BD, Dube SR, Giles WH. The enduring effects of abuse and related adverse experiences in childhood. A convergence of evidence from neurobiology and epidemiology. Eur Arch Psychiatry Clin Neurosci. 2006;256(3):174–86. https://doi.org/10.1007/s00406-005-0624-4.
2. Chapter 13: Pilgrimage to nonviolence. The Martin Luther King, Jr. Research and Education Institute. n.d. https://kinginstitute.stanford.edu/publications/autobiography-martin-luther-king-jr/chapter-13-pilgrimage-nonviolence
3. Jeffrey R. Temple-entry movement in travancore, 1860–1940. Soc Sci. 1976;4(8):3–27. https://doi.org/10.2307/3516377. p. 6.
4. Groemer G. The creation of the Edo outcaste order. J Jpn Stud. 2001;27(2):263–93. https://doi.org/10.2307/3591967. p. 265.
5. Gordon JA. Caste in Japan: the Burakumin. Biography. 2017;40(1):265–87. http://www.jstor.org/stable/26405020. p. 266.
6. Donoghue JD. An eta community in Japan: the social persistence of outcaste groups. Am Anthropol. 1957;59(6):1000–17. http://www.jstor.org/stable/666461. pp. 1000-1001.
7. Sunda M, Milner R. Japan's hidden caste of untouchables. BBC News Asia. 2015, October 23. Retrieved September 17, 2023, from https://www.bbc.com/news/world-asia-34615972
8. Alabaster J. Old Japanese maps on Google Earth unveil secrets. 2009, May 2. Retrieved September 17, 2023, from https://phys.org/news/2009-05-japanese-google-earth-unveil-secrets.html
9. Minority Rights Group. DALITs—Minority Rights Group. 2021, February 5. https://minorityrights.org/minorities/dalits/
10. Kramer S, Pew Charitable Trust. Religious composition of India: all religious groups show major declines in fertility rates limiting change in the country's religious composition over time. 2021. p. 7.
11. Klostermaier KK. A survey of Hinduism: Third edition. 2007. p. 289. https://doi.org/10.1353/book5195.
12. Monier-Williams M. A Sanskrit English dictionary: etymologically and philologically arranged. Oxford: Clarendon Press/Oxford University; 1960. p. 966.
13. Pew Research Center. Religion in India: tolerance and segregation. 2021, June 29. p. 26.
14. Wadia AR. Philosophical implications of the doctrine of karma. Philosophy East West. 1965;15(2):145–52. https://doi.org/10.2307/1397335.
15. Patyal HC. The term dharma: its scope. Bull Deccan Coll Res Inst. 1994;54(55):157–65. http://www.jstor.org/stable/42930466
16. Pew Research Center. Religion in India: tolerance and segregation. 2021, June 29. p. 7.
17. Srivastava VK. Speaking of caste: merit of the principle of segmentation. Sociol Bull. 2016;65(3):317–38. http://www.jstor.org/stable/26369539

18. Badrinathan S, Kapur D, Kay J, Vaishnav M. Social realities of Indian Americans: results from the 2020 Indian American attitudes survey. Washington, DC: Carnegie Endowment for International Peace; 2021.

19. Wang F-L. Brewing tensions while maintaining stabilities: the dual role of the Hukou system in contemporary China. Asian Perspect. 2005;29(4):85–124. http://www.jstor.org/stable/42704524

20. Mumtaz Z, Jhangri GS, Bhatti A, Ellison GTH. Caste in Muslim Pakistan: a structural determinant of inequities in the uptake of maternal health services. Sexual and reproductive health matters. 2022;29(2):2035516. https://doi.org/10.1080/26410397.2022.2035516.

21. Sen A. More than 100 million women are missing. The New York Review of Books. 1990, December 20. Retrieved September 10, 2023, from https://www.nybooks.com/articles/1990/12/20/more-than-100-million-women-are-missing/

22. Iftekhar N, Zhitny VP. Overview of skin bleaching history and origins. Dermatology (Basel, Switzerland). 2021;237(2):306–8. https://doi.org/10.1159/000509727.

23. Sukirtharani. Nature's fountainhead. Poetry and Sangam. 2013. Retrieved September 10, 2023, from http://poetry.sangamhouse.org/2013/09/natures-fountainhead/

24. Kaur N, Byard RW. Bride burning: a unique and ongoing form of gender-based violence. J Forensic Leg Med. 2020;75:102035. https://doi.org/10.1016/j.jflm.2020.102035.

25. Pew Research Center. Religion in India: tolerance and segregation. 2021, June 29. p 25.

26. Pew Research Center. Religion in India: tolerance and segregation. 2021, June 29. p. 27.

27. Adur SM, Narayan A. Stories of Dalit diaspora: migration, life narratives, and caste in the US. Biography. 2017;40(1):244–64. http://www.jstor.org/stable/26405019. p. 254.

28. Leichsenring F, Sarrar L, Steinert C. Drop-outs in psychotherapy: a change of perspective. World Psychiatry. 2019;18(1):32–3. https://doi.org/10.1002/wps.20588.

Assessment of Potential Harm in Eastern Religions: The Influence Continuum and the BITE Model of Authoritarian Control

Steven Alan Hassan and Jon Atack

"Man is made by belief. As he believes, so he is."
Bhagavad Gita [1]

Over the millennia, alongside genuine inquiry, many groups have used spirituality as a pretext for controlling and harming society. Among the most extreme examples are the Thuggees in India and the sacrificial cults of Central America. Elsewhere, spiritual teachings have brought civilization and harmony.

The same fundamental teachings are found in the Franciscan Order, which cared for the poor, and the Flagellants, bands of penitents who wandered around Europe beating themselves with leather thongs studded with nails. [2] Anti-social leaders can turn any teaching to bad ends.

European interest in Eastern ideas began with incursions into India and China in the eighteenth century C.E. Eager scholars collected and translated Taoist, Buddhist, and Hindu texts, some of which might otherwise have been lost, as many Pali Buddhist texts were under the Moghuls.[1]

---

[1]For instance, the Pali Text Society, founded in 1881, https://palitextsociety.org/; for Sanskrit scholars, see https://en.wikipedia.org/wiki/Category:Sanskrit_scholars_by_nationality, retrieved 04-07-23.

S. A. Hassan (✉)
Freedom of Mind Resource Center,
Newton, MA, USA

Member of The Program in Psychiatry and the Law,
Harvard Medical School, Newton, MA, USA
e-mail: center@freedomofmind.com

J. Atack
Nottinghamshire, UK

By the late nineteenth century, scholarship had spawned quackery. The first investigation of the scientifically rigorous British Society for Psychical Research clearly demonstrated the fraudulent methods of Helena Blavatsky, but this did little to hinder the influence of her Theosophical Society. [3] There is strong evidence that the "bishop" of Theosophy, Charles Leadbeater, was a pederast. Nevertheless, the cult burgeoned before its supposed messiah or "World Teacher," Jiddhu Krishnamurti, renounced his title and dissolved its central order. [4]

The two authors of this chapter have spent most of their adult lives helping thousands of former members of extreme authoritarian sects in their recovery. Steven Hassan, Ph.D., was deprogrammed from a leadership position in the Moon Organization in 1976. He has authored four books, including *Combating Cult Mind Control* and *Freedom of Mind* and created an online CE course, Understanding Cults, A Foundational Course for Clinicians. Jon Atack wrote the first history of Scientology, *Let's Sell These People a Piece of Blue Sky*, published in 1990. He has a lifelong interest in eastern philosophy from his brief time in a Soto Zen monastery in his teens to the publication of a version of the *Tao Te Ching*. His other books include *Opening Our Minds: avoiding abusive relationships and authoritarian groups.*

It is often challenging to separate genuine from fraudulent spirituality. Teachers may be sincere in their belief in dangerous ideas. As Martin

Gardner said of Anton Mesmer, it is possible to be both a charlatan and a crank. [5] Our concern is not the teacher's sincerity but the adoption of harmful methods to adherents or society. It is essential to differentiate between expert and rank authority when choosing a teacher. In the same way, it is vital to be able to differentiate evidence from opinion or feelings of knowing.

Even a well-respected spiritual leader can make errors of judgment. Over the years, the Dalai Lama has endorsed Aum Shinrikyo, [6] Osho (formerly known as Rajneesh) [7],[2] and NXIVM.[3]

In this chapter, we will examine models developed by Steven Hassan, Ph.D., and Jon Atack's ideas relating to human predators. We have spent more than four decades helping survivors of authoritarian groups and researching the framework in which such groups have developed. Through the lens of this research, it is possible to estimate possible harms in the behavior and techniques of contemporary spiritual groups.

As Dr. Koenig points out in this volume, the western Mindfulness movement has severed Buddhist meditation from its roots in the eightfold path of the Buddha. Such luminaries as Jon Kabat-Zinn [8] and Daniel Goleman [9] have asserted that compassion is the inevitable outcome of meditation, rendering the other seven aspects of the Buddhist Dhamma unnecessary [10].[4] We need only look to the daily use of zazen meditation in the Japanese military after the Meiji Restoration in 1868 through the horrors of the Korean and Manchurian occupations and WWII to see that meditation must be allied to an ethical code [11]. The same is probably true of all mind-altering techniques.

Yoga has similarly been detached from its original spiritual form. Like Buddhist meditation, it has been repurposed for relaxation, destressing, and health rather than as the "yoke" (yoga's literal meaning) to the divine. These are powerful techniques needing competent supervision, especially for beginners. It is sobering that Heinrich Himmler, the architect of the Final Solution, led retreats for the S.S. in both meditation and yoga.[5]

It is also often the case that practitioners will interpret normal physiological responses as transcendent experiences. So, for instance, the fixation of visual perception leads to an altered state of perception known as the Ganzfeld Effect.[6] Meditators will usually experience distortions in the visual field and a sense of euphoria. They may attribute this to a spiritual rather than a neurological change and believe it to be the gift of their teacher. In fact, the Ganzfeld Effect is a shift from wakefulness to light sleep – from alpha or beta waves to theta waves.

We strongly agree that practices such as Mindfulness should be linked to a positive moral outlook to achieve their full benefit. This need not be theistic or spiritual in its base but can be atheist, agnostic, or humanist. Mindfulness practitioner and clinical psychologist Professor Willoughby Britton offers advice to would-be meditators based upon sound research funded by the U.S. National Institute of Health at the Clinical and Affective Neuroscience Laboratory website.[7]

For some people, meditation can cause a sense of unease known as "relaxation-induced

---

[2]Fingerprint. "Osho is an enlightened master, who is working with all possibilities to help humanity…"

[3]The Vow, series 1, asserts that the Dalai Lama received $2 million from NXIVM. HBO Original.

[4]"Kabat-Zinn and a number of his secular teachers have argued that an ethical framework would be an imposition."

[5]Purser [10], op. cit. (p. 225f) citing The International Business Times, retrieved on 04-07-23 from https://www.ibtimes.com/heinrich-himmler-nazi-hindu-214444 and a Yoga Journal review of Mathias Tietke's *Yoga In National Socialism*, retrieved on 04-07-23 from https://www.yoga-journal.com/yoga-101/history-of-yoga/nazi-leaders-fascinated-by-yoga/

[6]Ganzfeld Effect: retrieved on 04-07-23 from https://www.psychreg.org/ganzfeld-effect/

[7]Retrieved on 04-07-23 from https://sites.brown.edu/britton/

anxiety."[8] One commonly reported adverse effect of meditation is triggering intense emotions or traumatic memories, known as "emergence reactions." For a few people, a single session can provoke a psychotic episode [12].[9] Some practitioners use meditation to achieve bliss states and relinquish real-world responsibilities. Even the editor of the Oxford Handbook of Meditation, Dr. Miguel Farias, admits to having become a "meditation junkie."[10] He warns us, "Contrary to its Buddhist roots, individualism is at the heart of modern mindfulness."[11]

Some groups use rapid breathing to cause hyperventilation. This will cause respiratory alkalosis which generates a different state of consciousness.[12]

It is possible to subject any practice or belief system to the models we present to determine how much a practitioner has lost the locus of control to a teacher or guru.

Of course, guru traditions in the East are comparable to the vow of poverty, chastity, and obedience common to Christian monastic tradition.

Such submission may be held to be a necessity for the getting of wisdom. We would argue that the novice has the right to understand the nature and extent of submission before setting foot on the path and the right to withdraw if ethical violations occur. There is tremendous danger in a world so full of spiritual counterfeits. We should be able to assess the virtue of a teacher before following her or his path. We do not believe that abject submission is a requisite for development.

As Viktor Frankl pointed out, psychotherapists need to understand the belief system of their clients [13]. All too often, escapees from authoritarian cults are treated to a cookie-cutter approach that can do more harm than good. Jon Atack refers to the "cultic shell" through which a damaged former believer will continue to view the world [14]. The therapist will be dealing with the constructed cult identity rather than the submerged authentic self in such a situation. It is important to understand the worldview of a client before embarking upon psychotherapy.

Any group can be examined through these models, and the practitioner must determine whether to continue on the path offered to them. However, we would recommend a deeper understanding than we can outline here for those seeking an immersion in religious practices. It should also be noted that some extreme techniques, especially those relating to sexual behavior, such as Tantra, should be approached with significant caution.

---

[8]Retrieved on 04-07-23 from https://psychology-spot.com/paradoxical-anxiety-induced-by-relaxation/; Purser [10], *op. cit.* (p. 199f)

[9]Purser [10], op. cit.

[10]Farias and Wikholm [12], op. cit., p. 118.

[11]Farias and Wikholm [12] op. cit., p. xi.

[12]https://my.clevelandclinic.org/health/diseases/21657-respiratory-alkalosis

The Influence Continuum

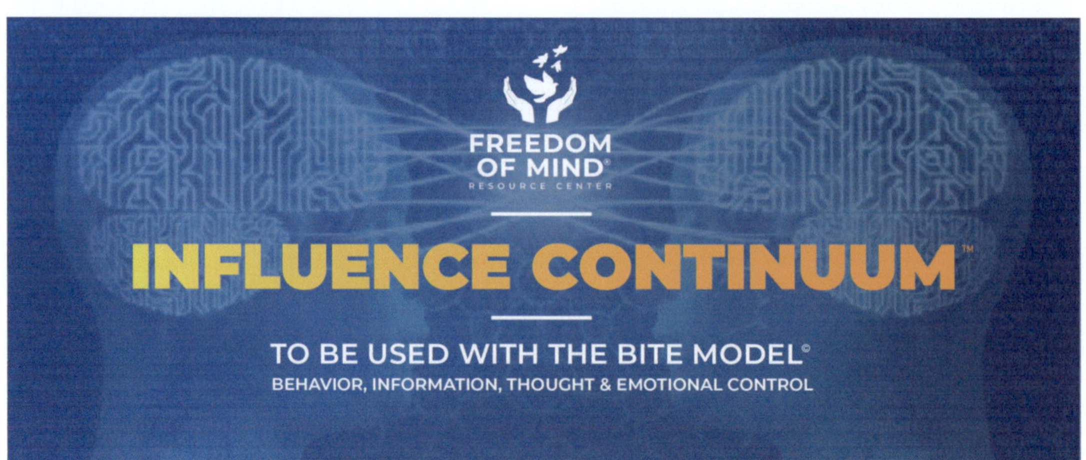

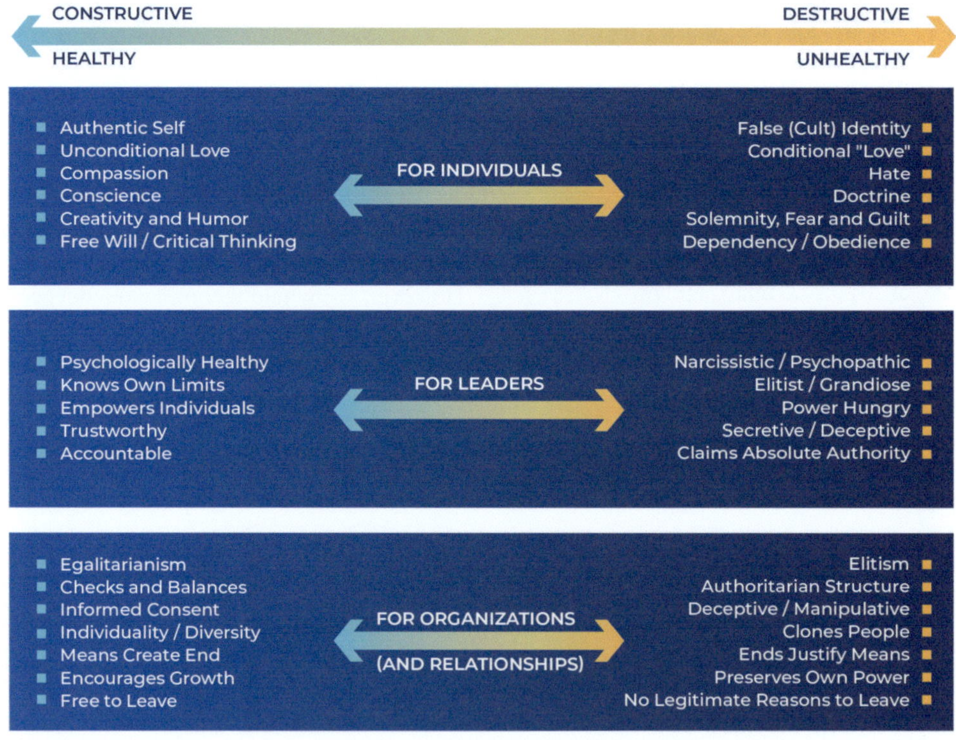

FROM COMBATING CULT MIND CONTROL (2018) BY STEVEN HASSAN

Steven Hassan developed the Influence Continuum to examine the dynamics of involvement in authoritarian cults, showing the essential distinctions between ethical and unethical influence. Ethical influence is based on informed consent. No sensible person joins a group with the expectation that they will be exploited and abused. People are deceptively recruited into authoritarian cults [15].[13] There is no informed consent because these cults hide their actual beliefs and practices from recruits until they are locked in. Information is distorted, exaggerated, or hidden, and outright lies are told.

Usually, the workings of the inner circle will be hidden from raw recruits. Core practices and beliefs are concealed unless and until the recruit is fully immersed in the cult. The true nature of the cult is deliberately withheld. Instead, a promise of enlightenment, liberation, or a future paradise hides the intent to enslave.

The group surrounding the leader will zealously conceal immoral behavior from followers. For instance, Ma Anand Sheela and others in the ruling group surrounding Rajneesh maintained his pretense of a vow of silence and said nothing of his daily use of large doses of diazepam and nitrous oxide [16].[14] The closer they are to the leader, the more willing followers become to hide corruption and deceit. A proposed solution to groupthink acceptance of immorality can be found in Ira Chaleff's "Courageous Followership." [17]

The BITE Model of Authoritarian Control [18]

The BITE Model[15] derives from the work of eminent psychologist Leon Festinger. His model of cognitive dissonance is perhaps the most thoroughly investigated of all psychological models. [19] Dr. Hassan took the aspects of control of behavior, thought, and emotion and added control of information to create a robust model that takes its name from the initials of the forms of control: Behavior, Information, Thought, and Emotion.

Obedience and dependency upon the leadership and its dogma are the essential criteria of behavior control. A follower who acts independently without permission from a superior will be criticized and sanctioned. Permission may be required for any leave from the group or for communication with non-believers. Communication with critics will be forbidden with a policy of ostracism (also known as *shunning, disfellowshipping,* or *disconnection*).

Individual expression is censured, and surrender to the group and its doctrines is demanded. Rules–often petty in nature—are strictly enforced. Dissenting thoughts, feelings, and actions are censured and must be reported to superiors.

The group often demands uniformity in clothing and hairstyle. The dress code may include a single item—the Scientology "Clear" bracelet or the Kabbalah red string—or an entire way of dressing—as with militant Islamists or Krishna monks. Followers may be prohibited from following fashion trends or even forced to dress in "traditional" clothes that separate them from non-believers. Such uniforms become dangerous if they violate the free choice of the follower [20].[16]

Behavior control often includes a restricted diet. NXIVM's Keith Raniere demanded that female members follow a strictly calorie-controlled diet that verged on anorexia [21]. Prohibitions of diet may be arbitrary. Live-in members often subsist on a high-carbohydrate diet. Some groups enforce fasting for days on end, which can lead to hallucinations and dissociation.

Members tend to confirm their behavior to group norms, which will often seem eccentric—and even destructive—to outsiders. Behavior is judged by the cult's rules: compliant behavior is rewarded (particularly making new recruits, especially wealthy new recruits), and non-

---

[13] Atack, Opening Our Minds [14], op. cit.

[14] Sheela, M.A. [7], *op. cit.*

[15] Due to AI misuse concerns, BITE Model™ and Influence Continuum™ are both trademarked

[16] Hussein was surprised to find on his visit to Syria that the garb adopted in London actually belonged to the Christian community there.

compliant behavior is censured—frequently in front of other members—and penalized. Some groups use the "hot-seat" technique developed in the Chinese thought reform program [22], where the assembled group loudly and harshly criticizes the individual for some perceived deviation.

Behavior often includes derision for non-believers and elitism that verges on narcissistic veneration of the group. Followers often perceive themselves to be superior to outsiders. This contempt for others is also an aspect of emotional control. Behavior can escalate to Robert Jay Lifton's "dispensing of existence,"[17] where any harm that befalls outsiders and critics gives satisfaction to the believer. The most extreme example of this is the perversion of the Buddhist doctrine of *poa,* or fulfillment of karma, by Aum Shinrikyo. This group planned to use sarin nerve gas to annihilate the population of Japan, to release it from negative karma-vipaka [23]

Anti-social behavior is the hallmark of authoritarian cults. The fundamental principle of Stefan Molyneux's Free Domain Radio internet cult is to "defoo" or divorce the "family of origin," even if that family had not been in any way abusive. The group is seen as the "real" family, rejecting parents, childhood caregivers, and siblings in preference for fellow believers. Members of the Unification Church or Moonies refer to Sun Myung Moon as "True Father." [24]

Information Control

Authoritarian cults restrict and misinterpret information to exploit others. It is vital to differentiate the ethical and unethical use of information. An ethical group is open about its doctrine, history, and expectations of new members. Believers are encouraged to analyze and debate doctrine.

Recruits of the military are aware that their lives may be at risk. An honest belief group openly describes cultural restrictions–such as abstinence from beef or pork, vegetarianism, or veganism. A dishonest belief group restricts, dis-

torts, or conceals essential information or simply lies. Moonies justify their "heavenly deception" by citing Jacob's deception of his father Isaac to receive a blessing.[18] The story of Rahab's protection of Israelite spies is used as a justification for deception by Jehovah's Witnesses.[19]

Believers are often expected to spy on their fellows and anyone critical of the cult, including family and friends. Scientologists submit "knowledge reports" about any deviation from the group's dogma. [25] Any thought, feeling, or activity that deviates from the group's beliefs must be reported in what Robert Jay Lifton calls "the cult of confession."[20] These reports violate the sanctity of the confessional because they may be made public.

Authoritarian cults are expert at propaganda. With the rise of the Internet, such cults can saturate their members with a constant flow of information, misinformation, and disinformation. Web sites and videos are available 24/7; meetings can be live-streamed to believers. Larger groups have whole departments which produce all forms of media, from traditional print to podcasts and apps.[21]

Independent thinking relies upon access to reputable sources, the ability to determine credibility, and knowing how to make free choices. Unfortunately, these skills rarely feature in school curricula, and most people are ill-equipped to determine the veracity of material or the authenticity of teachers.[22]

In an authoritarian cult, leaders decide what information members are allowed. Media may be prohibited or derided. Rajneeshis speak of the "poodle press," [26] and QAnon members ridicule the "mainstream media." [27]

---

[17]ibid.

[18]ibid.

[19]ibid.

[20]Lifton, R.J. [22]. *Thought Reform and the Psychology of Totalism,* op. cit.

[21]For instance, Scientology's New Era Publications and Bridge Publications, its Golden Era Productions and online TV channel.

[22]Atack, *Opening Our Minds,* op. cit.; vide The Institute for Propaganda Analysis, retrieved on 04-07-23 from https://en.wikipedia.org/wiki/Institute_for_Propaganda_ Analysis.

As an aspect of information control, members are indoctrinated to dismiss any negative report without considering it. Groups may completely deny access to all public media. Aversion is aroused,[23] so members avoid or dismiss any negative evidence. All too often, members' time is taken up so thoroughly that they have no liberty to consider anything outside the group's own material or to meet with anyone who questions the group's beliefs. In this "echo chamber," only material that reinforces group doctrine is ever considered. Search engines tend to reinforce this echo chamber phenomenon, assisting the burgeoning of web-based cults, such as Free Domain Radio and QAnon.

Groups may even control believers through frequent texting, calls, or even through their cell phones' GPS tracking. Inner group members of NXIVM were enjoined to answer calls from their "masters" within minutes, day or night [28]. Scientology distributed programs to members that surreptitiously included net nannies stopping access to critical websites.[24]

The echo chamber of the World Wide Web makes it possible for untrained minds to exclude differing opinions and evidence. Often, information control is self-imposed: members of authoritarian cults simply refuse to study anything that criticizes the group's doctrine and instead make an ad hominem attack upon the source of criticism.

Thought Control

There are many ways of controlling and directing thought. Former members are usually surprised when they listen to the tedious, self-aggrandizing lectures that enchanted them when they were believers. Monotony can distort reasoning. Speakers will often use the group's special or "loaded" language;[25] talks are peppered with difficult, redefined, or invented terms.[26] Believers are expected to regurgitate strings of words – sometimes in a language unknown to the chanter – without any appeal to their comprehension or any practical application.

Repetitive drumming, clapping, dancing, and marching can lock people into unison. Chanting mantras, spinning prayer wheels, rounds of prayers, speaking in tongues, rocking back and forth (*davening*), or long periods of immobile silence can all induce mental states that inhibit or even suspend analytical thinking and rational evaluation. Repetition, mimicry, and perceptual fixation often override critical thinking.[27] All can create states of the mind altered by variations in brain chemistry.

People can become addicted to sports and exercise because it stimulates the human analog of morphine—the "endogenous morphine" or "endorphin"—so vigorous exercise can lead to dependence and blunted reasoning. Techniques that employ repetition, fixation, and mimicry will produce euphoric states—with the release of neurochemicals and hormones— that can also cause dependency. Some Transcendental Meditation practitioners report 12-hour meditation days, and many meditators speak of being "blissed out."[28] Unfortunately, bliss states are not conducive to rational thinking—or even rational perception.

Authoritarian cults use methods that induce euphoria and elation. Variations of these methods are used in established religions. It is for believers to decide if they are being controlled in any way. However, visualization and "guided meditation" techniques often heighten suggestibility, making it easier to slip past reasoning and implant thoughts, beliefs, and even false memories into believers [29].

---

[23] Atack, J. [14]. *Opening Our Minds*, op. cit.

[24] Retrieved on 04-07-23 from https://www.xenu.net/archive/events/censorship; retrieved on 04-07-23 from https://markrathbun.blog/2012/05/29/scientology-inc-internet-nannies/.

[25] Lifton, R.J. [22]. *Thought Reform and the Psychology of Totalism*, op. cit.

[26] Ron Hubbard explained the use of such distortion in his Policy Letter, Propaganda by Redefinition of Words, HCOPL 5 October 1971. His Scientology group has published two 600-page dictionaries of his redefinitions.

[27] Atack, J. [14]. *Opening Our Minds*, op. cit.

[28] 12 hour meditation: Jon Atack interview with former TMer, 1991.

Authoritarian cults eliminate subtle discrimination and paint the world as a simplistic division between that which is good and that which is harmful. In this polarized world, everything is good versus evil, black or white, all-or-nothing, us versus them. There is not even the slightest possibility that there are shades of gray, let alone colors. The teachings are seen as the final "Truth" and are considered both sacred and scientific or "sacred science,"[29] meaning that there is no further need for scientific, rational, or real-world evidence. Believers are insulated from criticism via self-activated "thought-stopping" techniques.[30] They learn that they must follow the rules exactly to retain–or achieve–purity and be protected from "evil" thoughts or influences. For instance, ISKCON Krishna devotees learn to chant the "Hare Krishna" mantra to drown out cognitive dissonance [30, 31]. Destructive cults fence members in with their special argot or "loaded language,"[31] which is often incomprehensible to outsiders. As all conceptual thinking is mediated by language, it can become impossible to think coherently; especially in an environment of sleep deprivation [32], constant work, harsh conditions, inadequate nutrition, and perpetual humiliation.

An authoritarian cult avoids or prohibits doubt or unwelcome questions about its doctrine or leadership. Any deviation from the doctrine is seen as a failure of faith. Believers are persuaded to use their critical thinking skills purely in defense of the group, the leader, and the teachings. Even the most constructive criticism may be considered sinful or immoral simply because it disagrees with the preferences of the leadership.

All other faiths and belief systems are rejected as mistaken, evil, or harmful—despite public protestations to the contrary. Objective thinking and scientific analysis are rejected. Beliefs rigidify beyond correction; they become "truths." In William James's terms, these are actually "feelings of knowing," a sense of certainty without objective evidence to support it [33]. Insights and information connected to the group are beyond question.

Like information control, thought control can be self-imposed. Believers exclude any thought that questions the dogma they fervently accept as inviolable truth. We should encourage our educational institutions to shift from memorizing and regurgitating data to develop critical thinking and intelligent disobedience (as described by Ira Chaleff) [34].

The appendix to George Orwell's *Nineteen Eighty-Four* posits the idea that thinking can be inhibited by restrictions of language—making a "thoughtcrime" impossible [35]. Loaded language limits and controls thinking— the thought control aspect of the BITE model. Lifton's "loaded language"[32] upsets rational thought and allows the ideas of the only authoritative source in the believer's mind—the founder or leader of their cult. The cult's echo chamber limits access to truthful information and instills the determination to scorn and reject anything different from the party line. Without access to information, there is much less chance that the believer will realize the true intention of the leadership–to dominate and control others into adulation and submission.

Emotional Control

The Moonies gave us the term "love-bombing"[33] for deliberate flattery designed to quickly forge an emotional bond and bypass reasoning. The recruiter is your new best friend and offers a dazzling vision of the group, its noble aims, and its leader's genius. This mock friendship is bolstered by constant agreement with the target's opinions. An Al Qaeda recruiting manual explains, "Don't criticize the candidate's behavior. Thank him for any help, even if it is just a little. Caution: don't disregard his opinion or his manner of thinking

---

[29]Lifton, R.J. [22]. *Thought Reform and the Psychology of Totalism*, op. cit.

[30]ibid.

[31]Lifton, R.J. [22]. *Thought Reform and the Psychology of Totalism*, op. cit.

[32]Lifton, R.J. [22]. *Thought Reform and the Psychology of Totalism*, op. cit.

[33]Hassan, S. [24]. *Combating Cult Mind Control*, op. cit.

but let him express his opinion even if it opposes yours … Be close to him in order to get to know more about his character." [36]

Newcomers join because they are tricked about the nature of the group and because of the warm welcome always offered to raw recruits. More experienced group members will love-bomb them with compliments—especially if they announce a realization based on the dogma. This helps to maintain the "honeymoon" phase of membership.

Some groups have a strict division between the leader's entourage and the worshiping (and paying) public. Scientology differentiates these as "staff" and "public." As Hassan's Influence Continuum shows, the closer to the authoritarian leadership, the stronger the fervor. Cults often recruit by teaching a method of experiencing feelings of euphoria—wonder or awe. Under the influence of this euphoria, people often believe the teacher to have a special understanding and bow to the teacher's direction as an authority figure. The teacher may become a pseudo-parent. Some believers will be in high fervor, others less so [37].

As the honeymoon phase fades, membership is maintained by creating frustration and dependency. The bursts of euphoria will be wider apart and less intense. The pursuit of euphoria will generate constant frustration, as will the demand for purity[34] and the failure to achieve it. Legitimate concerns will be dismissed, and sinfulness or impurity will be given as the rationalization for any discontent. Self-esteem shifts to be based upon an almost childlike submission to the leadership, the cult, and the doctrine rather than to the individual's own achievements. Guilt, fear,[35] and aversion or disgust[36] are the most often used emotional control techniques.

Phobia induction and indoctrination are integral parts of destructive cults.[37, 38] Besieged by phobias, normal life is impossible. As Alexandra Stein points out, members have a disorganized attachment to the leadership, which quickly shifts between acceptance and rejection, between encouragement and dismissal [38]. This behavior is akin to a parent who switches from doting to scolding. Ironically, believers become dependent upon the group and its dogma to defend them from the very fears that the group's dogma has instilled.

Phobia becomes a route along which a destructive cult can infiltrate programmed responses and generate an overwhelming belief that life outside the cult would be impossible.

Guilt focuses the believer's attention inward; it inverts the usual fundamental attribution error, where we tend to justify our own shortcomings through extenuating circumstances but believe others are deliberately falling short. In a destructive cult, the fundamental attribution error justifies the group's excesses and amplifies the member's shortcomings. Many cults believe that we are all entirely responsible for everything that happens to us; even catching a cold can be seen as an inference of guilt.

Believers may come to inhabit the group's illusory world to such a profound extent that they become dependent upon the group for their emotional well-being.

Human Predators

Authoritarian cult leaders share certain characteristics, as listed by Jon Atack in *Opening Our Minds* [39].[39] They are red flags that should alert caution for followers.

Human predators:

- are mean.
- are utterly selfish.
- pretend friendship and love but feel absolutely nothing for others.
- are charming and good at flattery, but don't mean a single word of it.

---

[34] Lifton, R.J. [22]. *Thought Reform and the Psychology of Totalism*, op. cit.

[35] Hassan, S. [24]. *Combating Cult Mind Control*, op. cit.

[36] Atack, J. [14]. *Opening Our Minds*, op. cit.

[37] Hassan, S. [24]. *Combating Cult Mind Control*, op. cit.

[38] Atack, J. [14]. *Opening Our Minds*, op. cit.

[39] Atack, J. [14]. *Opening Our Minds*, op. cit.

- brag and boast and make up outrageous lies. When challenged, they blame others.
- don't feel anxiety or fear - or are deeply anxious and cowardly.
- are impulsive and easily bored. They demand thrills and take dangerous risks. They enjoy pushing others into taking dangerous risks, too.
- are bullies with explosive tempers.
- are cunning and manipulative.
- enjoy humiliating people.
- weaken people with insults and putdowns.
- hate it if anyone else has power or is praised. For the predator, life is a competition and they want to WIN.
- lie easily and think nothing of breaking a promise.
- are without conscience: they do not feel remorse or guilt.
- often boast about the harm they've done other people.
- are parasites and lazy, living off others, giving as little as possible in return.
- are control freaks, stopping others from taking control of anything if they can.
- force petty rules on others – rules that are impossible to follow.
- boast about tricking other people and breaking the law.

Of course, leaders may not believe themselves to be in the least predatory but have the sincere belief that they are helping their followers. However, it does not matter how well-meaning a physician is if the medicine they are enthusiastically offering is actually poison. And there are all too many instances of this in medical history. The same is most certainly true for spirituality.

Conclusion

Gautama Buddha urged rationality in opposition to supernaturalism. In the Kalama Sutta he said, "Don't go by reports, by legends, by traditions, by scripture, by logical conjecture, by inference, by analogies, by agreement through pondering views, by probability … When you know for yourselves that, 'These qualities are skillful; these qualities are blameless; these qualities are praised by the wise; these qualities, when adopted & carried out, lead to welfare & to happiness' — then you should enter & remain in them."[40]

In a pluralistic world, we should be tolerant of other cultures and religious traditions. We should allow freedom of belief – and freedom of disbelief – and accept the right to develop our own individual metaphors for the great unknown. However, where practices are harmful, they should be exposed to public view, and where they are criminal, the perpetrators should be legally prosecuted.

In the twenty-first century, neuroscience and social psychology can help to unpick false and dangerous beliefs. Freedom of mind and our other essential human rights demand that mental health professionals use discretion and do not blindly accept dysfunctional systems that may affect their clients negatively. Our commitment is to help people to make healthy decisions for themselves and those they love.

The very word "religion" comes from words meaning "to bind together." Religion can be a binding force for a community. It can motivate the most noble behavior and inspire the highest art. However, religion—or indeed any belief system—can be corrupted to anti-social and even anti-human ends. We hope to have pointed out some of the many pitfalls that believers must negotiate to find the faith that best suits them and most profits the world.

References

1. Mascaró J. transalator. The Bhagavad Gita. Middlesex: Penguin Classics; 1962.
2. Cohn N. The pursuit of the millennium. London: Martin Secker and Warburg; 1957, 1970.
3. Blum D. Ghost hunters. London: Arrow; 2007.
4. Tillet G. The elder brother: a biography of Charles Webster Leadbeater. London/Boston/Henley: Routledge and Kegan Paul; 1982.

[40] translated from the Pali by Thanissaro Bhikkhu (1994), courtesy of the Pali Text Society. Retrieved on 04-07-23 from https://www.accesstoinsight.org/tipitaka/an/an03/an03.065.than.html

5. Gardner M. Fads and fallacies in the name of science. London: Constable; 1957. p. 9.

6. Hogendoorn R. Knave or fool? The Dalai Lama and Shōkō Asahara affair revisited. Research Gate. December 2020. Retrieved on July 04, 2023, from https://www.researchgate.net/publication/346718565_Knave_or_Fool_The_Dalai_Lama_and_Shoko_Asahara_Affair_Revisited

7. Sheela MA. Don't Kill Him. New Delhi; 2012.

8. Kabat-Zinn J. Coming to our senses: healing ourselves and the world through mindfulness. London: Piatkus. Citing Thich Nhat Hanh; 2005. p. 138.

9. Goleman D, Rinpoche T. Why we meditate: 7 simple practices for a calmer mind. London: Penguin Life; 2022.

10. Purser RE. McMindfulness: how mindfulness became the new capitalist spirituality. London: Repeater Books; 2019. p. 79f.

11. Victoria BD. Zen at War. Lanham: Rowman and Littlefield; 2006.

12. Farias M, Wikholm K. The Buddha Pill: Can Meditation Change You? London: Watkins; 2015.

13. Frankl V. The doctor and the soul: from psychotheray to logotherapy. London: Souvenir Press; 1969.

14. Atack J. Opening our minds. Colchester: Trentvalley Limited; 2021.

15. Atack J. Scientology: the cult of greed. Colchester: Trentvalley Limited; 2014.

16. Milne H, Hodgkinson L. Bhagwam: the god that failed, 1987. Middlesex: Penguin; 1987.

17. Chaleff I. The courageous follower: standing up to and for our leaders. Williston: Berrett-Koehler; 2009.

18. Hassan S. The BITE model of authoritarian control: undue influence thought reform brainwashing mind control trafficking and the law. December 2020. Retrieved on July 04, 2023, from https://www.proquest.com/docview/2476570146/

19. Harmon-Jones and Mills. Cognitive dissonance: progress on a pivotal theory in social psychology. Washington, DC: American Psychological Association; 1999.

20. Husain E. The Islamist: why I joined radical Islam in Britain, what I saw inside and why I left. London: Penguin; 2007.

21. Seduced: Inside the NXIVM Cult. Santa Monica: Lionsgate Television; 2020.

22. Lifton RJ. Thought reform and the psychology of totalism. New York: Norton Library; 1963.

23. Lifton RJ. Destroying the world to save it: Aum Shinrikyo, apocalyptic violence, and the new global terrorism. New York: Henry Holt; 2000.

24. Hassan S. Combating cult mind control. Newton: Freedom of Mind Press; 2015.

25. Atack J. Let's sell these people a piece of blue sky. Colchester: Trentvalley ltd; 2018.

26. My Dance is Now Complete. London: Gizmo Productions; 1989.

27. Beverley JA. The QAnon deception: everything you need to know about the world's most dangerous conspiracy theory. Concord: Equal Time; 2020.

28. Edmondson S, Gasbarre K. Scarred: the true story of how i escaped NXIVM the cult that bound my life. San Francisco: Chronicle; 2019.

29. Hassan S. Freedom of mind: helping loved ones leave controlling people, cults, and beliefs. Newton: Freedom of Mind Press; 2012.

30. Muster NJ. Betrayal of the spirit: my life behind the headlines of the Hare Krishna Movement. University of Illinois Press; 2001. retrieved on 04-07-23 from https://www-jstor-org.fgul.idm.oclc.org/stable/10.5406/j.ctt5hjjjv

31. Bryant, Ekstrand, editors. The hare Krishna movement: the postcharismatic fate of a religious transplant. New York: Columbia University Press; 2004.

32. Walker M. Why we sleep: the new science of sleep and dreams. London: Penguin; 2017.

33. James W. The varieties of religious experience: a study in human nature. Boston: Longmans, Green and Co; 1917.

34. Chaleff I. Intelligent disobedience: doing right when what you're told to do is wrong. Oakland: Berrett-Koehler; 2015.

35. Orwell G. Nineteen eighty-four. London: Penguin; 1949.

36. Al Qa'idy A. A course in the art of recruiting. No publisher; undated.

37. Yuval Laor Y. Fervor: what cults teach us about the evolution of religion, unpublished manuscript; 2023.

38. Stein A. Terror, love and brainwashing: attachment in cults and totalitarian systems. Abingdon: Routledge; 2017.

39. Hassan S. The cult of trump. New York: Simon and Schuster; 2019.

Omnism: A Religion for All

30

Rama Rao Gogineni, Shridhar Sharma,
and H. Steven Moffic

For a considerable portion of humanity today, it is possible and indeed likely that one's neighbor, one's colleague, or one's employer will have a different mother tongue, eat different food, and follow a different religion than oneself. . . It is by moving beyond narrow self-interest that we find meaning, purpose, and satisfaction in life. [1]
Dalai Lama

This chapter conveys first author's evolutionary learning or religion, faith, and spirituality, the development of Omnism, some well-known Omnists, and life experiences that contributed to believing he is an omnist and a co-authors' responses.

Evolution of Religion, Religiosity

Generally speaking, and with the current state of our knowledge, it seems as though organized religion can be traced back at least 11,000 years to the near East with the development of farming, as a means to provide moral, social, and economic stability with a central authority. Anthropologists have found that most societies justify political power through divine authority. There are over 4200 religions globally, and all differ from one another over time and across places but fall into the following categories [2–4].

Theism refers to the belief in the existence of one or more gods. Islam, Christianity, and Judaism have a monotheistic belief in one God, whereas a polytheistic religion such as Hinduism encourages belief in more gods. Deism closely resembles theism, but the God of Deism has made the world and set up the laws governing how it is run rather than being involved with human beings in a personal way [4].

Pantheism is the view that the world is either identical to God or an expansion of God's nature. The pantheist God is not a personal God, but rather a non-personal divinity that pervades all existence. There remains some uncertainty about just how pantheism is to be understood and who is and is not a pantheist. Some well-known historical figures who may have been pantheists are Plato, Lao Tzu, Spinoza, Emerson, Walt Whitman, Beethoven, and Martha Graham [4].

Atheism is often thought to refer to a denial of, or opposition to theism. An atheist is one who denies the existence of a personal, transient creator of the world. In psychiatry, Freud, though he identified as being Jewish culturally, did not do so religiously, and would be an example [4].

R. R. Gogineni (✉)
Developmental Psychiatry,
Cooper Medical School of Rowan University,
Camden, NJ, USA
e-mail: gogineni-rao@cooperhealth.edu

S. Sharma
National Academy of Medical Sciences, Delhi, India

H. S. Moffic
Private Community Psychiatrist,
Milwaukee, WI, USA

Agnosticism argues that there is no firm basis on which to judge that theism, pantheism, or atheism as intrinsically more probable than the other. An agnostic believes that the answers to the basic questions of existence are unknown or unknowable [4].

Baha'ism emerged from Islam and holds to the unity of God as revealed by the prophets [4].

Spirituality

Spirituality refers to a personal sense of connection to something larger than oneself that provides meaning to life. It may or may not come out of—or include—religions. Science can be a source of spirituality, when it provides a cosmic perspective on an interdependent whole. Religiosity and spirituality are associated with several neurobiological correlates, e.g., greater cortical thickness, and several physiological brain functions involving the left-anterior middle frontal gyrus, left superior parietal lobule, and others. Prayer may reduce alcohol cravings and increase attention and control processes in the brain [5, 6, 7].

Neurotheology refers to the advances in brain research studies. These suggest that spirituality and religion map onto a common brain circuit centered in the periaqueductal gray area, a brainstem region implicated in fear conditioning, pain modulation, and altruistic behavior. Lesions in the area can influence spirituality and religion to the extent of delusions [8].

Almost all religions try to explain death, the dying process, and any afterlife. Spiritual death, or sallekhana, is an Eastern preparation for physical death by which dying with dignity and control come from relinquishing passions through a process of meditation. This process begins while the person is conscious and realizes that life is about over but does not extend to suicide [9].

Faith

Pew Research Center study of the ways religion influences the daily lives of Americans finds that people who are highly religious are more engaged with their extended families, more likely to volunteer, more involved in their communities and generally happier with the way things are going in their lives [10].

Scientific reductionism, "I think, therefore I am" goes totally against the integral nature of the human person where the spiritual component is an essential part. A broader perspective is to integrate science and faith. That is, natural sciences collaborating with theology, and theology collaborating with the natural sciences are useful concepts for advancement [11].

"Values cannot be justified by the intellectual process alone. Faith must be involved." as said by Professor Klaus Schwab, Founder and Executive Chairman of the World Economic Forum, 26 October 2015. Eighty-four percent of the world believes that faith communities represent a key ingredient to a flourishing society. Faith possesses, the wisdom of long memory, as well as the desire to do the right thing by future generations, faith communities have always contributed to an inter-generational common good [12].

Omnism

There term omnism came into use in the 1800s but can be traced to prehistoric times when people likely intermixed beliefs, seeing the good in everything. It originated in a verse in the book by the Festus poet Philip Bailey in 1939. He believed in all religions. The term is now used not to describe a religion, but rather spirituality [13, 14] (Fig. 30.1).

The American actress Ellen Burstyn popularized omnism as a spiritual opening to the truth in all religions. Each religion thereby holds a fragment of the "truth." Consequently, Omnism has also been described as a syncretistic religion, allowing individuals to combine features of different religions with each other, often when their cultures are combining. Thousands of religions are available globally from which to choose [13, 14].

This uncertainty of the definition of Omnism is the point. Omnism does not have a fixed sys-

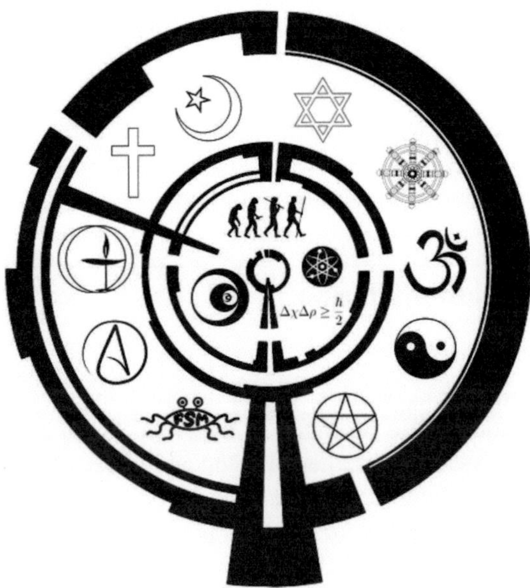

Fig. 30.1 An omnist symbol containing symbols of other religions such as Christianity, Islam, and Hinduism. This symbol emphasizes a belief in scientific knowledge in its inner ring. Is there some religious and spiritual conception that can tie all these variations together? Perhaps it is monism [13]

tem of beliefs, a holy book, or a set of mandatory rituals. Often, an Omnist follows a few sets of practices of the major faiths, while continuing to follow many rituals of their childhood faith. Sometimes people practice Omnism without knowing of the term. There is limited research into Omnism, which is often practiced in small groups [13, 14].

There may have been many notable Omnists besides the poet Philip Bailey and the actress Ellen Burstyn. The jazz saxophonist John Coltrane could be one, when he overcame substance addictions by an epiphany involving belief in all religions, most notably expressed in his famous recording, A Love Supreme. The basketball star Shaquille O'Neal identified as believing in every religion, saying he was Muslim, Jewish, Buddhist, and more. The author Celeste Ng describes an unconventional path for herself. Raised is atheist household, she found Omnism

to be the most liberating and fulfilling discovery she ever made. Despite an atheistic theology, she admired how her religious peers seemed to feel so happy and safe [13, 14].

Rama Rao Gogineni's Journey to Omnism

I was born into an upwardly mobile middle class in Southern India. I spent most of my school years in village culture. My parents were like most of the rest of middle-class families, with visits to the temples, places, and events of Hindu culture and rituals. I was exposed to Muslims and Christians at the age of 14 after my family moved to a town. In medical school I made many friends, immigrating to the United States at the age of 26. I completed a psychiatry residency and fellowship in child and adolescent psychiatry in Philadelphia, and later psychoanalytic and family therapy training. I married a woman of Quaker faith and fathered a son and an adopted daughter.

Several salient events shaped my religious and spiritual life. In the various training programs, I was taught mostly by Christian and Jewish teachers who were kind and helped me to grow up, feeling good in America. I appreciated the religious, spiritual, and humane aspects of my teachers. I formed friendships with individuals from multiple religious and ethnic groups, including Jewish, Christians, Muslims, Sikhs, Hindus, and others.

Three experiences impacted my spiritual life. After hearing about my admission to medical school, I was biking to a village farm where my father was residing. On my way, I uncharacteristically stopped at a roadside temple and placed a rupee in the worship bin, thanking God for giving me an opportunity to go to medical school. I was surprised by my act. The second episode occurred while my mother was visiting me in Philadelphia. I took her to visit a Hindu temple which was considered very sacred. While she was inside the temple and I was standing outside, I suddenly felt that I understood acceptance, surrender, and the concept of a higher power referenced in Alcoholic Anonymous. The third spiritual experience occurred while I was attending a World Association of Social Psychiatry meeting in the Ashoka Hotel in New Delhi. I was walking in a park outside the hotel. A Temple in the park was playing spiritual songs. I felt nostalgic, emotional, and a connection to the spirituality that was wafting in the air as well as inside me. Feeling good, I stopped in front of the temple, at the same time surprised at the power of spiritual connection.

These experiences made me realize that despite my belief in the scientific explanation of the way things work, I am also internally connected to a spiritual universe. These experiences along with relationships with people from other religions and friends, through attending Passover celebrations, Thanksgiving, and Christmas, provided me the same kind of feeling good, grateful, and connected to something more than humanness. As I am growing biologically older and many of my elders have passed, I have entered the self-actualization phase of my life. There has been a shift in my connection to the world; I have grown into the role of elder in my self-representation and my relationship to the outside world. I have started listening again to Telugu songs of worship that have connected me to my roots and something more than a material world. Thus, when Dr. Moffic asked me, "Rama Rao, What is your religion?" I thought about these earlier experiences and concluded with a sense of gratitude, and that I am blessed with a potpourri of relationships that come from such different religious backgrounds and an ethereal connection to a spiritual universe.

To connect the dots of the psychosocial life stages, the evolution of my early life in a small Hindu Village and eventually becoming an Omnist is a complicated task. Being a favored, idealized special grandson of the extended family made me feel special which gifted me with gratitude and a recognition of the fortunate life I had been given. This followed me into professional life. The scientific understanding of human nature, as well as positive and negative vicissitudes of life contribute to a further humility of what is an unknown, unthinkable "force," a higher power. Unable to explain many aspects of life, I have found some comfort in Omnism.

Shridhar Sharma

I was born in a traditional Hindu family, and my father was a high school teacher and social reformer. He belonged to the Arya Samaj sect. Arya samajists believe in God and Vedas and no idol worship. Right from childhood I would not eat or drink before I did my prayers, "Sandhya" chanting, Vedas worshipping God. When I reached college, we had to be there early in the morning. After 6 months of speeding through the morning prayers, I realized that rituals are not essential but one's religion is what one thinks and contemplates when alone. If you have good ideas and no hatred, it is a good religion. This belief was crystallized after I became a psychiatrist and read various philosophies and psychoanalysts. India's long tradition of spiritual teaching is based on individual spiritual experiences which help one to attain individual salvation. Truth is obtained by illuminated insight, and through identity with all pervading spirit. For most, higher knowledge is arrived at through faith, effort and reflection. Practice in pursuit of these qualities is most likely to be effective.one must have some belief in what one is doing when the results aren't yet self-verifying. Which is to say faith in another's ideas as worth consistently pursuing. This effort can't be indiscriminate; rather, it must be focused, thoughtful. In other words, coupled with what is directly translated as 'memory'. For, it can only be through reflecting on past experiences that we can clearly come to see the mistaken ideas we have about the nature of our being [15]. J Krishnamurti has aptly remarked, "truth cannot be given to you by somebody, you have to discover it and to discover there must be a state of mind in which there is no direct perception." In Indian culture

"Dharma" is one of those Sanskrit words that defy all attempts at an exact rendering in English or any other language. Dharma is not equivalent to religion. It is beyond that having passed through several vicissitudes. The dictionaries set out various meanings of Dharma such as ordinance, usage, duty, right, justice, morality, virtue, religion, good work, etc.

It is generally though not invariably assumed that there is only one "reality"; however, the nature of this reality is expressed differently by different traditions. Veda is the source of Dharma, and the tradition and practice of those who know the Vedas further virtue and self-satisfaction. The author of Dharma sutras was justified in looking to the Vedas as a source of Dharma.

Religion may sometimes act as a driving force. Religion is accessible at a church/mosque/temple. Spirituality does not depend on institutional affiliation. Spirituality is a personal way of relating to the divine, self, people, and the world. Spirituality offers autonomy from institutions and provides open ground for exploration. Spiritual people share an ability to communication flow, without doctrines, dogmas, and intellectual argumentation. The core of spiritual philosophies lies a focus on understanding the purpose and meaning of life, and a search for truth. Science provides us physical comforts, whereas spirituality brings us mental peace, and raises our consciousness. Belief in scriptures and prophets may be essential in all religions but humanism is the essence of all religions. As human beings we have to be humane with every human being irrespective of his religious background [16].

H. Steven Moffic's Response

When I heard that Rama Rao considered himself to be an Omnist, I said to myself: What!? I didn't know what Omnism meant, having assumed he would describe himself as Hindu. So much for superficial surface assumptions about how a person feels about themselves. This reaffirms the necessity to always check with the other, whether a stranger, colleague, patient, or friend.

On composing myself, I no longer felt surprised. Of course, Rama Rao could have achieved a more universal, transcendent religious and spiritual identity because he always looked to find the good in others. Among the religious and spiritual complements, contrasts, and contradictions, Omnism seems to provide multiple paths to finding these meaningful jewels of life. At its essence may be the so-called God particle, the fundamental particle that permeates the universe and gives mass to other fundamental particles.

In a way, it seems as though our scientific and healing field of psychiatry has paralleled the development of Omnism. From ancient understandings of people from religion, literature, and philosophy, our organized field of psychiatry has emerged in recent centuries. At its best, psychiatry brings together multiple other fields, including general medicine, neurology, social work, sociology, anthropology, and others.

For me personally, I still firmly identify as a Jewish American or American Jews, but seem to have bits and pieces of Omnism in me, hoping that the world is moving toward an overlay of Omnism that will help unify us.

Conclusion

In conclusion, belief in multiple supernatural, pagan beliefs were prevalent prior to organized religions. Beliefs and/or practices grounded in religious texts still exist in most religions. Neuroscience has led to theories about the evolution of spirituality. As the world is becoming one, in spite of some setbacks, many people are acting and incorporating practices and beliefs from many religions along with science in practicing Omnism. For an Omnist who is a believer of all religions, all religions are true in part, none in totality.

> I came to the conclusion long ago that all religions were true and that also all had some error in them, and while I hold by my own religion, I should hold other religions as dear as does Hinduism. So we can only pray, if we were Hindus, not that a Christian should become a Hindu but that a Hindu should become a better Hindu, a Muslim a better Muslim, and a Christian a better Christian. MK Gandhi [17]

Science investigates, religion interprets. Science gives man knowledge which is power, religion gives man wisdom which is control. Science deals mainly with facts, religion deals with values. The two are not rivals. They are complementary. — Strength to Love –ML King [18]

References

1. Dalai Lama, Alexander Norman. Beyond religion: ethics for a whole world mariner books, December 6, 2011.
2. Diamond J, Ordunio D, et al. Guns, germs and steel: the fate of human societies. Book 1 of 3: civilizations rise and fall series. 1st ed. New York: W. W. Norton & Company; 1999.
3. Peoples D. Marlowe hunter-gatherers and the origins of religion. Hum Nat. 2016;27:261–82. https://doi.org/10.1007/s12110-016-9260-0.
4. Archer, Religion 101: From Allah to Zen Buddhism, an Exploration of the Key People, Practices, and Beliefs that Have Shaped the Religions of the World Adams Media; Illustrated edition (November 29, 2013) 5. Rosmarin DH, Kaufman CC, Ford SF, Keshava P, et al. The neuroscience of spirituality, religion, and mental health: a systematic review and synthesis. J Psychiatr Res. 2022;156:100–113.
5. Ferguson MA, et al. A neural circuit for spirituality and religiosity derived from patients with brain lesions. Biol Psychiatry. 2022;91(4):380–8.
6. Sri Sri Ravi Shankar Spiritual Leader and Founder, Art of Living Foundation on Jul 16, 2010 wrote.
7. Galanter M, et al. An initial fMRI study on neural correlates of prayer in members of Alcoholics Anonymous. Am J Drug Alcohol Abuse. 43(1):44–54. https://doi.org/10.3109/00952990.2016.1141912.
8. David Eckel M, Jain M, Kumar VS. Spiritual death according to Hinduism, Jainism, and Buddhism. Boston University.
9. Goswami S. Spiritual dimensions of Indian culture. J Sociol Soc Work. 2014;2(1):241–56. 01. https://www.google.com/search?q=coversion+to+omnism-serp#:~:text=Omnism%20101%3A%20A, 7/30/2023.
10. Pew Research Center. Religion in everyday life. https://www.pewresearch.org/religion/2016/04/12/religion-in-everyday-life/. Research Topics April 12th, 2016.
11. World Economic Forum. The role of faith in systemic global challenges. https://www3.weforum.org/docs/WEF_GAC16_Role_of_Faith_in_Systemic_Global_Challenges.pdf
12. Cortés ME, del Río JP, Vigil P. The harmonious relationship between faith and science from the perspective of some great saints: a brief comment. Linacre Q. 2015;82(1):3–7.
13. Allia Luzong Omnism 101: A Full Guide to the Omnist Belief https://www.alittlebithuman.com/omnist-info-guide-to-ominism/ Source www.alittlebithuman.com was first indexed by Google in January 2020.
14. Omnism. Unionpedia, the concept map. https://en.unionpedia.org. Omnis 8/2/23.
15. Ten most important yoga sutras. https://www.keenonyoga.com/most-important-yoga-sutras/ Aug 3, 2021.
16. Sharma S. Titled spirituality, yoga, religion and mental health. Rom J Psychiatry. 2009;11(4):137–41.
17. Sean Dragon. An interview from beyond with Mahatma Gandhi! Medium. https://medium.com
18. Quote by Martin Luther King Jr.: "Science investigates, … Goodreads. https://www.goodreads.com/quotes/701891-science-investigates-religion-interprets-science-gives-man-knowledge-which-is.

Part V

Conclusions

Afterword: Lessons Learned on the Eastern Religions, Spirituality, and Psychiatry

H. Steven Moffic, Rama Rao Gogineni, John R. Peteet, Neil Krishan Aggarwal, Narpinder K. Malhi, and Ahmed Hankir

In *The Location of Culture*, the cultural theorist Homi Bhabha writes, "We have to learn to negotiate 'incommensurable' or conflictual social and cultural difference while maintaining the 'intimacy' of our inter-cultural existence and transnational associations." Drawing from his experiences as a member of the minoritized Zoroastrian community in India as well as from contemporary psychoanalytic interpretations of literature, Bhabha encourages us to view incommensurability and intimacy in our relationships as complementary, not oppositional.

We have taken a similar approach in this volume. Like Bhabha, contributors belonging to Eastern religious/spiritual traditions have articulated their understandings of mental health and illness. As providers committed to practice, all have written with an acute recognition that intimacy must be fostered in each inter-cultural clinical encounter. In chapters from those who do not see themselves as belonging to these traditions, authors have grappled with the legacies of European colonization and the challenges of encountering worldviews that differ fundamentally from their own. New immigration policies, revolutions in information technology, and the decreasing costs of travel worldwide have reconfigured transnational associations to render the geographical boundaries between the "East" and "West" obsolete. As proof, one need only look at our contributors residing in multiple continents who have found ways to collaborate.

Rather than reify, exoticize, or minimize cultural differences, we have chosen dialogue to explore what connects us all as humans. More than any specific method or approach, the psychotherapeutic tradition in mental health offers all of us the capacity to negotiate differences toward greater understanding. The courage to listen is often as crucial as the courage to speak, and we hope that our work promotes interreligious dialogues in mental health.

H. S. Moffic · J. R. Peteet
N. K. Aggarwal (✉) · A. Hankir
New York State Psychiatric Institute, Columbia
University Medical Center, New York, NY, USA
e-mail: Neil.Aggarwal@nyspi.columbia.edu

R. R. Gogineni
Developmental Psychiatry, Cooper Medical School of
Rowan University, Camden, NJ, USA

N. K. Malhi
Department of Behavioral Health, ChristianaCare,
Wilmington, DE, USA

Index

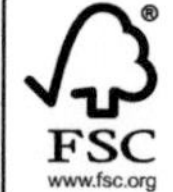